UNNATURAL HISTORY

Unnatural History explores the change over the last two centuries from isolated, private fears to an immense individual and collective risk of breast cancer. The book begins with the experiences of a Quaker woman diagnosed with breast cancer in 1812, and ends with our problematic era in which almost every woman is waiting for "the axe to fall." In between, the book traces changes in the beliefs and values of women and their doctors, medical knowledge and technology, clinical and public health practices, and the biological impact of the disease.

The picture that emerges from *Unnatural History* is that our clinical, public health, and societal responses to breast cancer have radically transformed the experience of disease and its apparent societal impact, without necessarily having had much effect on the disease's biological devastation.

Unnatural History suggests that we have oversold both the fear of breast cancer and the effectiveness of screening and treatment, leading to miscalculation at the individual and societal levels.

Robert A. Aronowitz studied linguistics before receiving his M.D. from Yale. After finishing residency in internal medicine, he studied the history of medicine as a Robert Wood Johnson Foundation Clinical Scholar at the University of Pennsylvania. Dr. Aronowitz is currently Associate Professor in the History and Sociology of Science Department at the University of Pennsylvania. He holds a joint appointment with the medical school's department of Family Medicine and Community Health. Dr. Aronowitz was the founding director of Penn's Health and Societies Program. He also codirects the Robert Wood Johnson Health and Society Scholars Program, a postdoctoral program focused on population health. In 2005–2006, he was a Fellow at the Wissenschaftskolleg zu Berlin.

Dr. Aronowitz's central research interests are in the history of twentieth-century disease, epidemiology, and population health. He is the author of *Making Sense of Illness: Science, Society, and Disease* (Cambridge, 1998). He is currently working on a historical project on the social framing of health risks, for which he received an Investigator Award in Health Policy from the Robert Wood Johnson Foundation.

Unnatural History

BREAST CANCER AND AMERICAN SOCIETY

Robert A. Aronowitz, M.D.

University of Pennsylvania

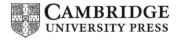

CAMBRIDGE UNIVERSITY PRESS
Cambridge, New York, Melbourne, Madrid, Cape Town,
Singapore, São Paulo, Delhi, Mexico City

Cambridge University Press
The Edinburgh Building, Cambridge CB2 8RU, UK

Published in the United States of America by Cambridge University Press, New York

www.cambridge.org
Information on this title: www.cambridge.org/9781107651463

First published 2007
First paperback edition 2013

A catalogue record for this publication is available from the British Library

Library of Congress Cataloguing in Publication Data
Aronowitz, Robert A. (Robert Alan), 1953–
Unnatural history : breast cancer and American society / Robert A. Aronowitz.
p. ; cm.
Includes bibliographical references and index.
ISBN-13: 978-0-521-82249-7 (hardback)
ISBN-10: 0-521-82249-1 (hardback)
1. Breast – Cancer – United States – History. 2. Breast – Cancer – Social aspects –
United States. I. Title.
[DNLM: 1. Breast Neoplasms – history – United States. 2. Attitude to Health – United States.
3. Breast Neoplasms – epidemiology – United States. 4. Breast Neoplasms – psychology –
United States. 5. History, 19th Century – United States. 6. History, 20th Century –
United States. WP 11 AA1 A769U 2007]
RC280.B8A783   2007
614.5'999449 – dc22   2007006339

ISBN 978-1-107-65146-3 Paperback

For Jane

Contents

Acknowledgments

During the many years I spent on this book, I have received help and support from many friends and colleagues. Katrina Armstrong, David Asch, Alan Brandt, Britta Cusack, the late Alvan Feinstein, Chris Feudtner, Steve Feierman, Zehavit Friedman, Dominick Frosch, Melissa Kulynych, Ilana Lowy, Dietrich Niethammer, Ilana Pardes, Rosemary Stevens, Janet Tighe, and Keith Wailoo read and commented on parts of earlier drafts. Knud Lambrecht and Clifford Hill read a few chapters very closely. They have been my most demanding nonmedical readers, whose high standards I have tried to but could never reach. Charles Rosenberg read the entire book in different iterations. Like a good cancer doctor, he has carefully balanced critical reading with sustaining hope.

Friends, relatives, and colleagues have supported my unusual medical and social science career. Over the years, I have also profited from discussing with them my evolving views about the history of breast cancer. Fran Barg, David Barnes, Mike Berkwits, Chuck Bosk, Marjorie Bowman, Charlie Brown, Andi Casher, Ruth Cowan, Pete Cronholm, Steve Gluckman, Bob Hedley, Kathleen Hill, Bob Hornik, Pat Johnson, Ralph Kaufman, Riki Kuklick, Susan Lindee, Jun Mao, Ohad Parnes, Harriet Power, Jean Rabinowitz, Scott Schlegel, Joe Straton, Tom Sutton, Ed Viner, and Larry Weisberg have each contributed to the writing of this book. I have also learned a great deal from discussions and close working relationships with too-many-to-mention faculty and fellows at the RWJ Health and Society Scholars Program at Penn and nationally.

Over the years, I have also benefited from comments and suggestions made after talks and presentations. At Penn, I presented parts of this book to the Family Medicine Fellowship seminar, the Religious Studies

Colloquium, the Nursing History Center, the Annenberg School, Presbyterian Hospital Grand Rounds, and the History and Sociology of Science workshop. Other venues outside of Philadelphia have included the Institute for Health Care, Health Policy, and Aging at Rutgers University; the Social Medicine Program at the University of North Carolina; the Foundation Merieux in Annecy, France; the Center for Health and Well Being at Princeton University; the History of Medicine program at the University of Kansas; CERMES in Paris; the National Institutes of Health; the Wellcome Institute for the History and Understanding of Medicine in London; and the Wissenschaftskolleg zu Berlin.

I am grateful for the help I received at each of the archives and libraries listed in the reference section. John Bailar not only talked extensively with me about his recollection of events described in Chapter 10, but also lent me a copy of his Freedom of Information Act search of NCI documents.

Frank Smith and before him, Alex Holzman, shepherded the book at Cambridge. Kennie Lyman read through an earlier version of the entire manuscript, offering many valuable suggestions.

Part of the time working on this book was generously supported by the NIH (R01 HG01837) and the Robert Wood Johnson Foundation's Investigator Award in Health Policy. I spent the 2005–2006 academic year at the idyllic Wissenschaftskolleg zu Berlin. There are simply too many fellows, staff, and administrators there to thank individually, but the disparate parts of this book would not have come together without their help.

One consequence of having a project with such a long gestation period is that students who once worked for me as research assistants are now scholars in their own right, such as Elizabeth Toon and Carla Keirns. Elizabeth taught me, an interloper in history from clinical medicine, a great deal about working in archives and organizing research data. She independently researched a lot of material for Chapters 4 and 5, and my ideas about "life at risk" and truth telling evolved partly as a result of our joint efforts to select and prioritize Halsted's vast clinical correspondence. Other students who have worked with me in archives and libraries include Sejal Patel, Tiffany Behringer, Dominique Tobell, Caroline Todd, and Corinna Schlombs.

Part of what I hope is valuable about *Unnatural History* is the close examination of the patient experience of cancer and the doctor–patient relationship. Those parts of the book could not have been written without the experiences I have had as a doctor and friend to many people struggling with cancer. For reasons of privacy and space, I cannot mention their names, but I will remember here Dianne Barton, Michael Powell, and Marty Bloch. Dianne was the doctor who gave everything to her patients, and she expected the same from the vast network of health care professionals she consulted but never quite let take charge of her care. Michael let me and others who cared for him into the most intimate places. Even at the most desperate moments, he remained a gifted teacher. Both Dianne and Michael came as teachers to my undergraduate classes at Penn and generously imparted a great deal of what they experienced and learned. Marty died before I started this book but his life and struggle with cancer have shaped every part of this project.

My family members have put up with a lot over the past few years and have helped me enormously. My parents Nat and Eve Aronowitz have selflessly supported everything that I do. My father died just as this book was completed. Up until his last illness, I gave him a progress report in our daily calls that I now miss so much. Over the years, I have learned a great deal from discussing the issues raised in this book with my brother Jerry Aronowitz and sister Sandy Katz. Daniel and Sara, my children, read parts of the book and let me inject risk and cancer into dinner conversations and family vacations. Over the years, they have given me all kinds of frank and often smart advice, more of which I should have heeded. My wife, Jane Mathisen, made too many sacrifices to mention. She read every word of the book and gave me her honest but always supportive suggestions. I dedicate this book to her.

ONE

Introduction

I

Breast cancer is all around us: cutting down lives, causing fear, and presenting difficult, often impossible, dilemmas. In the week in which I first drafted this introduction, both my 80-year-old uncle and his 50-year-old daughter-in-law (my cousin's wife) were diagnosed with invasive breast cancer. My then 12-year-old daughter did not think men had breasts; most adults similarly do not know that men get breast cancer. My cousin's wife could have chosen a limited excision of her small cancer but instead decided to have both breasts as well as her ovaries removed. Her mother had died at about her age of ovarian cancer, and her younger sister had recently died of breast cancer. She was "taking no chances." I understood her reasons for this decision and would not second-guess them. But I also knew that even such radical surgery would not entirely extirpate the danger or her fear of cancer.

American women fear breast cancer much more today than they did a hundred years ago when there seemed to be less of it, and it was not such a visible – and contested – public concern. In today's way of talking about and experiencing the fear of breast cancer, we characteristically speak of the increased *risk* of the disease. The central development I analyze in *An Unnatural History: Breast Cancer and American Society* is the historical change over the last two centuries from isolated, private fears of breast cancer to immense individual and collective concern over the risk of breast cancer. I will detail how and why our biological understandings, epidemiological perceptions, clinical and public health interventions, and personal experience and fears of breast cancer have changed so radically.

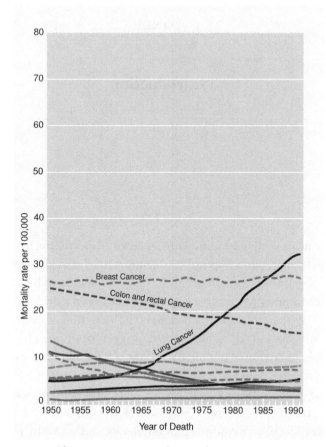

Figure 1.1. Changing patterns for twelve major cancers in U.S. females 1950–1991. Death rates for females, per 100,000, for twelve sites, 1950–1991, age-adjusted to 1970. (Adapted from SEER Data, public use files.)

The change from a disease that was hardly visible to anyone who was not directly affected by it to the highly publicized statistic that women in the United States have a lifetime risk of 1:8 of being afflicted with the disease is not simply a reflection of more and worse disease. Epidemiologists have observed that the age-specific mortality from breast cancer – the odds of women of a given age dying from breast cancer – in the United States remained essentially unchanged from the time minimally adequate aggregate data were first collected in the 1930s until around 1990 (see Figure 1.1), when it began to decline.[1] Epidemiologists use age-specific mortality to make valid historical comparisons – in this case, to factor out the increase in breast cancer deaths due only to more people surviving into older ages (when breast cancer is more common). It is possible that efforts at early detection and progress in treatment had just kept up with an increasing tide of new breast cancer cases, resulting in a mortality standoff for most of the twentieth century. A more economical explanation is that we have detected a large amount of disease not destined to seriously harm or kill and – until quite recently – have not made significant progress in treating cancer.

Unnatural History's terrain is the chasm between our medical and cultural understandings of breast cancer and its direct biological impact. Starting with the experience of breast cancer in the early nineteenth century, I examine the *social* forces and developments that led to a radical transformation of breast cancer's impact and meaning in American society.[2] Some readers and medical colleagues will probably be surprised and challenged by my emphasis on underlying social rather than biological causes of the historical shift in both the perception and lived experience of breast cancer in the United States. For example, I will argue in Chapter 6 that the widely perceived improvements in breast cancer survival rates in the middle decades of the twentieth century largely resulted from changed health-seeking behavior and diagnostic practices rather than more effective means of prevention and treatment. I want to redress an imbalance that follows from the priority generally given to biological over social explanations in cancer and many other diseases. Pushing social explanations as far as they might plausibly go also has considerable heuristic value. Cancer and other diseases look different when social factors are in the foreground, rather than evoked only to explain what cannot be attributed to biologically mediated changes.

At the same time, I do not assume that breast cancer, as a purely biological process in the bodies of American women, has had an unchanging clinical expression or population impact. It is highly probable, for example, that the real incidence of breast cancer (number of new cases in a given time period) was rising during the nineteenth and early twentieth century America. This change most likely resulted from social and economic shifts that led to earlier onset of menstrual periods, older age of first childbirth, fewer children, and later menopause.[3] Neither do I assume that our clinical and public efforts have had little or no impact on breast cancer as a biological process. The declining breast cancer mortality in the United States since 1990 has probably resulted from more use of effective treatment, especially hormonal therapy and chemotherapy given to women who do not have clinical evidence of cancer spread, and to a lesser extent, the identification of cancers through screening.[4]

Unnatural History is not a polemic about medical and popular misunderstanding of breast or other cancers' natural history and epidemiology, and the exaggerated claims of efficacy by supporters of current efforts at prevention and treatment. There already exists a sizeable literature that uses the tools of clinical epidemiology and "evidence-based medicine" to critically analyze current concepts and practices.[5] While this literature often points out important limitations of many beliefs about cancer and treatment practices, it does not try to systematically account for how we arrived at our present situation. *Unnatural History* is a *history* of how we incrementally arrived at our present state of belief and practice. This narrative involves choice, change, and continuity in medical and lay beliefs about cancer and the body, the felt experience of cancer and fear of cancer, the nature of relations between patients and doctors, and the assumptions patients and doctors have used in making clinical decisions.

The narrative alternates between detailed "grain of sand" case studies of individual patients and overviews of important developments in medical thought and clinical and public health practice, from the early nineteenth century to the third quarter of the twentieth century. I do not consider in any detail case studies or medical developments after 1977. This is in part arbitrary, but also reflects my belief that the major elements of what I consider to be our current era of breast cancer risk (subject of the concluding chapter) were in place at that time. The detailed case studies give texture to the felt experience of affected women. I similarly use the writings and clinical records of selected doctors to provide a close up view of the often subtle continuities and changes in medical assumptions about breast cancer. The larger picture that emerges is thus potentially distorted by my selective sampling, but I hope that this limitation is balanced by the book's wide historical sweep and the advantages of examining in detail how breast cancer was experienced and decisions were made in different eras.

In the many casual historical overviews of breast cancer, which have appeared in such diverse places as patient accounts, newspaper articles, medical review articles, and grand round talks, there are typically three recurring motifs: (1) the post–World War II movement away from radical mastectomies toward more localized surgery, led by a few researchers who tested their original ideas in robust clinical trials whose results then influenced practitioners to change their practice; (2) the important role women played in this and other changes in cancer treatment; and (3) the declining paternalism and increased honesty in doctor–patient interactions surrounding breast and other cancers. While these overviews capture some important developments, they are incomplete and partly reflect the problematic assumptions, priorities, and visions of their narrators. They assume a basic stability in what breast cancer is and means as well as that significant therapeutic progress has and is being made. They tend to ignore countervailing contemporary trends, such as the increased frequency of radical surgery for breast cancer risk, and deeper continuities, such as the desire of both physicians and patients to maintain hope and avoid stark confrontations with mortality.

Apart from a skeptical reading of epidemiological trends, there are reasons to believe that the many historical changes in the magnitude, meaning, and significance of the risk factors for breast cancer are not a simple reflection of the disease's increased deadliness. Risk, as many anthropologists, sociologists, historians, and others have reminded us, is a cultural construct that bears a problematic and often indirect relationship to death rates or other "objective" markers of danger and bad outcomes.[6] In our contemporary response to breast cancer, risk is an elusive term with different meanings and uses. It may be used to describe a quantitative assessment of disease incidence or mortality in a defined population upon which policies such as annual screening mammography are built or it may describe a highly individual, subjective sense of danger, which might influence lifestyle "choices" such as the timing of a first child, the use of oral contraceptives, or starting a low fat diet.

Epidemiologists, doctors, and laypersons often use terms such as *risk factors*, *risk reduction*, and *risk assessment* in a way that implies or assumes that the important causes of breast cancer are mostly a matter of individual – rather than social or communal – concern and responsibility. There is also often a problematic quantification in some risk-factor discourse that makes it appear that we know more than we do about the precise causes of breast cancer and the relative impact of different putative risks. While existing risk factors sometimes help mediate the gap between aggregate data and individual decision-making, they are hardly an unfailingly wise guide to lifestyle, clinical, and policy choices. They can obscure as much as clarify.

Thus we should not understand breast cancer risk ideas and terms as a merely logical or self-evident way of conceptualizing and communicating about danger, choice, cause, or responsibility. Modern risk discourse often reveals more about our present and past assumptions, priorities, and investments than it expresses new etiological, preventive, or therapeutic insights.

Nothing seems more new, objective, and insightful than recent developments in the genetics of breast cancer. In the early 1990s, molecular biologists identified mutations in two "susceptibility" genes for hereditary breast and ovarian cancer (BRCA1 and BRCA2), and epidemiologists began to correlate genetic mutations with particular ethnic groups, most notably the association between specific mutations and Ashkenazic Jewish women.[7] These discoveries have already led to widespread genetic testing and risk assessment, prophylactic surgery for some genetic mutation carriers, and ethnicity-based disease advocacy and community programs. It is likely that lay and biomedical interest – as well as finite economic and intellectual resources – will shift in a problematic and disproportionate manner from the much more common sporadic cases of breast cancer to the seemingly more certain, mechanistically rationalized, "genetic" cases. The test for a breast cancer susceptibility gene is likely to be one of the first of many such tests that will transform our view of individual health from a complex group of consequences of one's heredity, environmental exposure, lifestyle choices, and chance to a more specific, precise, and frightening "at risk for" consciousness.

Yet, however profound these changes may appear, they cannot be understood as direct, unmediated consequences of new genetic knowledge. There are many continuities between the seemingly revolutionary impact of genetic insights and earlier experimental, pathological, epidemiological, and clinical insights. For example, the enthusiastic medical and popular reception of genetic insights and the rapid deployment of genetic tests reflect a historically familiar calculus of change. Clinicians and laypersons have often made fundamental decisions – to encourage or consent to some type of cancer surveillance, to consult a doctor for a breast lump, to choose one type of therapy over another, or to promote this or that educational message – because of the vision of the future with which they most closely identify. Promise more than evidence from clinical trials or the lived realities of disease and clinical practice has repeatedly played a determining role in many personal, clinical, and policy decisions and developments concerning breast cancer. Knowledge of these historical continuities can help clinicians and patients respond more thoughtfully to the many clinical and policy conundrums presented by genetic tests, screening mammography, lifestyle interventions, and prophylactic surgery and chemotherapy.

II

But why an *Unnatural History*? The choice of title partly goes against – and distinguishes my approach from – the more fashionable trend of emphasizing the natural, that is, the biological and adaptive, basis of complex behaviors and social structures, in paper, book, and lecture titles, for example, the natural history of parenting, sex, alcoholism, fear, and so on. But the history of the meaning, perception, and experience of breast cancer in the nineteenth and twentieth centuries can be thought of as "unnatural" in several other ways. First, for much of breast cancer's modern history, we have radically transformed breast cancer's epidemiological, clinical, and personal meaning, often without significantly changing its natural history, that is, its destructive course within the body. Second, the most important initiators and mediators of these transformations are best understood as social (e.g., lowered thresholds for seeking medical attention for breast lumps or expanding definitions of cancer) rather than biological/natural. Finally, there is the historical contingency of the natural history concept itself. In each era and setting, researchers, clinicians, and laypersons have often meant, assumed, or focused on different basic identities and definitions of breast cancer – macroscopic or molecular, one disease or many, constitutional or local, a disease from within or without, predetermined or treatable, discrete from or continuous with "premalignant" and benign conditions. "What *is* breast cancer?" has been a recurrent, central, if often unarticulated, question just below the surface of so many controversies about cause, prevention, treatment, prognosis, and policy. It also lies just below the surface of many individuals' difficult decisions.

Students frequently ask me how physicians and patients could use the word *cancer* in the era before microscopic descriptions of abnormal cells and in clinical situations where nothing remotely like twentieth- or twenty-first-century diagnostics were done. They also question any historical comparisons between whatever we mean by cancer today and these older entities. I often respond by pointing out that categorizing and diagnosing cancer is contingent on tools, medical knowledge, and the social and medical uses of labels, in the past and now. To bring this point home, I imagine a future medical world where students wonder how early twenty-first-century physicians and patients accepted chemotherapy for small "breast cancers" and surgery for some "prostate cancers" when they did not yet have the XYZ test that predicts with a high degree of certainty which tumors will be lethal and which will be slow-growing and unlikely to metastasize.

I am a doctor as well as an historian, and my clinical experiences and training have shaped my historical approach. I have been influenced by teachers and mentors who have had a skeptical, empirical, and quantitative "evidence-based" approach to clinical practice and health policy. My clinical experiences and those of my patients, friends, and family members, some of which are discussed in this chapter, have often reinforced my skepticism about many existing public health and clinical strategies in breast and other cancers. But at the same time I worry about the implications of this skepticism. It has been personally difficult, for example, to reconcile my belief that past and present prevention and treatment efforts in breast cancer are less effective than widely believed with my responsibility for the health of patients, friends, and family. I recently talked with a friend in her 40s who said that she was still not getting screening mammograms "thanks to you." I immediately protested that our previous conversations were about my historical research and not meant to suggest specific courses of action in the here and now. But I also knew that I was on thin ice. Like the many historical actors whose actions and beliefs I closely examine here, I would like to eat my cake (in this case, draw general historical implications for the present) and have it too (not be tied to specific clinical recommendations, especially since the evidence is often unclear and almost always changing). One result of this awareness has been to redouble my efforts to approach the different actors in historical and contemporary controversies in an empathetic, balanced, and nonpolemical manner.

III

Naming and Classifying Breast Cancer

My friend Janet was 47 years old when she made an appointment for a screening mammogram. Although her family doctor had told her that medical opinion was divided over whether women in their 40s needed mammograms, she had been feeling guilty about not having had one. A few minutes after her mammogram was done, a radiologist asked Janet to come into a consultation room and showed her a 1-inch suspicious mass on the just developed film. The radiologist then called Janet's family doctor, who arranged for her to see a breast surgeon a few days later. The surgeon reviewed Janet's mammogram and then examined her. She thought she could feel something that corresponded to the suspicious area on the mammogram. She did a needle biopsy in the office, which turned out to be benign. After these results became known, the surgeon suggested to Janet, and a few days later performed, an excisional biopsy both to remove any doubts about malignancy and to make it easier to evaluate future screening mammograms.

Janet was shocked when the surgeon called a few days later and told her she had something called "lobular carcinoma in situ (LCIS)." Janet's surgeon explained that LCIS was a kind of precancer, which in her case was probably an accidental finding unrelated to the abnormal mammogram. She explained that "carcinoma in situ" in Latin roughly means "cancer in position" and describes the presence of abnormal, cancer-looking or cancerous cells that are contained within the normal boundaries of the epithelial tissue from which they arose. In LCIS, the abnormal cells are confined to the breast lobules (one of the small masses of tissue within the breast).

Janet was even more puzzled when her surgeon explained that Janet was not "cured" by her excisional biopsy, since the precancerous condition could be present diffusely in both breasts. Her treatment options included doing more vigilant screening, taking an antiestrogen medicine called Tamoxifen, which might help but which would probably bring on menopause and increased her risk of uterine cancer, enrolling in a clinical trial of new agents, or having "prophylactic" bilateral mastectomies (in an earlier era, shortly after LCIS was first "discovered," many physicians recommended mastectomy without reservation). Janet's overriding emotion was regret over having had the mammogram in the first place. But there was no going back, only a series of disturbing questions for which her doctors could not give her satisfying answers: What exactly is LCIS? What were her chances of dying from cancer if she did nothing? Took Tamoxifen?

While Janet's predicament had its origins in medical knowledge and technology, existing medical evidence provided little guidance about what she should do. Some clarification might have come from understanding the history of the conflicting values, perspectives, and interests that have contributed to how we classify and name breast and other cancers. Throughout the nineteenth and twentieth centuries, this history has been contentious: What is the proper definition of cancer? What is the relation between clinical and pathological diagnosis and cancer's clinical behavior? Who gets to decide? What is cancer's natural history? How should the circumstances of discovery, diagnosis, and treatment affect the way we name and classify cancer?

Some researchers and clinicians have come to understand LCIS as a risk factor for future invasive breast cancer more than as a pathological entity in itself. In this view, the meaning of a positive biopsy is in what it signifies about future risk rather than the dangers emanating from a localized entity. LCIS thus helps bring breast cancer into the borderland between disease and risk, joining company with many contemporary – and controversial – entities such as osteoporosis and hypercholesterolemia.

In almost every site-specific cancer, there are similar risk/disease complexities. Urged on by her family doctor, a relative of mine in her 70s decided to undergo a full colonoscopy as a screening test for colon cancer. Her gastroenterologist took out a few polyps, one of which was a small villous adenoma, which, while having some definite malignant potential, does not uniformly progress to colon cancer. Shortly after her colonoscopy, she received a letter in which the gastroenterologist congratulated my relative for her decision to undergo screening, since it resulted in the discovery and removal of cancer. With continued vigilance, the doctor continued, she could remain cured of colon cancer. The use of the words *cancer* and *cure* to describe my relative's polyp and polypectomy exaggerated and gave a pseudoprecision to the danger and drama of her screening test and the cancerness of her premalignant condition. This conflation of risk and disease, problematic under ideal circumstances, is especially troublesome when linked to the provision of preventive services, which bring economic rewards to their providers.

In looking at the history of the emergence of such entities as LCIS, I question the taken-for-grantedness of the basic terms and concepts different actors have used to conduct research, structure public health campaigns, and understand their own problems and decisions. Social norms and attitudes, not only clinical and technological developments, have determined how we classify and diagnose cancer. Like the popularization of risk factors for coronary heart disease, the promulgation of breast cancer risk factors has led to many contested questions for individuals and policy makers: What constitutes a risk factor? Are these risk factors diseases in themselves? Should we test for risk factors in clinical practice? What level of evidence might justify interventions?

The juxtaposition of "carcinoma" with "in situ" to form a name for an uncertain probability of future cancer is part of a larger phenomenon in which the terms used to denote, modify, or describe cancer and cancer risk carry problematic connotations, which influence our clinical and policy responses. Some observers have strongly objected to using "carcinoma" to denote cells that have not invaded adjacent tissues and only have a weak statistical probability of ever doing so.

Another contemporary example of the importance of how cancer and risk are named and classified can be seen in debates over the privacy of genetic information. These debates often pivot on fears of losing health insurance because of a "preexisting condition." In what sense is knowledge of some portion of an individual's DNA sequences any more "preexisting" than knowledge of that individual's family history? In what sense is a particular genetic sequence "a condition" when it produces no symptoms and has only a statistical correlation with some adverse endpoint? We cannot answer these questions in some abstract sense since virtually no one inside or outside of biomedicine offers explicit definitions of what constitutes a legitimate disease or risk. Historical study of the ways these terms are used can help us understand different groups' norms for labeling variation a "risk" or a "disease." A deeper understanding of these norms is essential to understanding and resolving debates about the meaning and definition of genetic risk and genetic disease.

Idiosyncrasy and Ontology

During my first year of medical school, more than a generation ago, my friend Ruth felt a lump in her breast. Ruth was in her late 30s at the time, recently divorced, raising her young daughter by herself and trying to build a career that would put her Ph.D. in biochemistry to productive use. Ruth's surgeon performed a biopsy that showed cancer. He recommended that Ruth have a mastectomy along with a dissection of the lymph nodes in her armpit. If the lymph nodes contained cancer, she would receive chemotherapy. Ruth was skeptical of the surgeon's recommendations and his authoritarian style. The proposed treatment plan seemed too focused on destroying cancer rather than nurturing the body's "natural" defenses. With a critical eye informed by her scientific background, Ruth read the medical literature on breast cancer treatments. She was also interested in healing outside of orthodox medicine. She read widely in this area and talked with healers and cancer patients who had used unorthodox treatments. Ruth believed that her cancer was largely caused by the way she had lived her life so far, especially the stress she experienced during her failed marriage and difficult divorce. She wanted to attack her cancer largely by rededicating herself to making important changes in the way she lived.

Her reading of the medical literature and discussions with medical people led her to conclude that treatment beyond an excision of her primary tumor was not going to significantly improve her chances for survival. After her limited surgery, she planned to seek alternative treatments and make changes in the way she lived that would strengthen her own immune defenses against cancer.

I remember my frustration over Ruth's decision to forego dissection of the lymph nodes in her armpit and thus the possibility of chemotherapy if her nodes proved positive for cancer. My oncology teachers taught this standard approach and expert opinion in the medical literature agreed with them. I conceded to Ruth that there was a great deal we did not know about the true efficacy of standard approaches to breast cancer, but I believed the plan proposed by her doctor was the right one given these uncertainties. I also believed that better treatments for breast cancer might be imminent and feared the consequences of Ruth's decision to leave standard medical care after her limited surgery. I was at the time – and remain – more skeptical about many alternative therapies than about treatments for which there are at least some data to use in clinical decisions.

While I smugly predicted that Ruth would eventually see the wisdom of at least combining standard medical approaches with her pursuit of holistic ones, she never swayed from her course. Her quest for alternative healing took her to different healing traditions, a new career in health promotion, and to injections of serum pooled from individuals who had "beat" cancer. She lived a good and active life for another 12 years – empowered by, and enthusiastic about, her quest to live with and perhaps survive cancer in her own way. She never suffered any of the side effects of orthodox treatments or symptoms from cancer until she died suddenly from a blood clot in her lungs, a common complication of cancer, when she was 50.

How Ruth chose to live her life raised difficult questions for me about medical knowledge and practice. Was Ruth's fate fixed at the time of diagnosis? Was she courageous or foolish? How was I – as I underwent my training as a physician – going to respond to my patients' "why me?" and "why now?" questions about cancer and the deep personal searching and unconventional decisions that often follow from trying to answer these questions?

Ruth's quest was a challenge to medicine's authority to determine the best ways to treat cancer. It also challenged the notion that the accumulated clinical, pathological, and epidemiological knowledge about breast cancer as a disease was the most relevant knowledge for her particular situation. Like Ruth, I also have wanted to see breast cancer less as a standard "thing" common to all people with a certain tissue pathology and more as a unique problem for different individuals. We generally take it for granted that the category breast cancer describes a limited set of physical abnormalities whose defining criteria can be spelled out and applied in a uniform way. Historians of medicine and others have sometimes called this way of categorizing sickness "ontological," that is, diseases are specific entities that unfold in characteristic ways in the typical person. They can be said to exist in some platonic sense outside of their manifestations in any particular individual. The complementary perspective on sickness is sometimes labeled "physiological" or "holistic," and emphasizes individual idiosyncrasy and individual adaptation to a changing environment.[8]

The question of idiosyncrasy is at the root of many contemporary clinical and policy controversies in breast cancer. For example, the controversy over whether women between the ages of 40 and 50 should have screening mammograms is typically understood as one over evidence and its interpretation. There is a large body of evidence that suggests that screening in this age group either does not save lives or has a very small and costly benefit. Nevertheless, many people support screening mammography for women under 50 because it seems only logical that such a practice should save or extend some lives. Breast cancer can affect women in their 40s. Mammography should be able to identify at least some small cancers that have malignant potential but have not yet spread. For many people, extrapolating from no good evidence to not screening means suspending an entire belief system about cancer. Not to screen means accepting the idea that women in their 40s suffer breast cancers that are idiosyncratic, either so "good" or so "bad" that early detection adds little to the eventual outcome. (This idiosyncratic dimension is important even when one considers the influence of more conventional explanations for mammography's poor efficacy in younger women such as age-related changes in the mammographic appearance of the breast and lower prevalence of disease in younger women.) Thus, the most important dividing line in this controversy may be whether one is willing to suspend belief in the dominant ontologic model of disease – that breast cancer has an orderly and predictable natural history – and accept a more idiosyncratic view of breast cancer.

Cancer, Fear, and Time

Maria is a 42-year-old colleague who had started to get annual mammograms at age 40 "just to be on the safe side." Her most recent mammogram showed some new, small, suspicious calcifications in her right breast. On the same afternoon of her mammogram, Maria's radiologist did a fine needle aspiration biopsy of the suspicious area. Two days later, a pathologist interpreted the biopsy as ductal carcinoma in situ (DCIS), a kind of pre-cancer similar to LCIS in that its natural history, clinical significance, and proper treatment have long been the subject of controversy (in DCIS, the cancerous-looking cells are confined to the breast ducts).[9] At the same time, DCIS is a more localized process than LCIS and is generally treated very similarly to "bona fide" cancer (tumors that have spread beyond the normal tissue boundaries), that is, with surgery, radiation, and often hormonal therapy. Over the next few days, Maria consulted a general internist, a medical oncologist, and a surgeon who specialized in breast cancer. She talked with a number of friends and friends of friends who had personal experiences with breast cancer, some of whom had DCIS, and read about breast cancer in books she took out from the library. Maria focused her energies on the most pressing decision – whether her initial surgical treatment should be a wide excision, unilateral mastectomy, or bilateral mastectomy.

Although none of her close relatives had breast cancer, Maria had always felt that it was not a question of whether she would get breast cancer but when she would get it. Maria's doctors told her that DCIS increased the probability that she might later develop invasive breast cancer. They stressed the great scientific uncertainty surrounding specific probabilities, the lack of data directly comparing treatments for DCIS, the high probability that any future breast cancer could be detected early and treated successfully, and that, no matter what Maria decided to do, her absolute risk of dying from breast cancer was low. Maria struggled with the meaning of the statistics presented to her and came to an understanding that they were an abstract reality that was of limited help – she had only one flip of the coin and it was going to land either heads or tails. Faced with a small, uncertain, but "real" possibility of not being able to live to see her children grow up, Maria chose to have bilateral mastectomies, the option she believed would best guarantee that she would not die from breast cancer. She underwent surgery exactly 1 month after her screening mammogram.

Maria's experience of breast cancer at the beginning of the twenty-first century – her mammograms, precancer diagnosis, heightened sense of risk, struggle with statistics, surgical options, "radical" decision, and the rapidity of events – seems very different from the experiences of women with breast cancer at the beginning of the twentieth century. Yet in many ways her experience is continuous with, and a direct consequence of, a century of ideas and practices surrounding the prevention and treatment of cancer, especially breast cancer.

Throughout the century, there has been a war against time fought on a series of fronts – public education campaigns to get women not to delay in seeking medical attention for lumps and other suspicious breast changes, technological innovation aimed at developing new ways of early diagnosis, new pathologic knowledge about "earlier" stages in the natural history of breast cancer, and – as in Maria's case – aggressive treatments aimed against the possibility of future disease. We can gain some critical insight into Maria's difficult decision and those faced by many other women today by a more detailed historical understanding of the complex interactions between clinical and public health practices and fear of cancer.

Doctor–Patient Relationship: Honesty, Trust and Hope

Robin was a 40-year-old physician who felt a new pelvic pain. She was not satisfied when her gynecologist could not find anything abnormal on physical examination and attributed her pain to work stress. She ordered a pelvic ultrasound for herself, which revealed an ovarian mass. A week later, a gynecological oncologist operated on Robin and removed the mass. The mass turned out to be ovarian cancer that involved the adjacent tissues and lymph nodes. Both Robin's gynecological and medical oncologists suggested a standard chemotherapy protocol as the next step, but they supported Robin's desire to get a second opinion about a much riskier and more toxic higher dose chemotherapy regimen, which would require a bone marrow transplant.

Robin was referred to a leading clinical researcher who specialized in such regimens. This expert reviewed Robin's history and did a cursory physical examination. He prefaced his discussion of treatment options by stating that Robin should not ask any question to which she was not ready to hear the answer. He first asked Robin about her current thinking. Robin said that she understood that her long-term odds of survival were less than 50 percent and so she was willing to take some increased risk of more toxic treatment now if there was reason to believe that such treatment would change these terrifying odds.

The ovarian cancer specialist explained that while the medical literature on ovarian cancer typically describes different stages along with subtypes and borderline categories, he generally divided patients into two categories, optimal and suboptimal. Robin was visibly shaken as she understood that she had a number of different reasons for being in the suboptimal category. He said there was no evidence that the more extreme treatment protocols were better than the standard approach for women with "suboptimal" cancers.

When pressed by Robin, the expert further explained that the great majority of women in Robin's suboptimal class will soon die of their cancer no matter what the treatment. Robin then asked even more specific questions about her own odds of surviving ovarian cancer. In some frank, difficult, and awkward give and takes, the expert said that her odds of surviving were "much, much less" than fifty-fifty. "So we're talking Gilda Radner?" Robin asked after a long silence (Gilda Radner was a prominent television and film comedian who had died from ovarian cancer a few years earlier). "Yes, we're talking Gilda Radner," the expert replied.

Robin chose the standard chemotherapy regimen. On the basis of a strong family history of breast and ovarian cancer, she was later tested and found positive for the "breast cancer gene." One year after her ovarian cancer diagnosis, she had bilateral, prophylactic mastectomies. She lived for 7 years after her initial diagnosis, ultimately dying from cancer but far outliving the expert's or the textbook's prognosis.

Robin would recall the "Gilda Radner" moment as one of the lowest points in her struggle with cancer. She felt that the expert had extinguished her hope for survival at a time when she was not ready to have this hope shattered. She wondered if the expert had strayed from the more usual pattern of softening or evading a "hopeless" prognosis because she was a physician-patient. At the same time, she acknowledged that the exchange might have been pivotal in her decision to not pursue experimental treatment, a decision that seemed wise in hindsight. Was the expert wrong to have been so "honest"? A contemporary bioethicist might find this a straightforward case. Was Robin's autonomy respected? Was the expert beneficent? But such a *principled* approach glosses over the tragic conflict that often exists among competing goods, such as truthful communication, trust between doctor and patient, and hope for survival.

We often act as if we live in an era in which the patient–consumer has a right to truthful information, which he or she will use to make autonomous medical decisions. Physician's evasion of cancer diagnoses and other less-than-truthful exchanges around cancer seem an embarrassment from a distant age. Yet looking at the history of doctor–patient interactions one sees more continuities than discontinuities. While I do not think that a deep historical awareness of these currents makes judgments about honesty, trust, and truth any easier, it might make us more skeptical about the idealized patient–consumer role and more aware of the complexity and tragedy of action when hope and honesty are in conflict.

Women at Risk

The last contemporary "case" I will recount concerns a woman who not only does not have cancer but has neither name nor face – just a lacy bra and a number. A few years ago she appeared in a print advertisement for the drug Nolvadex (tamoxifen) in general newspapers and magazines all over the United States (see Figure 1.2). Nolvadex is a synthetic female hormone that has been shown in clinical trials to be an effective treatment for some women with breast cancer. In more recent years, it has been tested – with mixed and controversial results – as a means of

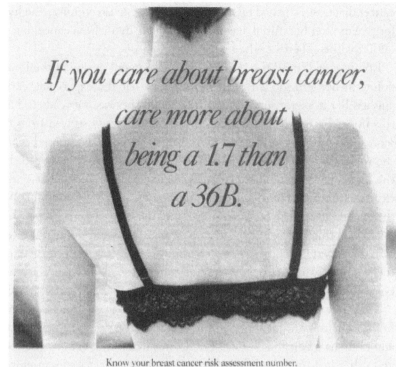

Know your breast cancer risk assessment number.

Know that NOLVADEX® (tamoxifen citrate) could reduce your chances of getting breast cancer if you are at high risk.

Figure 1.2. NOLVADEX(r) (tamoxifen citrate) direct-to-consumer advertisement. (Reproduced with permission of AstraZeneca.)

preventing breast cancer among "high-risk" women. The advertisement encourages women to "know their risk assessment number" and asserts that Nolvadex can reduce their chances of getting breast cancer if their risk assessment number is equal to or greater than 1.7.

The number 1.7 turns out to be the predicted relative risk of breast cancer that was used as an entry criterion in one of the most positive Nolvadex prevention trials (drug manufacturers are allowed to make claims about their drug's efficacy for populations that resemble the group tested). In that trial, different characteristics of individual women, such as their age, family history of breast cancer, previous benign biopsies, and other factors, were entered into a complicated formula that resulted in a risk assessment number. The number 1.7 means that a woman is 1.7 times more likely than a woman at average risk to develop breast cancer in her lifetime. Many women have a relative risk of greater than 1.7 on the basis of single factors such as having had a diagnosis of lobular carcinoma in situ or a combination of more innocent factors such as being postmenopausal and having had a first child after 30. Many American women today, if so assessed, would thus turn out to have a high enough risk to be eligible for preventive drug treatment. If such risk assessment were to take hold in American popular and medical culture, there would be a huge new market for a drug that has serious side effects such as premature menopause and menopausal symptoms, blood clots, and even uterine cancer, and whose role in prevention is still contested.

The woman in the advertisement is one representation of breast cancer risk among contemporary American women. Her existence makes sense only in a world in which breast cancer evokes a devastating blow to sexuality and femininity as well as more universal fears of pain, suffering, and loss of life. The modern American woman's concern for a desired breast size and shape (36B), the advertisement suggests, is trivial (and perhaps egotistically self-destructive) compared to what she really needs in light of the danger she may be in of having breast cancer.[10]

The many other problematic assumptions and messages in this advertisement – the quantitative and pseudoprecise style of risk assessment, the focus on individual responsibility, the leap from uncertain aggregate data to individual behavior, the stoking of cancer fears, the problematic role of the profit motive in research and prevention, the link between the physician's prescription and his or her role as risk assessor, and more – did not arise de novo. *Unnatural History* traces the developments in American society and medicine that led to present beliefs about and responses to breast cancer risk.

IV

Unnatural History is not an argument to cleanse distorting social influences from current breast cancer ideas and practices so that we more objectively see and respond to breast cancer's true, biologically based natural history. There is nothing about breast cancer's biology that strictly determines where pathologists should draw the boundary between benign and malignant or what balance of individual risk factor and population-based prevention works best or even if women should fear breast cancer more than coronary heart disease. These are perceptions and judgments resulting from interacting social and biological factors, past and present.

Breast cancer's social history and identity would not suddenly become irrelevant if scientists discover some clarifying etiological insight or develop extremely effective therapy. Past and present beliefs, interests, and investments would continue to influence how Americans view and respond to the disease.

Unnatural History is also not an argument for specific clinical or policy actions or a polemic about what really causes cancer. This history is nevertheless relevant to present and future policy, clinical, and existential problems raised by breast cancer, but in more indirect ways. For example, it makes sense to evaluate the promise of genetic research to transform our clinical and public health approaches to cancer through the prism of over a century of unfulfilled promises about detection, prevention, and treatment, which share with the imagined genetic future an emotional appeal to the transcendent value of cancer prevention and cure. Such claims about the future have often served to brush aside contemporary doubts about the effectiveness of specific practices, questions about their potential costs and consequences, and alternative visions of the cancer problem. Awareness of these interactions and other aspects of breast cancer's history in American society can help us make wiser decisions and set more reasonable priorities and policies.

TWO

Cancer in the Breast, 1813

In exploring the effects of past attitudes and practices on the current experience of breast cancer, early-nineteenth-century American society is a strategic place to begin. Many medical and popular beliefs and practices surrounding what was then referred to as cancer in the breast that had been essentially unchanged for centuries were beginning to shift as were the demographic patterns that shaped the population impact of the disease.[1]

I will structure my analysis of early-nineteenth-century American (and to a lesser extent, British) beliefs about and responses to cancer in the breast around the experiences of Susan Dillwyn Emlen, who died at Oxmead, her family home in Burlington County, New Jersey, on November 24, 1819 after a 6-year struggle with the disease. Emlen was born March 31, 1769 in Houghton, New Jersey to William Dillwyn (1743–1824) and his first wife Sarah Logan Smith (1749–1769), who died soon after her daughter's birth. Emlen's father later moved to England where he married his second wife, Sally Weston, and had eight children. Emlen was raised in Oxmead by her maternal aunt Susanna Dillwyn Cox. She grew up within a tightly knit group of prominent New Jersey and Philadelphia Quaker families. One great grandfather on her maternal side was James Logan, William Penn's secretary.

Emlen's obituary writer noted her "patience and resignation under the most severe sufferings and long protracted anguish."[2] These personal characteristics and the events that tested them are well documented in a rich correspondence among Emlen's tightly knit but far flung family, friends, and Quaker associates as well as in other personal papers and writings.[3] These different perspectives on Emlen's life and illness provide a scaffold upon which to hang an inquiry into the early American experience of cancer in the breast. What did medical men and ordinary people understand about cancer in the breast? How did these ideas and other influences shape the diagnosis and treatment of women with suspected cancer? How were decisions, treatments, and the disease itself experienced? What was the texture of afflicted women's hopes and fears for the future?

In late 1813, at the age of 44, Emlen recognized that there was something wrong in her left breast. In a series of letters written in 1814 to William Dillwyn, Emlen's father who had moved to England to pursue his interests in Quaker education, abolitionism, and other causes, Emlen and her husband Samuel Emlen gave several slightly different accounts of when she recognized she had a tumor and told her husband and others about it.[4] Emlen's initial perception of something wrong in the breast gradually and haltingly turned into an apprehension that she had a cancerous tumor. The lump was "about the size of a partridge egg," typical of the size at which most nineteenth-century women recognized there was a problem and sought medical attention (if they ever did).[5] Emlen's tumor was initially painless, but later produced a "slight pressure." "My terror when I had fully ascertained the fact is not to be expressed," she wrote her father. Only "after some weeks of anxiety," did she mention her discovery to her husband and her "dear Aunt Cox."[6]

While Emlen's "terror" reflected the fact that many Americans knew that tumors could be cancerous and feared cancer, cancer in the breast or at other sites was not an especially prominent or visible danger. The decline in infectious and epidemic diseases that would lead to more people alive to die of chronic conditions like cancer was just beginning in the early nineteenth century. One can also infer that the incidence of cancer in the breast was significantly lower at the beginning of the nineteenth century than at the end because of the later age of menarche (onset of menses) and menopause, lower age of first childbirth, greater number of children, and increased breast feeding.[7] As a result of these different influences, many other diseases besides cancer were mortal threats to middle-aged men and women. For example, Samuel Emlen broke the news of his wife's cancer to her father only after recounting the details of the illness, deaths, and funerals of a number of close friends from typhus.

Americans in this era could read about the possible causes of cancer in the breast in the few medico-popular accounts that devoted some attention to cancer and related ailments. For example, William Buchan's 1785 edition of his popular *Domestic Medicine*, probably the most widely read popular health book in late-eighteenth- and early-nineteenth-century America, offered a variety of causes for cancer. Buchan wrote of a generalized disease cancer that affects men and women in many places, while mostly drawing his description from, and aiming his advice at, women with breast tumors. According to Buchan, cancer could be caused by tight stays, hereditary disposition, and "barrenness." He noted that tumors often appeared after "the menstrual flow ceases."[8]

Fear of cancer was itself often held to cause cancer and thus deserving of intervention. Scottish surgeon John Rodman in 1815 argued that fear of cancer was the most potent etiological consideration, one that explained the many observed patterns of cancer distribution, including clusters of cancer cases in families. Rather than evoking heredity when "mother and daughter were its victims," Rodman thought it was more plausible that "fretfulness of temper and superfluous anxiety, which sharpen the mental feelings, are not uncommon as maternal legacies."[9]

"Does not this resemble the desires of mankind in many things of life?" Rodman observed of the plight of many women who suffered breast tumors and became anxious and desperate enough to ask for surgery. In Rodman's view, surgery often only made things worse by increasing mental distress (which was a fundamental cause) and further irritating the already vulnerable organs.[10] In addition to advising women with breast tumors to avoid exacerbating influences such as bruises and cold weather and to regulate their excretions, blood volume, and body temperature, Rodman depicted the physician's most important role as actively intervening in this causative cycle of cancer fear and worry.

In one 1797 case, a woman with an oval tumor in her left breast consulted Rodman after being struck by a man's elbow.[11] Rodman treated her with leeches and general blood letting to reduce local inflammation, chamomile preparations to reduce the swelling, and other medicines to strengthen the bowels. While the problem was subdued within 3 years, years later (in 1809) this woman's "mamma became firm and bulky" upon hearing of a friend's breast amputation. Rodman's successful intervention was to convince her "that there was positively no cancer in the breast."[12] Rodman believed that fear was not only the cause of cancer in individual women, but was a vector through which cancer spread between women. He observed that "many feel afflictive sensations of concern whenever they hear of another being distressed with a mammary tumor named cancer. They reflect upon the calamities of this distemper with feelings of horror, particularly because the extent of these calamities is unknown, and because obscurity involved every relative circumstance, while they anxiously compassionate the state of the patient. Their interest in her ailments gains upon them, and, brooding over ideal miseries unhinges the mind, till the frame is disturbed, and disorder commences in their own breast."[13] Rodman's case descriptions make clear that among women with breast lumps and those in their immediate circles fear of cancer could be all-consuming.

Emlen's "terror" when she realized she had cancer directly reflected popular knowledge and fears of cancerous tumors in early-nineteenth-century America. In Buchan's chapter on "scirrhus and cancer," for example, Emlen could have read an account that mirrored her initial presentation and predicted the most terrifying outcomes. "Occult cancer," the feared next stage after the more contained and often painless scirrhus, most frequently occurs in women after 45 and "seems often very trifling at the beginning ... a hard tumor about the size of a hazel nut, or perhaps smaller, is generally the first symptom ... The pain and stench become intolerable; the appetite fails; the strength is exhausted by a continual hectic fever; at last, a violent hemorrhage, or discharge of blood, from some part of the body, with faintings, or convulsion fits, generally puts an end to the miserable patient's life."[14]

Samuel Emlen's initial response to his wife's tumor was to urge her to consult her brother-in-law, Dr. Philip Syng Physick, arguably the most eminent surgeon in postcolonial America.[15] Emlen, however, chose first to follow the advice of her uncle and friends "whose affectionate interest in her welfare gave weight to their opinions, [and who] were desirous that she should make a trial of Logan's plaster which had often been found efficacious in cases apparently similar."[16] Emlen and her physicians rationalized the use of topical applications like "Logan's plaster" on empiric ("found efficacious") grounds rather than on humoral or any other theoretical ones. Emlen later told her father that these initial treatment decisions also put her mind at ease in part because she was leaving her fate to "that ever gracious power who afflicts not willingly."

Emlen may have feared breast surgery – three decades before the introduction of ether anesthesia – as much or more than cancer itself. No one in Emlen's family nor any of her doctors criticized her for not promptly consulting her surgeon brother-in-law. She discussed her initial reluctance openly at the time and in retrospect. "It now appears strange to me that I should have been unwilling to consult any Physician," Emlen reflected later to her father, "but I knew Dr Physick's preference of a surgical operation in such cases, and I had not yet suffer'd enough to endure the thought of so terrible a measure."[17] Surgery was a last resort, and time was needed both to test whether lumps might disappear on their own or be reduced by treatments less horrific than breast surgery without benefit of anesthesia. While there was a hint of regret in Emlen's recollection, it was not imbued with shame nor was it viewed with moral opprobrium by those around her.

Like Emlen, English novelist Fanny Burney, residing in Paris, did not immediately seek medical attention after discovering her tumor in 1813, even though her husband similarly urged her to do so. Burney recalled that she initially could not "make so great a conquest over my repugnance."[18] In contrast to Emlen, Burney did offer some regret over not immediately seeking medical attention. She later rationalized her recounting of the events surrounding and including her mastectomy in a letter to her sister Esther as a warning to her and to later readers of the dangers of this "false confidence," of keeping knowledge of a breast lump to oneself.[19] The danger of Burney's delay was not that it made surgical cure impossible, as would be widely believed 100 years later. After all, she had survived her breast tumor and surgery. Rather, Burney seems to have regretted her initial inaction as unworthy or cowardly in itself.

In addition to fearing the evident horrors of conscious breast amputation, Emlen and Burney may have also sensed their doctors' pessimism about the effectiveness of breast amputations in saving women's lives. Medical pessimism that surgery – or anything else – could cure cancer in the breast long pre-dated the nineteenth century. Hippocratic tradition taught that "it is better to give no treatment in cases of hidden cancer; treatment causes speedy early death, but to omit treatment is to prolong life."[20] "I for one never could cure one single case," mediaeval physician Paul of Aegina "gloomily" wrote, "nor do I know anybody else who succeeded in doing so."[21] "Cancer cannot be cured and will never be cured" Gui Patin wrote in 1665, "but the world wants to be fooled."[22]

One reason for pessimism about cancer surgery was the long history of medical speculation that cancer had seeds, ferments, or roots, invisible to the surgeon, that could sprout new disease even after tumors were excised. These ideas prefigured and foreshadowed the cellular theories of tissues and cancer that would become prominent later in the nineteenth century. In the seventeenth century, George Stahl speculated that cancer contained self-propagating seeds and ferments that often remained in the body after surgery, resulting in an operation in which "nothing has been accomplished."[23]

Like seventeenth-century doctors who posited invisible cancer ferments, nineteenth-century surgeons, working in the era just prior to the ascent of microscopic anatomy in clinical practice, often observed and imagined that the "roots" of cancer could be very deep, much deeper than the mass removed at surgery. Astley Cooper reflected in 1839 that "the scirrhus tumour is not all of the disease; there are roots which extend to a considerable distance … When you dissect a scirrhus tumour, you see a number of roots proceeding to a considerable distance; and, if you remove the tumour only, and not the roots, there will be little advantage from the operation: no glandular structure, nor any of the roots, should be allowed to remain."[24]

Surgical removal of breast tumors was rare in the early nineteenth century. The few extant accounts of the experience of such surgery derive almost exclusively from the experiences of middle- and upper-class American and European women. While partly reflecting the higher likelihood that letters from prominent writers and women of high social standing would be preserved, this social asymmetry might accurately reflect the financial and social resources required to gain access to surgeons and to overcome obstacles – such as the need to turn kitchens into surgeries, family members into nurses, and homes into hostels to care for the doctors, friends, and family members who provided care after surgery.

Some early-nineteenth-century observers believed that surgical cures were rare because women presented too late to surgeons. Buchan, for example, was pessimistic about surgery because the "unhappy patient conceals it too long … after the disorder has arrived at a certain height, it generally sets all medicine at defiance." While Buchan recommended a proper diet, mercury pills and ointments, and bleeding as initial treatment, if the tumor did not soon respond, he recommended extirpation, "either by the knife or caustic … the sooner it is done the better. It can answer no purpose to extirpate a cancer after the constitution is ruined, or the whole mass of humors corrupted by it." Buchan recognized, however, that "few people will submit to extirpation till death stares them in the face," leading to dangerous operations as well as the failure to cure.[25]

In one sense, this idea of "early" surgery reflects a timeless moralism about swift action against a feared danger ("the sooner … the better") as well as the wish to evade the bleak clinical reality of cancer. But however universal or compelling the logic, Burney's and Emlen's surgeons did not blame them for not coming sooner. There is little evidence that "the sooner … the better" rhetoric had deeply permeated medical or popular attitudes toward cancer surgery or the relationship between individual doctors and patients. For one thing, women with breast lumps and their physicians believed, or wanted to believe, in the efficacy of nonsurgical remedies. Such treatments had a better fit with reigning notions of humoral imbalance and other constitutional assumptions about the causes and nature of illness. Patients and physicians generally tried such remedies based on testimonies of efficacy by credible sources and evaluated for themselves whether there was any effect on the size and shapes of breast lumps.

In February 1814, after weeks of applying the Logan plaster "without any reduction in the size of the tumor," Emlen was ready to consult Physick.[26] But Physick was at the time too ill to see her.[27] So she consulted another doctor who advised her to confine herself "to a recumbent posture, a low diet, and submit to some depleting remedies." Samuel Emlen wrote William Dillwyn in mid-March that "whether these will have the desired effect of expelling the disease without recourse to a surgical operation is yet too early to determine, but I have some hopes they may as the tumor appears to have decreased in size."[28] But the hope that the tumor was decreasing in size proved illusory and in the middle of April 1814, four or more months after discovering her tumor, Emlen consulted Physick in his Philadelphia home, where she, her aunt Smith, and others also stayed.[29]

Three other prominent Philadelphia surgeons examined Emlen's tumor with Physick – Caspar Wistar, Joseph Parrish (married to Emlen's cousin), and John Syng Dorsey (Physick's nephew). They found a lump "to exceed the size of a large egg and that the increase had extended under the left arm and contaminated the gland there."[30] Elite physicians had long known that tumors that extended to the armpit had an even grimmer than usual prognosis.[31]

Since antiquity, surgeons had been removing breast tumors. Partly as a consequence, cancer in the breast has had a long pedigree as a localized, specific disease. In 1815, Rodman, who in addition to being a surgical practitioner was the medical superintendent of a dispensary and a house of recovery, recounted that he had learned through surgical experience and the observation of cancer patients over time to abandon his constitutional views of cancer in favor of the idea that cancer was a "local" disease. "Like many others," Rodman observed, "I had imbibed the notion of some cancerous diathesis existing in the patient's constitution, which, by being either innate or accidental, could influence the system in some mysterious manner. When the notion was weakened by a variety of occurrences, I began to regard the subject in another point of view, and to consider the cause of Cancer only of a local nature."[32]

Even those physicians who held the most humoral beliefs about health and illness necessarily had to pay some attention to cancer in the breast as a specific disease because breast tumors were visible, tangible, and external.[33] Surgeons had long observed anatomical details of different degrees of hardness, ulcerations, extent, size, and other external characteristics of breast tumors and often explained them by recourse to visible, physical, mechanical, and localized-to-the-breast mechanisms such as stagnation, fermentation, obstruction, and trauma.[34] Physicians and surgeons had also long made clinical observations specific to breast cancer such as that swelling in the armpit signaled a bad prognosis and that breast cancer tended to occur after menopause.[35]

Physick and the other surgeons were candid to Emlen and her family. They did not evade the cancer diagnosis nor Emlen's uncertain prognosis. Physick told the Emlens that "as the disease now pervaded the armpit, there was the probability of it having extended too far to be reached by the operation and whether this was the case or not could not be ascertained with certainty without the parts being laid open." Physick was also candid about the "difficulty of the case."[36] Dr. Parrish wrote straightforwardly to his father-in-law (and Emlen's uncle) that Emlen was "laboring under a cancerous affliction of the breast – which has extended itself some distance from the original tumor and contaminated other or more glands of the armpit." He described how he, Wistar, and Physick had deliberated "on the subject" and that the "removal of the diseased parts by the knife" was the only "probable plan ... to rescue the valuable life of this most lovely and amiable woman." This news was nevertheless difficult to deliver to Emlen. Parrish reported that "this conclusion had not been imparted to her when I left the house," and the recommendation for surgery was left to Physick to deliver.[37] Emlen later recalled that the other surgeons all "agreed with Dr Physick that it was unlikely to yield to anything short of a surgical operation. This awful sentence I had anticipated but it filled me with great distress."[38]

While Emlen pondered her options, the surgeons immediately prescribed "a strict regimen as to diet, evacuation by bleeding and other means with a confinement to a recumbent posture ... a number of leeches were applied to the affected part and soon it was blistered and then dressed with mercurial ointment and some day afterwards, the leeches were again applied." Bleeding and leeches were traditional therapies generally understood to redress humoral imbalance and were the stock and trade of regular physicians and surgeons in treating a wide range of diseases. Physick and Parrish, for example, had used and promoted them in Philadelphia's periodic yellow fever epidemics.[39] Since at least the time of Paracelsus (1493–1541), mercury was believed to have some efficacy against cancer. But these therapies were also understood in the specific, ontological, and local terms of the surgeon contemplating the physical removal of a tumor. "By this means in the course of three weeks," Emlen noted about the bleeding, leeches, and mercury, "the circumference of the tumor of the breast was rendered more distinct to the touch." These traditional treatments were thus understood to aid the surgeon's attack on the local disease by preparing the tumor for easier excision. In addition to the visible and helpful changes in the tumor, these treatments produced troubling side effects. Because her arm "was bled yesterday" Emlen wrote her aunt, she was "still unable to sew or knit without pain."[40]

In mid-May 1814, after nearly a month's residence in the Physicks' home, Emlen returned to Oxmead "in order to form a conclusion on the subject of an operation." Deciding whether to consent to surgery was difficult because Physick had not guaranteed success and had emphasized the diverse outcomes of cancer. Some people "exaggerated" symptoms, while others endured cheerfully and with "a capacity for social enjoyment"; some people's cancer went "thro all its several stages and end in death in the space of forty days," while other patients sometimes lingered for twenty years."[41]

Cure was rarely articulated as an explicit goal in medical and popular writings about cancer surgery in this period. Most stressed that breast amputations could remove ugly and disturbing local masses while aiding women in their struggle with the disease.[42] Surgeons were of course cognizant of how painful and mutilating the operation was and thus they avoided it, temporized, and tried to at least "do no harm" by choosing their cases wisely.

Medical reluctance to operate on breast tumors was evident in Philadelphia Quaker Joseph Bringhurst's account of his sister Elizabeth's 11-year struggle with a breast tumor at the end of the eighteenth century. Bringhurst generally emphasized his sister's piety and spiritual reflections rather than dwelling on the physical and medical details of her disease. The limited voice of physicians is heard at the beginning and end of her disease. Joseph began the narrative by noting that in 1780 Elizabeth "perceived a small tumor in her left armpit, which gradually increased, tho' for several years gave her no pain. On consulting a Physician, she was advised not to do anything to it; as at her time of life, there seemed a probability it might never prove troublesome or become the cause of her dissolution."[43] After pain began years later, she was told by her physician that "an attempt to cut it [the tumor] out would be dangerous. She now had reason to believe it to be what it afterwards proved, a real confirmed Cancer." Thus medical and lay fear and pessimism about surgery and cure of cancer in the breast led some physicians to advise patients in such a way that there was never an appropriate time to perform surgery. At the time of discovery of a breast mass, physicians could emphasize that their patients might live with or outlive their tumors and later when problems developed and new growth was observed, surgery had became too dangerous.

Given the pessimism that surgery could cure cancer, why did any nineteenth-century surgeons amputate breasts? Why did some women consent? Sometimes, both patient and surgeon articulated the logic of fighting evil with evil. After consulting a few doctors and considering her options, Burney wrote of her decision to undergo surgery that "this *experiment* [my italics] could alone save me from its jaws" suggesting not so much a sober weighing of known risks and benefits but an enduring, existential bet that only the most extensive and severe therapy might have some chance of warding off an evil that threatened one's existence.[44] "Yet I felt the evil to be deep, so deep," Burney wrote in another context, "that I often thought it could not be dissolved, it could only with life be extirpated."[45] Although by the twentieth century decisions to undergo breast amputation will be discussed in formally more anatomic and clinical terms, this underlying emotional logic of "evil against evil" has persisted.

Many cancer patients feared death from cancer so much that death from surgery might be preferable. Burney recollected that one of her pessimistic surgeons calculated that she "would far rather suffer a quick end without, than a lingering life with this dreadfullest of maladies: he finally, therefore considered it might be possible to save me by the trial, but that without it my case was desperate and resolved to make the attempt."[46]

Both Emlen and Burney believed that the decision about surgery, in all its awful dimensions, was theirs alone to make. Burney and her doctors negotiated the time of the operation and how information should flow among the different parties. Burney exercised a good deal of control in these negotiations, obtaining "with difficulty a promise of four hours warning, which were essential to me for sundry regulations."[47] The resulting ignorance of the time and date of her surgery may have served to lessen tension around a fateful encounter with certain pain and possible death, but the 4-hour interval was necessary as it was consumed with actions aimed at keeping the operation a secret from her husband.

"These things were useful in giving me a full view on every side of the subject," Emlen wrote of Physick's prognostication and recommendation to have surgery, but "one which I was alone and unaided, except for sympathy, to form a decision."[48] Samuel Emlen also believed that the decision was Emlen's alone to make because it involved "a responsibility so serious and indeed awful that I was incapacitate for giving a sentiment either way and our kind relatives were equally at a loss. The momentous decision was therefore of necessity left to herself."[49] Emlen was well aware of the cancer diagnosis, its threat to her life, and the limited expectations of surgery. She sought and received the advice of friends, physicians, and family members, but was by no means subservient to them.

In the end, Emlen decided to undergo amputation of her breast mass. The ultimate rationale she offered for consenting to surgery is strikingly familiar to those offered by many patients today who choose feared and risky treatments in the present in order to minimize hypothetical, future regrets about not having done everything possible to fight cancer. "It appeared best to me to endeavor to submit to an operation," Emlen concluded, "believing that if it should prove unsuccessful I should suffer with more patience from believing I had availed myself of those means of relief placed providentially within my power."

Having made her decision, Samuel Emlen wrote Physick to come up to Burlington to conduct the surgery. Among other needs, the Emlens had to prepare for the possibly prolonged stay of various friends and family members who would live with them for weeks after the surgery, the lodging of the three surgeons from Philadelphia, and their family doctor. Emlen hired new servants to help with these arrangements.

Physick arrived in Oxmead on May 18, 1814, with his sister Abby, daughter Sally, and a nurse. Almost immediately upon arriving, Physick became very ill. Instead of having surgery, Emlen, along with her friends and family, and the other doctors focused their attention on Physick over the next few weeks. Emlen would have liked "the business to proceed but the young men [Parrish and Dorsey] are hesitating to perform it."[50] In this unplanned interval, Emlen fell in and out of "sinking spells."[51] She thanked "the fullest of beings" for supplying her with patience to endure the wait.[52]

Members of the large network of friends and family continued to search for nonsurgical remedies and suggested them to Emlen during this interval. Deborah Logan, one of her cousins, recommended that Emlen try some simple remedies that cured two other women with cancerous lumps. In the case of a woman with a new lump in a breast that had been surgically removed 9 years earlier, an herbal tea infused into cloth and applied to the lump effected a cure. In the other case, an application of another herbal treatment "removed the complaint." Logan was ambivalent about urging these remedies, however, noting that "different applications are proposed by almost all with whom one converses" and that "thee [Emlen] has the advantage of a great interest with the highest medical authority [Physick] that our own or perhaps any country can boast."[53] While this was still an era of "every man his own doctor," the reputation of eminent doctors, especially as it concerned such a serious ailment as cancer, carried great weight.[54]

Physick eventually recovered from what was assumed to be a liver problem and performed the surgery in Emlen's home on June 4, 1814, with Drs. Dorsey, Parrish, and Tucker (a local family physician) in attendance. Emlen told her father 5 months after the operation that when Dorsey arrived the night before the surgery and said the operation would be the next day, it produced a "distress" she would never forget. Emlen's aunt G.M. Smith and Physick's nurse Hook were the only people "thought necessary beside the physicians" to be with Emlen during the operation. Nurse Hook put a handkerchief over Emlen's head and led her in, "hoping it might save me the sight of the preparations," but she nevertheless saw Dorsey with his apron on and his sleeves tucked up. While Tucker supported her arm and her aunt her head, the operation proceeded. "My suffering was severe beyond expression, my whole being seemed absorbed in pain – the tumor was taken out in 25 minutes but it was an hour before I was in bed." It was 14 hours before she became "easy enough" to sleep.[55]

Emlen's very brief account of the actual surgery contrasts with Burney's much more detailed and better known one. Fully conscious and an intimate of her surgeons and physicians, Burney's bloody operation in her home had, in her retelling, elements of a gendered, domestic battle. Burney herself drew the analogy to childbirth, which like her breast amputation occurred at home among intimates and caused great pain to women. One doctor at the time of surgery asked if Burney had cried or screamed during childbirth. "Alas I told him, it had not been possible to do otherwise; oh then, he answered there is no fear! What terrible inferences there were here to be drawn."[56] Soon after she was tied to her bed, "a silence the most profound ensued, which lasted for some minutes, during which, I imagine, they took their orders by signs, and made their examination."[57] Burney's ensuing, explicit description of the operation (including the sensation of the knife going through her chest) is almost unbearable to read, let alone to have been experienced.

After Emlen's operation, her surgeons told her that they thought that the "disease was completely eradicated."[58] Samuel Emlen wrote his father-in-law that since "the diseased parts of both the breast and armpit" were "entirely extracted ... so far the kindness of providence all looks favorable."[59] It is of course impossible to know how much faith any of the actors had in the truth of these pronouncements of eradication and completeness. Later developments suggest that Physick did not believe that his sister-in-law was cured. Shortly after the operation, family friend Margaret Allinson commented that Samuel Emlen's "hopes are strong that she [Emlen] will yet be restor'd – and may be tis necessary in order to keep him from sinking quite," possibly a wink by Allinson that Samuel Emlen had unrealistic but thoroughly understandable hopes for his wife to be cured by surgery.[60]

Emlen's tumor weighed a pound and left a great hollow that over the next weeks resolved. She was given strawberries, toast, and water to prevent fever but then given chocolate and milk when her temperature was thought to be too low. Her pain and restlessness were treated with laudanum (opium dissolved in alcohol).[61] Samuel Emlen began a letter to his father-in-law 2 days after the operation, not being able to write sooner because his mind had been in a "state of mental conflict." He observed that his wife had a "daily occurrence of a nervous affection producing a restlessness which is very trying," and that was allayed by opium. He continued to give a near daily account of her ever-increasing strength but a "general debility" on the fifth day after her surgery "awakened" his fears."

Emlen's surgeons had left Oxmead by the eighth day after surgery, but her family physician (a student of Physick's) stayed a month, checking and dressing her wounds (hourly in the first few days after surgery).[62] Two weeks after the operation, Emlen was able to ride half a mile.[63] Seven weeks after the operation, Emlen wrote her father that "all the unpleasant consequences that remain are a small part of the wound which in two days more will I think be completely closed." But her husband's mind remained "anxious and apprehensive."[64]

Samuel Emlen worried why his wife's wound had not yet completely closed, only partly reassured that the "medical men appear to consider these circumstances as nothing more than might occasionally be expected to follow an operation."[65] "Most of the time since [the operation,]" Samuel Emlen wrote his cousin, "a train of consequent apprehensions has kept my fears awake and my mind in a state of painful tension."[66] As time passed, Emlen wrote her father about her resigned acceptance of additional consequences of surgery. She suffered a permanent weakness in her left arm. Dorsey had told her that he was obliged – presumably because of the visible, extensive reach of her cancer – to cut a muscle that moved her arm. She also continued to have pain in the operative scar.[67]

We know little about the Emlens' lives after the immediate postoperative period. They were not filled with follow-up visits and medical treatments. Emlen's extensive surgery, which included a dissection of her axillary glands and at least partial removal of her pectoral muscles along with the 1-pound tumor, may very well have left the Emlens unable to discern any cancer in the chest, although very aware of the mutilating effects of surgery. Without any visible sign of cancer in the breast, the Emlens could sustain some hope for a cure.

This dormant stage of disease lasted for over 2 years. Emlen had "a accurance of some symptoms of the disease" sometime in the late fall of 1816, soon after arriving in England with her husband and friend Sally Sharpless for a long visit to her ailing father and English friends. Her first 5 months in England were marked, her husband noted, by "hopes and apprehensions" in which "the former preponderated."[68] Along with Sally Sharpless and William Dillwyn, the Emlens had moved from the Dillwyns' home in London to the better winter climate of Exmouth in Devonshire. Sometime in early winter, they consulted a local physician, "a man of principle and experience," who observed that Emlen's new chest tumor was "without color, heat, or pain" and who was able to offer hope that "the hardness will become a permanent indolent tumour," in part because "her general health is good."[69]

Emlen's Exmouth physician's prediction of an indolent tumor reflected the common medical emphasis on the potential of tumors to worsen or lessen in seriousness depending on the strength of individual constitution and future events rather than understanding tumors and other diseases in irreversible, categorical terms. Early-nineteenth-century Anglo-American medical texts generally emphasized a traditional mix of local and constitutional influences that might transform a tumor from innocent to evil (and sometimes back again). "However, it is right to observe that some of these swellings," prominent London surgeon Astley Cooper wrote in 1829, "when they have existed long in a dormant state, will have alteration produced in them by changes of the constitution, by which their extirpation may be rendered necessary: for malignancy may be lighted up in them by constitutional diseases ... by anxiety of mind ... and by the cessation of the menstrual secretion."[70]

Emlen's Exmouth physician also emphasized the look and feel of the tumor rather than the degree of its apparent anatomic extension that Physick and his surgical colleagues had stressed 2 years earlier. This different basis for prognostication might reflect differences in knowledge between doctors or the more surgical orientation of Emlen's American surgeons, but perhaps had more to do with Emlen's different clinical situation in England. As further surgery was not an option that she wanted to seriously consider (the 25 minutes of unimaginable pain in her home, followed by weeks of wound and personal care by an army of physician house guests was not to be called upon again), her Exmouth doctor could best sustain hope by speculating on the possible noncancerous nature of Emlen's chest problems.

In all probability, the avoidance of the cancer diagnosis and the talk of doing things to keep the "hardness" as an "indolent tumor" also reflected a code, shared by all concerned, in which hope was sustained in a fearful situation. Abigail Adams Smith, the daughter of President John Adams and his wife Abigail, suffered cancer in the breast, following a remarkably similar course to Emlen during the same time period. One exchange between her husband, Colonel Smith, and Abigail Adams is highly revealing of the indirectness used to frame the diagnosis and prognosis of breast lumps.[71]

On July 23, 1811, Abigail Adams wrote to her son-in-law from Quincy, Massachusetts where her daughter was visiting after an absence of $3\frac{1}{2}$ years, about Smith's recently discovered breast tumor. Smith's doctor had advised that "no outward application should be made and that Mrs. Smith's general state of health is so good as not to threaten any present danger. He does not pronounce it to be of the nature we feared, though he cannot say but what it may terminate in one, and he further says, that it may remain in the present state many years unless improper application should be made. He advised the use of Hemlocke pills."[72] By not "pronouncing" Smith's breast problems as cancer but as something that could terminate as one if "improper applications" were done, the Adams family's physician, like Emlen's Exmouth physician, emphasized that Smith's fate was not yet determined but could be favorably or unfavorably influenced by choices, applications, and therapies, such as Hemlocke pills, aimed at redressing systemic imbalances. Like Emlen's English physician, Smith's physician avoided a recommendation for surgery, instead urging caution (avoid "improper application"), contingency ("may terminate ..."), and overall accumulated health ("general state of health").

Colonel Smith's initial response revealed that the indirect communication used among the Adams family members and in their communication with doctors had eluded him. (Smith was generally a problematic son-in-law, frequently abandoning his wife and falling far short in other ways of the former President and first lady's expectations.) In his reply to his mother-in-law's letter, Colonel Smith wrote with evident self-satisfaction that he had read up on cancer in medical texts and had essentially broken the physician's code, revealing his wife's problem as cancer and demanding appropriate and specific treatment (and offering to move in with his in-laws to help manage his wife's illness):

> You say that [the Dr.] does not pronounce it to be a cancer, tho he cannot say, but it *may* terminate in one. But knowing as I do that hemlock is the principal medicine recommended in Cases of Cancer.... I have no doubt in my mind, but he conceives this to be the disorder. Mrs. Smith in her letter of the 11th of July says the doctors opinion is

that it is an obstructed Gland. But what is a cancer? it is a hard indolent tumour seated in some of the Glands; as the breast, arm pits etc. If
the tumour becomes loose unequal, of a livid, blackish or leaden colour
attended with violent pain, it is plainly called an occult cancer. When
the skin is broken and [illegible] is discharged it is plainly called an
open or ulcerated cancer...I am an advocate for prompt and decisive
experiments to ascertain the nature of the complaint, and its decided
character, this was to me the primary essential object of the visit. I hes-
itated to take it as a cancer...but if it is a cancer, let it promptly be
cured. [73]

But Abigail Adams had understood what the physician was signaling and thus her daughter's situation. Her son-in-law's intrusive letter
revealed his ignorance rather than hers, and she gently redirected him
from the unwelcome plan to move in with them. Colonel Smith was
chastised. "I may have expressed myself with too much solicitude and
given my opinion too decidedly in opposition to the professional men,"
he wrote back to Abigail Adams 2 weeks later.[74] Smith, like Emlen and
Burney, ultimately received the cancer diagnosis and after consultations
with Benjamin Rush and others underwent surgery. Like Emlen's, Smith's
surgeons told her that they had completely removed the cancer, but 2
years later the cancer recurred and she died a short time later.[75]

The Exmouth doctor's use of a similar code to emphasize hope contrasted with Emlen's own description of her reactions, a narrative that
began with depression, followed only later by a marshaling of spiritual
and other resources to cope with her fears of further surgery and cancer. Initially, the "discovery of my local disease" had her "sunk to the
earth" and in a "depression of mind" which was "impossible to describe,"
made worse by her being far from home and friends and the responsi-
bilities of taking care of her own infirm father. Nevertheless, with the
passing of weeks and drawing on her Quaker faith "all things wear a new
aspect. I am encouraged to trudge on contentedly tho the way be now
and then a little rough and sometimes hope it will all eventually con-
tribute to our real good as every dispensation of Providence is most certainly intended to do." Faith in God played a palpably comforting role
for Emlen. Her Quaker faith and community permitted and supported
her speculation about the possible beneficial effects of her struggle with
cancer.

According to Emlen, her Exmouth physician had initially prescribed,
"medicines one of which the warm sea bath is a pleasant remedy."[76] The

major thrust of this therapy was to "do nothing further for this tumor which had resisted all endeavors to lessen it but by watchful care to guard against everything likely to bring on an inflamation by which means he thought it likely it might never give me any more trouble than it had done."[77] Emlen was content to try mild therapies like warmed sea water, vigilance, and careful observation, rather than purgatives and bleeding, or more surgery.

The use of mild and often locally specific treatments as well as efforts to avoid anything harmful while supporting the individual's constitution – all done without much confidence in cure so much as avoiding "more trouble" – reflected common nonsurgical approaches to breast tumors. For example, in 1789, leading Philadelphia physician and American patriot Benjamin Rush corresponded with Dr. Elisha Hall after Hall sought advice about how to treat Mary Washington, the president's 81-year-old mother, who was suffering from a breast tumor.[78] Rush first lamented that "there does not exist in the vegetable kingdom an antidote to cancers." He then half-heartedly endorsed the use of arsenic because it might cleanse and therefore retard the progress of the disease, but said, "I am afraid no great good can be expected from the use of it." Rush concluded that it was worthwhile to "give anodynes when necessary, and support the system with bark and wine. Under this treatment, she may live comfortably many years, and finally die of old age."[79] Like Emlen's English physicians, Rush articulated a temporizing goal, a hope that some mild treatments might slow down disease, an especially reasonable goal in the case of an elderly woman who by such means might survive long enough to die of other causes.

During the late fall and winter of 1816–1817, English friends and relatives offered advice and comfort to Emlen and her family. The Emlens had sought advice about whether they should leave Devonshire and return to London to consult experts, especially about the need for further surgery. One friend, Mary Stacey, gave details of Emlen's recurrence to a prominent physician friend, George Birkbeck, who wrote Emlen in November 1816 that "no injury can arise from delay" so there was no need "to return hastily to London."[80] Birkbeck requested that Emlen send him "a written account of the case ... a description as minute as possible in regard both to the part affected and thy own health and if it be sent immediately, answers may be very soon obtained." He did not believe that Emlen would need "the severe expedient [surgery] adopted on a former occasion."[81]

After receiving a description of Emlen's tumor and her Exmouth physician's impressions and treatments, Birkbeck offered the diagnosis that "the tumour in Emlen's breast is not a true scirrhus but partakes rather of a common glandular affection." In accordance with age-old empirical and humoral concepts of breast tumors and consistent with the minimal to absent emphasis on the physical examination of patients, Birkbeck by post prescribed leeches to the circumference of the tumor (but in moderation), natural salts, and mercury.[82]

In February 1817, Emlen wrote her aunt G. M. Smith in New Jersey that she was in good spirits since her local disease "has not certainly made the least progress" since she started the sea baths and other therapies in Exmouth. She was also heartened by the encouraging opinions of her physicians who told her that "glandular swellings are in this country far more common than in ours and my sister Alexandra tells me that in speaking to her Physician at Ipswich of my case, he assured her that out of eighty cases that had come under his notice, but three had proven cancerous."[83]

Widely held beliefs in the determinative role of local climate and environment thus permitted Emlen and her doctors to make optimistic inferences about the meaning of swellings in England that might not have been possible in New Jersey. Whether diagnosing glandular rather than cancerous disease, scirrhus-like versus true scirrhus, inactive versus active disease, Emlen's doctors worked to mitigate her fear of cancer and possible cancer surgery by labeling her problem as something other than a definite, active cancer and fashioning treatments aimed at strengthening her constitution. "Our medical advisors continue to encourage our hopes of the tumour remaining in an inactive state," Samuel Emlen wrote a colleague around this time.[84]

But Emlen's friends and doctors also understood that the mass in her chest might very well be cancerous and growing and wondered if there might be more effective treatments than warm sea baths. Foreshadowing the more aggressive search for "second opinions" and new means of combating cancer and cancer fear that were to become commonplace among middle-class Americans suffering cancer recurrences a century later, Emlen's husband and father urged her to consult a surgeon in London whom they had previously visited. Emlen wrote her friend Sally Dickinson that she preferred to continue with the Exmouth physician's mild treatments, "but I cannot suffer alone. I must consult also those who would suffer most with me and it is the wish of both my father and S. Emlen that Pearson [the surgeon] in London should be again consulted and that I should see him after which we can better judge and form our plan for the summer."[85] In this and other decisions, Emlen often acted out of concern with their impact on her family and friends.

Samuel Emlen had also sought Physick's expert opinion soon after they discovered the new breast tumor. Physick wrote back from Philadelphia a few months later that he was "very sincerely grieved...that another tumour has formed in sister Susan's breast." He had confidence in the "measures employed" against the tumor and supposed that her doctors believed that "The disease is of a scirrhus nature...I hope they are correct in this opinion." Physick then added that "you may possibly be asked why the whole breast was not removed when the operation was performed here. Should such a question be proposed I have a very satisfactory answer which however owing to the explanations necessary for understanding it I have not time at present to communicate."[86]

Physick presumably brought up that he had reasons for not entirely removing Emlen's left breast to head off any criticism of his surgical performance. Physick may have protested that he had "not time" to explain his surgical rationale, but more likely, he was shielding the Emlens from the disturbing interoperative findings. When the "parts were laid open" in 1814, Emlen's tumor was probably too advanced for a complete resection of all visible cancerous material. Physick's use of the term *scirrhus* was probably offered to allay fears as well, as the term historically denoted "a perpetual disposition to undergo one or another form of corruption," that is, a tumor that was not (yet) an ulcerating cancer but could easily turn into one.[87]

Emlen, her husband, father, and Sally Sharpless returned to London in April 1817. Samuel Emlen believed the journey, "tho slowly and certainly performed in 9 days, seemed to rouse the tumour into a more active state and its size increased. On our arrival here no time was lost in seeking medical assistance, and a mode of reducing the tumour by compression which had been introduced with success within the last few years, being advised, was adopted."[88] The change in tumor size and an "uneasiness of the tumor led to a suspicion that it might prove to be something more serious than a mere enlargement of the glands, under which opinion we had for some time taken shelter from our anxieties. This suspicion was converted into no small degree of sorrowful certainty when two medical men of this City (one an eminent Surgeon) whom we consulted very early after our arrival gave an explicit opinion that it was of a cancerous nature." Compression therapy was chosen "in preference to excision, this ever soon concluded on by Susan."[89]

The particular compression technique that Emlen submitted to (attributed by Emlen's circle to Samuel Young) was enjoying a high degree of popularity in England and was considered novel.[90] Young's technique, as described in his collection of cases that testified to the treatment's effectiveness, involved "plaister straps, sheet lead forming shields of various thicknesses, tin plates, linen compresses, and the use of appropriate rollers." The lead plates were cut to "the figure of the tumor."[91] As was the case with most specific and localized treatments in this era, Young also administered medicines acting on the patient's constitution, such as digitalis. He understood compression to work by both mechanical pressure, mimicking nature's way of absorbing hernias and growths, and by obstructing the arterial supply to the tumor.

Young's testaments of success took the form of case histories in which compression therapy greatly reduced or eliminated breast tumors. Most of the testaments, however, ended with the death of the patient. This at best limited or ambiguous definition of success foreshadowed the myopic definitions of therapeutic success that would be claimed for radical surgery a century later (see Chapter 4). "The tumor still very much reduced," Young characteristically wrote about the definite efficacy of compression in one of his case histories, but quickly added that she was "fast approaching dissolution."[92] After the patient's death, autopsy confirmed the reduction in the tumor's size. To further emphasize the efficacy of compression, Young included a testament by "Mr. Pulley, surgeon, attendant on the Bedford House of Industry" who wrote that the patient's death should not to be blamed on Young or compression therapy because the patient "could scarcely have had a more unfortunate constitution for his operations."[93]

Emlen's own compression therapy was difficult. It lasted 6–8 hours a day and was "followed by a considerable degree of pain."[94] The Emlen clan found accommodation close to their West End surgeon Joseph Pearson, leaving them feeling "lonely amidst the surrounding thousands." Emlen wrote her aunt G. M. Smith in June 1817 of the physical hardship of the tight bandages, applied in home visits by Pearson every 2 days, but recognized that the "inconvenience and pain are gentle indeed when compared with the extreme measures [surgery] to which I had recourse before." But having already suffered through the anxiety and horrifying pain of an earlier episode of cancer and surgery, Emlen admitted to her aunt the "gloomy anticipations of the pains, the helplessness, the tediousness, and all the evils in which my malady might involve myself."

Surgical and other interventions may not have prolonged Emlen's life but they altered her experience of the disease. She had lived for over 2 years after surgery without visible evidence of local disease, allowing her to believe she had been cured. This period led to a difficult final act in which the return of cancer deflated these hopes and during which Emlen gloomily anticipated the malady's "evils."

In this final act, Emlen increasingly drew on her considerable spiritual resources and Quaker faith. Her goal was "to cherish a spirit of submission and confidence that no affliction can ever be assigned to any of us but what is found necessary for our most important interest."[95] Until her last days of life, however, Emlen also maintained a pragmatic focus on the treatment options and did not discuss her personal salvation or life after death. She frequently wrote about her acceptance of her fate. Her friends and family frequently evoked a God who acts unwittingly vis-à-vis the individual, a tenet of Quaker theology that seems particularly well adapted to an increasingly secular and medicalized world in which individuals bore more responsibility, certainly in terms of decisions and their consequences, for illnesses such as cancer in the breast.[96] "That you have been enabled to yield a calm and quiet submission to these and many other privations, during a season of trial and affliction, while the laboring mind is passing thro' many changes," one of Emlen's New Jersey friends tellingly wrote about a God who doesn't cure cancer but supports people in times of suffering, "is an evidence of the consoling support and cheering influence of the gracious and benevolent Being," who is "touched with the feeling of our infinities," and "ministers to all our wants in the time of need."[97]

But even among Philadelphia Quakers suffering cancer in the breast, the spiritual dimension varied, not only by individual personality and faith, but also in terms of the pace, chronicity, and stage of disease and degree of medical intervention. Elizabeth Bringhurst continuously articulated her hope for personal salvation and life after death. From the time of her diagnosis, her brother depicted her as preparing for "a house eternal in the heavens when this tabernacle of clay should be dissolved," concerned whether she was worthy enough for that "house," and persistently questioning whether her "afflictions would work for her everlasting good."[98] Bringhurst's focus on the status of her spiritual preparedness was as adapted to the absence of medical interventions and decision-making in her illness as Emlen's occasional evocation of God's "unknowingness" was adapted to a life filled with difficult, secular, medical decisions and their consequences.

Samuel Emlen believed that the compression therapy was working against his wife's tumor. In the first weeks of compression treatment, "a very rapid reduction was apparent, it has since been more slow as the surgeon early informed us he expected would be the case, but I believe not less certain, and the size I think is now [4 months into treatment] not more than about one fourth of what it was at the commencement of the process."[99] Emlen herself was skeptical of her husband's and surgeon's assessment of progress against the tumor. "The progress of the cure which our friend Pearson [her London surgeon] believes to be going on is so very slow," Emlen wrote her friend Sally Dickensen in the same month as her husband's assessment that the tumor had shrunk to one quarter of its original size, "that I can form no clear idea when I can hope for that pleasure [i.e., some progress]."[100]

These different perspectives on the efficacy of Emlen's compression therapy reflect both a timeless subjectivity in assessing success as well as a more specific-to-cancer continuity. Did Emlen's tumor shrink or did vicissitudes of perception and small variation in symptoms and signs permit the perception of progress? The perception and interpretation of the signs and symptoms of the cancerous body in real time was and is often disputed and ambiguous, the sum vector of an unstable mix of observation, theory, and knowledge, shaped by the desperate need for hope that has often been set against accumulating, if temporarily refutable, evidence of progression to further disease and death.

Patients and their friends, family, and physicians judged the efficacy of compression therapy from the reputation of its enthusiasts as well as by evaluating the technique and its results. Such judgments were shaped by the limited information available about a new technique, the difficulty of ascertaining change in tumor size, and the strong desire to believe that something was working. John Cox, a close friend of Emlen's, wrote to another family friend that the compression therapy "had often been attended with success" in others and had reduced Emlen's tumor size by half. He also related that while the bandages "occasioned considerable uneasiness for some hours" they gradually permitted "the dear patient" to "enjoy the pleasures of social intercourse."[101] Emlen's cousin Ann Cox wrote to her in September 1817 with the hope that the compression treatment, building on earlier reports of great reductions in size, "had perfected a cure." Cox lamented that Sally Sharpless, having learned to help administer Emlen's compression therapy, was not in New Jersey because another woman in the family was suffering "a cancer in her breast that is likely to prove a very serious one, and she has been repeatedly advised to take some advice from a professional man, but whether it is from an apprehension of surgical operation or some other reason, I have not learn'd, she still declines it."[102]

Emlen consented to compression because it was not surgery, was endorsed by her surgeon, and "had been introduced with success within the last few years."[103] The Emlens read a convincing testament of its utility in Young's book on cancer, which Samuel Emlen sent to Physick in Philadelphia for review. Physick thanked Samuel Emlen for the detailed description of "the manner in which compression has been applied for the removal of the tumour and also the book in which the whole treatment is detailed." While Samuel Emlen wanted him to spread the word among Americans, Physick wrote that he had "pleasure of informing you that the idea of causing the absorption of scirrhus tumours in the breast is by no means new to me having actually had recourse to such a measure in the case of Miss Wilson from Baltimore in the year 1803–1804."[104] Despite Physick's claim that there was little new for him in this therapy, compression therapy was novel enough that doctors from outside London visited the Emlen household to inspect it.[105] Anne Cox wrote Emlen about how Dr. Parrish back in Philadelphia had recently proposed compression treatment to a woman with an apparent recurrence after excision and about another mutual friend who was "going to try the new mode of treatment." She also noted that "Young's book has been so much in demand among our Doctor medical friends."[106]

American friends wrote the Emlens about other treatments and offered to arrange for medicinal herbs to be sent to England. Joseph Bringhurst suggested and offered to send Pyrole umbellate, a plant remedy for cancer. Upon hearing about Bringhurst's suggestion, Emlen was able to find a letter in a medical journal suggesting its efficacy against dropsy. Pearson, Emlen's surgeon, said that he would try Pyrole on Emlen if it could be obtained from America in extract or powder form.[107]

As part of the same transatlantic effort to research and find effective treatment, Anne Cox wrote to Emlen that she read a clipping from a Liverpool paper that stated the "wonderful effects" against cancer in the breast of a piece of dough "thoroughly mixed with a lump of Hoyslase (?) of the same dimensions (the older the better) so as to form a kind of salve, spread on a piece of white leather and applied to the diseased part." But then Cox added that she had heard of this remedy a while ago and "I should have told thee of it sooner, but from the improbability of the fact. For if it was really so can we suppose that it would remain untried in a number of cases, and by this time the truth confirmed, and the remedy brought into general use?" As eager as Emlen's friends were to offer news of cancer cures, they often retained a healthy skepticism about isolated reports that were not tried and tested by credible observers and found to be effective.[108] As with the compression therapy, Emlen and her circle actively evaluated an eclectic mix of evidence on the efficacy of proposed and tried treatments, whose credibility was subjected to intense, transcontinental social negotiation.

By the fall of 1817, the Emlens were preparing for their return trip to America. Their doctors continued to give them optimistic reports about the compression therapy's effects on Emlen's cancer but it is unclear whether Emlen or her husband still believed them. Samuel Emlen wrote in his diary that Pearson had examined the tumor with another physician and remarked, "from present appearances he thought that in the course of another month the tumor would be so far removed as to render his attendance unnecessary."[109] But this was a constantly receding horizon, as Samuel Emlen noted a month later that Pearson "expressed his hope that by the close of the year the tumor which has so long affected my dear Susan would be removed."[110] Increasingly, Emlen's activities were restricted because of her treatments as well as breast symptoms. Samuel Emlen noted that he, Susan, and Sally went riding but "after riding for about 3/4 of an hour, the motion producing some uneasy feelings in her breast we returned home, she walking part of the way."[111] By the middle of December 1817, Emlen wrote her aunt G. M. Smith in New Jersey that the end of the month was the "limit of the surgeons' every other day visits" and that Pearson "should sometime see me" after he "resigns me to Aunt Sally."[112] Talk of limits and resignations suggest that the end of this long process of treatment evoked in Emlen feelings of abandonment and fears for the future. Letter writers from America also acknowledged that the year of hopeful announcements of progress had not added up to a cure. In February 1818, the cycle of rising and deflated hopes for the compression therapy led cousins John and Ann Cox to write the Emlens that they had "really felt greatly disappointed from time to time, when from preceding accounts we had reason to expect that the next letter would announce a perfect absorption of the tumor."[113]

The Emlens returned to America in the summer of 1818. Samuel Emlen noted that his wife "has been more indisposed since our arrival" and attributed it to the "excitement" of her reunion with old friends.[114] Letters between the Emlens and their friends continued to talk of treatments and progress, but much less so than before, while the references to the "kind and merciful being who will never leave or forsake those who put trust in him" increased.[115] In January 1819, Emlen wrote her friend Deborah Bringhurst that she was going to continue with the Pyrola but framed its use in spiritual terms: "[pyrola] remarkably suits my constitution and if it pleases the great Physician to add his blessings may at least alleviate my hitherto obscure and obstinate malady." She admitted that "now and then, however, when harassed by pain I have faltered in my resolution to persevere and as I have seen no beneficial change in the tumor been tempted as has my beloved Husband to listen to the many suggestions offered with benevolent kindness by sympathizing friends and with such variety that without more medical skill than we can pretend to we should be at a loss which to choose."[116]

Friends and family increasingly acknowledged among themselves Emlen's slow decline. "She is gradually weakening under painful sensations," wrote her cousin John Cox in October 1819, "without hope, on her part or ours, of a radical cure of the sore disease, under which she has long been a resigned and patient sufferer – or indeed of any thing more than the application of palliatives, to render the remnant of a life so dear and precious to many friends, a little more comfortable; and even these earnest and sympathetic efforts to smooth the way, are not at all times effective."[117] Sally Dickinson, having not seen Emlen in 10 weeks before October 7, observed "so great an alteration" that she was "not prepared for."[118] Samuel Emlen noted on November 11 that his wife was unable to move out of bed without assistance and "is often under great bodily pain" but looks forward "to the blissful exchange which awaits her."[119]

Emlen's friends Sally Sharpless and Margaret Smith recorded a spiritually framed, blow-by-blow account of her last weeks of life. Their report of

Emlen's words and conversations, filled with their prompting and interpretation, demonstrates the social shaping of cancer death among New
Jersey Quakers in 1819. They opened their narrative with the bleeding
from a "vein in the ulcer," reflecting a longstanding belief that when a
tumor ulcerates through the skin it is the last stage of life with cancer. "For
three days before her death, the sense of bodily suffering seemed absorbed
in the blissful enjoyment of thanksgiving and praise," they observed. In
the evening before her death, Emlen reportedly said:

> "I am done, what a wonderful – I am passing – I am passing – this
> moment passing – into an infin." "Infinitely happy state," said I. She
> answered "Yes" – repeating the words – "into an infinitely happy state."
> "Hast thou," said I, "an assurance of it?" "Yes I have." "Then thou does
> not regret all that thou hast suffered?" In an emphatic and animated
> tone, she replied, "That I don't."

In the midst of these spiritual epiphanies, Emlen complained about cold
and pain, asked for or refused laudanum, and had consciousness enough
to worry that the loved ones around her had missed meals. Susan Emlen
died on November 24 "about fifteen minutes before noon," surrounded by
her family doctor, husband, friends Sarah Sharpless and Sally Dickensen,
and family members Aunt G. M. Smith, Margaret Smith, Uncle Dillwyn,
Aunt Cox, and cousin Richard Smith.[120]

SUSAN EMLEN'S LIFE WITH AND DEATH FROM CANCER IN THE BREAST IN
early-nineteenth-century America exemplified some characteristic ways
that the disease was understood, feared, responded to, and experienced.
Her friends and doctors, despite their hopes and efforts, were not surprised
by the return of her illness and eventual death. Doctors and most lay
persons were deeply pessimistic that surgery – or anything else – could
cure cancer in the breast.

Cancer in the breast was generally defined by its behavior over a
sustained period of time rather than its clinical appearance in a single moment. It was a disease that often began as a localized lump but
quickly or slowly caused much more harm. Along with its emphasis on
the idiosyncratic and contingent nature of health and illness, this definition meant that the cancer diagnosis was often haltingly and flexibly
attached to individuals, revealed in the course of time, and often only at

the end of life. The inability to cure cancer was a defining feature in this way of understanding the ailment, so much so that if surgery resulted in an apparent cure, surgeons often believed that they had removed a non-cancerous lump. Cancer was not yet a disease of errant cells, but there was already a long history of medical speculation that cancer had seeds, ferments, or roots, invisible to the surgeon, that could sprout new disease even after tumors were excised.

Emlen's experience helps explain why breast amputations were rare occurrences. Suffering was severe beyond expression. Many women with breast lumps feared "conscious" breast surgery as much or more than cancer itself. Despite lasting only minutes, breast surgery was a major production as families needed to turn homes into hospitals, kitchens into operating theaters, and relatives and friends into nurses. Given these fears and obstacles, many physicians advised women with breast lumps in such a way that there was never an appropriate time to perform surgery.

But like Emlen, some women did have their breast lumps removed by the knife. In addition to the evident benefits of removing an often offensive growth, medical and lay persons believed that some women who underwent surgery early enough might be saved, reflecting in part a very old belief in swift action against a feared danger ("the sooner...the better"). In some cases, both patient and surgeon articulated a goal of cure, not so much based on experience or theory, but a deeper emotional logic of "evil against evil." Emlen also articulated a rationale of *anticipated regret* behind her decision to have surgery – and it was *her* decision – in which the choice of surgery in the present might mitigate any regrets about having not done everything possible to fight cancer if and when cancer recurred. Surgery was the antithesis of resignation. The attached pain and suffering made consenting to surgery an even more powerful statement of hope for continued survival.

Since antiquity, surgeons had been removing breast tumors. As a consequence, cancer in the breast has had a long pedigree as a localized, specific disease in addition to being understood in more traditional constitutional terms. Patients often received locally specific treatments as well as efforts to support their general constitution. These efforts were typically done not so much for cure but to avoid "more trouble."

The doctor–patient relationship in cancer was shaped by the desperate need for hope that was often set against accumulating, if temporarily refutable, evidence of progression to further disease and death.

Doctors were often intimates of patients, as Physick was with Emlen, or tightly tied to local communities, like Emlen's British Quaker physicians. Women exercised a good deal of control in deciding the choice and timing of treatments. Family and friends helped evaluate the credibility of putative cures, were part of the negotiated and ever-shifting acts of diagnosis and prognosis, helped find and prepare materia medica, and sometimes administered treatments.

There was no absolute taboo against uttering the word *cancer*. In any event, there were few revelatory moments in which the physician offered the definite diagnosis to the patient. The gulf between doctor and patient in knowledge about the body and health was generally narrower than it would be later in the century. Doctors' speculations on the possible noncancerous nature of chest problems were not so much evasions of a well-accepted reality as a reflection of medical understandings of disease as idiosyncratic and contingent and as part of a larger effort – that involved the patient herself, as well as family and friends – to maintain hope.

Cancer in the breast was also not a very visible societal problem in early-nineteenth-century America. More attention was understandably paid to epidemic diseases, childhood fevers and diarrhea, and other ailments that were more prevalent causes of death. Women generally recognized and made doctors aware of breast lumps when they were as large as partridge and other bird eggs. Fear of surgery presumably led many women with breast lumps to never seek medical attention at all.

Surgical and other interventions may not have prolonged Emlen's life but they had changed her experience of the disease. She lived without local recurrence for over 2 years although she and her husband appeared to have been very apprehensive about the return of problems during that interval. When she developed new chest problems, Emlen's physicians actively worked to understand them as noncancerous and tried a variety of local treatments aimed at improving her general constitution. Some of these postsurgicaltreatments, like her compression therapy, were rationalized by reports of empirical success, vested with hope and expectation, and were seen as working for as long as hope could be plausibly sustained. As eager as Emlen's friends and physicians were to offer news of putative cancer cures, they often retained a healthy skepticism about isolated reports that were not repeatedly tried and tested by credible observers.

Although cancer in the breast had a long history as a humoral disease and there was some contemporary speculation about inciting and exciting causes, these notions did not seem to impinge very deeply on medical treatment or patients' self-understanding of the disease. The "why me?" and "why now?" questions of greatest significance to the Emlens, their doctors, and their circle of friends and family members, at least in their correspondence, were spiritual ones, especially about the relationship between God and the suffering due to cancer and those questions emanating from the search for spiritual growth in cancer suffering. While there was something timeless in the way Emlen initially responded to her worsening disease with depression, the ways that Emlen and her doctors, friends, and family marshaled spiritual resources to make sense of her illness and to cope with fears for the future were more specific to the time and place in which Emlen lived. As her disease progressed, she increasingly drew on her considerable spiritual resources and Quaker faith.

Throughout the rest of the nineteenth century, this reliance on spiritual resources was haltingly and gradually eclipsed by a growing faith that doctors and medical science might soon develop effective responses against what was increasingly understood as a more specific disease with a more characteristic, uniform, and predictable natural history. By the end of the nineteenth century, *cancer in the breast* would yield to *breast cancer*. These shifts had much more to do with broad social change and medical insights and responses to infectious disease than to developments specific to cancer. As we shall see, rising expectations of progress coexisted awkwardly and problematically with the largely unchanged clinical and lived experience of women with breast lumps and the perception that cancers of all types were becoming more prevalent.

THREE

Pessimism and Promise

In the time between Emlen's death and the technological changes that would later transform surgery (beginning with general anesthesia in the mid-nineteenth century and later antisepsis), there was little change in the way patients experienced cancer or doctors treated it. For example, Mary Shipley, a 66-year-old woman from Wilmington, Delaware, experienced cancer in the breast in 1844, just prior to the first demonstrations of ether anesthesia, in ways largely unchanged from previous generations. Shipley had showed her breast tumor to female relatives but did not consult a surgeon until 6 years later when arm swelling developed. Because of her age, the apparent extent of disease, and her resignation to her fate, the surgeons did not recommend a breast amputation, but urged traditional measures such as leeches and plasters. Letters from friends and family about Shipley's impending death from cancer were clear and unimpeded by euphemism and denial. While Shipley and her family desperately wanted a cure, they were well aware of the limits of medical knowledge and treatments. They maintained some hope that she might have less-than-feared suffering, dignity in the face of advancing disease, and spiritual reckoning at the end of life.[1]

While the medical attention Shipley received was hardly different from earlier periods, Anglo-American medical ideas about cancer were undergoing a profound shift in the mid-nineteenth century. This shift was part of a larger change in medical thought that historians have argued foreshadowed and paved the way for the late-nineteenth-century emergence of the germ theory of disease.[2] Before germs were causatively linked to illnesses such as cholera and tuberculosis, there was a more fundamental change in the *style* of etiological thinking about, and meanings attached to, infectious and other illnesses. Important aspects of this style included thinking about illness in terms of specific disease entities, the use of quantitative arguments and data, and the acceptance of hidden physiological and chemical processes as possible causes of disease.

Many of these same changes constituted a new reductionist temper in mid-nineteenth-century medical thought about cancer. I use *temper* to emphasize a largely attitudinal or mood change that did not directly follow from new discoveries or insights. This reductionist temper is well illustrated by the writings of Anglo-Irish pathologist and clinician W. H. Walshe (1812–1892) in his 1846 text on cancer. Walshe emphasized that modern medical ideas about cancer represented a dramatic and clear break from the past.[3] He caricatured the pathological understanding of "earlier times" as "fanciful." Until recent times, he claimed, definitions of cancer merely "imitated" their predecessors.[4]

Walshe's belief in a radical disjuncture preceded a strictly cellular understanding of cancer. Although Walshe wrote, "some portion of every specimen of every variety of cancer consists of certain hollow *spherical* bodies, termed cells," he also believed that cancer consisted of other tissue elements (granules, nuclei, fibrous substances, etc.). Cancer growth might be a matter of something akin to cellular reproduction (Walshe noted that the nucleus served as a kind of embryo for the cell) or perhaps might derive from particulate matter.[5]

Part of this changing temper was a relentless empiricism. Walshe disapproved of any causal inference that was not based on direct observation. For example, he attacked as mystical the widely held notion that cancer's spread throughout the body reflected a "sympathy" between different organs (e.g., between the mamma and the uterus) because such connections could not be visualized. Walshe derisively dismissed a possible germ etiology of cancer because no germ had ever been identified. He similarly dismissed chronic irritation as an etiological factor because this process had not been directly observed by gross or microscopic examination. Even Walshe's rationale for his cancer text was empirical, eschewing theory and philosophy. He "patiently sought out all available evidence bearing upon the propriety of extirpating cancers, as a means of either curing the disease, or of ensuing advantages of a less substantial character." His "sober" review of this evidence produced a result of "unexpected character," namely skepticism about the surgical curability of cancer.[6] Skepticism about cancer surgery was hardly new but sober review of multiple levels of evidence, including statistical data, was part of a new style of medical thought.

Walshe emphasized that cancer was a specific and unitary disease rather than a nonspecific kind of degeneration. He modeled his classification of cancer on the plant and animal kingdom, deploying the language of genus and species in his descriptions of cancer's specificity. Ultimately, Walshe viewed cancer as a specific disease that united knowledge drawn from chemical analysis, pathological anatomy, physiology, and clinical observation.[7] This view of cancer was a programmatic statement as Walshe and his contemporaries had not reached consensus on any specific anatomical, chemical, or physiological understandings of cancer. Walshe was anticipating that clinical and laboratory science would soon provide a detailed mechanistic picture of cancer's natural history, including distinct boundaries between cancerous and noncancerous conditions, and a predictable and orderly relationship among the different levels of description.

Walshe understood that establishing such precise relationships among these different levels would necessarily involve numbers and statistics. Having trained with Pierre Louis in Paris, he held up numerical analysis of aggregate data as an ideal, even if his own view of cancer derived from qualitative clinical and pathological impressions rather than the few extant statistical investigations of the disease. Walshe wrote, for example, that suckling breasts "probably" exposed women to less danger of cancer but this presumption "requires to be numerically proved."[8] At mid-century, medical faith in numbers often preceded the existence of numbers.

And where numbers existed, Walshe demonstrated a sophisticated skepticism and critical temper in an era before there was an adequate epidemiological vocabulary for routinely expressing and evaluating aggregate data on disease. After noting the increased number of cancer deaths in England and Wales since 1837, Walshe cautioned that "the real causes of the augmented ratio are, there cannot be a doubt, the decrease of mortality from epidemic diseases, and the greater accuracy of diagnosis, as respects carcinomatous affections." Walshe criticized the increased cancer mortality reported by Rignoni Stern in northern Italy, attributing it to changes in diagnostic practice. Walshe noted, for example, that in one decade at the end of the eighteenth century in northern Italy, no uterine cancers were reported while in another decade 113 such deaths were reported, a result explainable only by changes in diagnostic practices.[9]

"What Is Cancer?"

Despite the changing temper of the times and the expectation of a new synthesis, cancer was not easily reconfigured in reductionist terms. At the same time, debates about how best to define and classify cancer (especially cancer in the breast) had assumed new importance because of changes in clinical practice at mid-century. The introduction of ether in the 1840s and the widespread use of antisepsis in the 1860s meant that breast amputations were no longer dramatic and painful events and much more cancer surgery could be and was done. This increased surgery made problems with diagnosis and treatment much more visible and important, especially the challenge of distinguishing benign from malignant tumors and the question of whether surgery was effective.

This, in turn, affected the debate about what cancer actually was. On the one hand, surgery's continued failure to cure reinforced older con-stitutional formulations of cancer, which posited an important role for hidden systemic processes – emotions, heredity, predisposition – besides the visible localized tumor that could be removed with the knife. Cancer remained idiosyncratic, disorderly, and unpredictable. At the same time, new clinical and pathological insights and the more reductionist temper of the era encouraged a more mechanistic, orderly, physical, and localized view of the disease.

While cancer, especially cancer in the breast, had long been under-stood as a specific disease, the idiosyncratic and disorderly progression toward death in many patients suggested a general breakdown of the body. D. Hayes Agnew (1818–1892), one of Philadelphia's leading surgeons, evoked the nonspecific, degenerative character of cancer by comparing it to a decaying nation whose "monarch from decrepitude and age is no longer able to hold firmly the reins of authority, insubordination and anar-chy are developed, so in the realm of vital processes, with the decline of function, as when the force which regulates orderly or physiological cell life is weakened or lost, there begins a monstrous and aimless accumula-tion of tissue elements which observe neither order or form."[10]

Agnew and other late-nineteenth-century elite American surgeons were quick to state that this general "decline of function" was neverthe-less a carefully orchestrated rebellion resulting from a specific, internal physical process of cancer spread. A related challenge to cancer's speci-ficity was how these very general processes "which observe neither order or form" could be set in motion by a specific agent or a localized pathological process. Prominent British surgeon Sir James Paget (1814–1899) argued that many of these observed degenerative changes in cancer "only make the parts less able to maintain themselves, less able to resist the invasion of any morbid material in the blood, which is brought into contact with them." In other words, cancer did not result from a general falling apart of the body but from the interaction of some specific internal or external agent and a weakened or perhaps merely unlucky body or body part. This contact led to what Paget called a "selfish" and unruly "life apart" that characterized both cancer and other specific diseases.[11]

But this characterization of cancer posed an important challenge for cancer diagnosis and definition. In many ways, cancer's "selfish" "life apart," its propensity toward total body breakdown and death, was the core definition of cancer, more so than any static morphological and/or clinical criteria. This meaning of cancer was so central that a cancer diagnosis was often suspect if a patient lived for years after the surgical extirpation of a tumor. In 1860, New York surgeon Willard Parker (1800–1884), whose clinical experiences will be analyzed in some detail later in this chapter, saw a 70-year-old woman whose left breast he had amputated 8 years earlier.[12] The tumor had been attached to muscle, an unfavorable prognostic sign, so the lack of further problems was surprising. "Was the disease cancer?" Parker asked himself in his casebook.[13] In another case, which apparently did not go to operation and where the patient lived "several years" anyway, Parker noted that "left breast I have some doubts about cancer."[14]

Pathologists studied microscopic findings in patients who died from cancer and extrapolated criteria that could define cancer prior to the late clinical stages in which the diagnosis was obvious. One criterion was microscopic evidence of cancer cells invading otherwise healthy tissues. "All persons up to the present time would agree," one nineteenth-century pathologist argued by common sense, "in describing as cancer a growth which, whatever its minute character might be, had already begun to infect or infiltrate a neighboring part." Extrapolating from this clear-cut situation, this pathologist further argued that the cancer diagnosis should also not be held back from "any growth which did not infect, merely because it had not yet arrived at that state, but which might do so hereafter."[15] The definitional problem remained just how to distinguish tumors that "had not yet arrived" from those which might never "infect." Criteria were proposed and used, but they had little bearing on the decisions whether to operate because tumors were not yet sampled and examined microscopically prior to surgery.

Many nineteenth-century pathologists and clinicians understood that there were no perfect static criteria with which to discern growths that were malignant in this predictive sense. Some believed that the very concept of malignancy was too vitalistic, not in keeping with the reductionist temper of the times. Paget recognized that the term *malignant*, which captured this destructive potential, was

> sometimes treated with disrespect, as being figurative and without scientific meaning. Yet, as an expression of certain qualities shown in the method and course of diseases to which it is applied, it is neither unfit nor I think, unmeaning. For the qualities which the name "malignant" indicates are far more distinctive, more surely diagnostic, of this group of diseases than the minute structure and chemical composition of the diseased parts, or even than the method of their growing; and in this is an example of what we must hold in the study of all disease, for pathology is a part of biology, and not derived chiefly from the study of anatomy and chemistry.[16]

Paget's acknowledgment that a tumor's malignancy was not simply revealed by its histological and chemical properties represented a less tidy view of the relationship between clinical behavior and pathological observations than Walshe's vision earlier in the century. The imperfect correlation between "the structure and chemical composition of diseased parts" and malignancy meant not only that some benign appearing tumors would have to be classified as cancer because of their potential to do harm, but also that some tumors would be labeled cancerous that would never become malignant.[17]

In addition, many late-nineteenth-century observers recognized that there was a continuum of clinical and morphological features between cancer and noncancer, including those observed by microscopy, thus making difficult the reliable pathological diagnosis of cancer, even when using uniform, objective, and observable criteria. Paget wrote in 1887, "another indication of the relation between the innocent tumours and the cancerous appears in that it is impossible to mark any fair boundary line between them."[18]

Was Cancer a Local or Constitutional Disease?

Over a few months in 1873 and 1874, the distinguished members of the Pathological Society of London debated whether cancer was a local or constitutional disease. Campbell De Morgan began the conference by offering the generally accepted compromise that while "the disease has its origin in the constitution at large," cancer was mostly a local process.[19] What distinguished De Morgan's argument from Walshe's and other earlier ones was the vast array of clinical and pathological observations and protoepidemiological data used to construct the localist part of this compromise. These diverse data not only reflected the more advanced state of clinical and pathological science by 1873, but also the special vantage point of cancer specialists like De Morgan who could observe patients from cancer diagnosis to autopsy at Middlesex Hospital, a London cancer hospital.

De Morgan observed that the "common story" among cancer patients was the statement "I did not think there could be anything in the lump because I was feeling so particularly well."[20] If a general breakdown in health did not typically precede the onset of cancer, De Morgan argued, then cancer was less likely to result from some general constitutional process. In contrast to the cancer patient's general state of health, De Morgan observed that the look of cancer cells under the microscope was very revealing, "the more the structure of a tumor resembles a natural structure the less the power of doing harm."[21] De Morgan also noted the nonrandom pattern of cancer recurrences, which he believed argued against some general distribution of cancer in the blood or body. This specificity reminded him of other highly specific pathophysiological correlations such as "those strange phenomena observed by Dr. Brown Sequard in guinea pigs with partially divided spinal cords. As is well known they become epileptic, the fits occurring, however, only when a small area of skin near the angle of the jaw is pinched."[22] Also supporting the localist idea was the observation that secondary tumors resembled the organs in which the cancer was first localized rather than the organs to which they spread. Finally, De Morgan brought out Percival Pott's observation that chimney sweeps developed scrotal cancer to emphasize a more specific and localized environmental causation than what was usually meant by constitution.

By the last quarter of the nineteenth century, constitution had become more of a complementary perspective on cancer than one in direct opposition to localism, often serving as a placeholder under which many of the more untidy beliefs and observations about cancer could be organized. Constitutional arguments had also assimilated many reductionist assumptions and stylistic features. For example, constitution was increasingly linked to a putative morbid material in the blood that was the physical mediator of hereditary transmission, metastasis, general cachexia (wasting), and other aspects of cancer not readily understood as local phenomena.

The term *dyscrasia* was often used to refer to a specific morbid material or some poorly specified structural change in the body that mediated these difficult-to-localize phenomena. Agnew had summarized dyscrasia as "a peculiarity of organization extending not to the blood alone, but to all solids of the body, in consequence of which, when the proper excitant is applied, a new formation or morbid growth follows. This general constitutional stamp of an individual is capable of being transmitted from father to son."[23] Mr. Moxon, another speaker at the 1873 London pathology conference, argued that constitution was a "doubtful ambiguous word" that covered up differences more than illuminating anything. For Moxon, the issue of constitution and dyscrasia needed reformulation in materialist terms, that is, does "the first cancer that appears in the patient's body generate the cancers which appear afterwards? Does it precede them in every way? Or, on the other hand, is there a general state of the whole system which is ready to put out cancer anywhere, and puts out the first in the same way as it afterwards puts out the second and third?" Moxon had no reason to evoke constitution or dyscrasia since clinical and pathological observations about cancer could be economically explained as deriving from a single, localized, cancer cell.[24]

Demonstrating the important economic and professional motivation for surgeons to embrace a localist view of cancer, Mr. Jonathan Hutchinson remarked that only localism guaranteed a role for surgeons and surgery in cancer management. If cancer was "in the blood" or a generalized state of the body, it was not amenable to the surgeon's knife. For 15 years, Hutchinson "taught this [localist] doctrine to the students with whom I have come into contact as earnestly as I could, because I think that in the belief of the local origin of cancer rests our only hope of dealing satisfactorily with it as surgeons; and I also believe that our patients' interests are prejudiced most seriously by the sort of hesitancy in the acceptance of this doctrine which prevails in a large section of the profession."[25]

For others, embracing localism because it provided the rationale for surgery and surgeons in the management of cancer was circular, self-interested, and unscientific. William Jenner protested, "You are not to believe it because it is true, but because it is necessary that you should believe it in order to operate. Now, I think that is a very bad argument. It is true or false. If it be true that cancer is local, it would still be a question how far it could be removed by operation. That is a question of numbers – a thing to be settled, not by argument, but by fact."[26]

It would take, however, over a century for the faith in numbers, clinical experimentalism, empiricism, and skepticism about economic, professional, and other biases in evaluating efficacy to yield purposeful clinical experiments of cancer surgery. Nineteenth-century surgeons could draw only the most miserable conclusions about the efficacy of surgery from their own and others' clinical experiences. "We have failed in hundreds and thousand of cases; for years, for centuries past, we have failed to cure cancer as a local disease," Paget argued. "Every excision of cancer followed by return is a failure; even the largest, the roughest attempts to cure it as a local disease. If we can have any hope at all of curing cancer it must be in the study of it as a constitutional disease, for, so far as therapeutics yet have proceeded, nearly the whole power of therapeutics is that of constitutional remedies against constitutional diseases."[27]

In the decades after Paget and the London conference, American and British surgeons would reach consensus that cancer was a local disease. Cancer's constitutional nature would either be ignored or caricatured as a discarded myth (as in the myth of "cancer taint" in families). This consensus did not emerge because of new pathological insights or more efficacious therapies, but as part of an organized campaign to put medical and lay beliefs about cancer on a modern, scientific basis, ridding them of the prevailing – and diversely expressed – uncertainty, pessimism, and skepticism.

A key component of this solution was the articulation of a more localist meaning to a term long associated with the constitutional nature of cancer: *metastasis*. Metastasis had a long history of denoting a more general relationship between local and systemic manifestations of disease, especially those separated in space and time. Galen had distinguished between *apostasis* and *metastasis*, the former being a crisis that liberated the patient from illness and the latter "the flaring of an old sickness to a new focus."[28] In the eighteenth century, the term was largely used to denote the process by which a mild superficial complaint became a dangerous internal one, such as the way a skin problem could – if neglected or treated badly – spread to a vital internal organ.

For example, metastasis was a fundamental term in eighteenth-century debates about the nature and proper treatment of scabies, which was characterized clinically by localized rash, generalized itch, and other systemic symptoms. "Metastatic theory" was used by eighteenth-century elite physicians to assert their medical authority in the crowded marketplace of healers and surgeons. These physicians often claimed that they had specialized knowledge with which to understand and mitigate the danger that superficial processes would release morbid material into the body, leading to internal disease.[29]

The use of the term *metastasis* to denote the transmission of the morbid matter of cancer from a primary site to a secondary one has been most frequently attributed to Recamier at the beginning of the nineteenth century.[30] During the nineteenth century, this cancer-specific usage became more prominent and was increasingly understood as the transmission of the physical matter of cancer, which by the last quarter of the century meant cancer cells. But this later consensus had been anticipated. "The micrography of cancer," Walshe wrote presciently in 1841, "shows that the translation and deposition of a few cells only from the original nidus might lead to the development of the largest mass; each cell is in itself the possible embryo of a tumour."[31] Agnew in his 1881 text reviewed claims that cancer "juices" or other cancer products, rather than cancer cells themselves, might transmit cancer throughout the body but concluded that plugs of cancer cells traveled around the body.[32] This belief was not only consistent with the more materialist orientation of the age, but also drew on parallel understandings of embolic spread of infectious disease material and blood clots (sometimes the term "embolism" was substituted for metastasis) and the direct visualization of cancer cells in blood and lymphatic vessels. Agnew further argued that the accumulation of secondary cancer deposits was responsible for cachexia and general dissolution, phenomena that formerly were understood as constitutional processes.[33]

Late-nineteenth-century physicians explained the often long interval between the discovery of the primary tumor and the clinical appearance of metastasis (often many years after breast amputations) by analogy to syphilis, anthrax, and other infectious diseases that were newly discovered to have the capacity for latent, dormant, silent infection.[34] De Morgan argued for the plausibility of cancer's latency by analogy to the many normal physiological phenomena that await the right time in development and the life course to awaken, such as the changes of the female breast at puberty and the loss of children's teeth.[35] Prominent London cancer surgeon Herbert Snow (1847–1930) described this latency as resulting from an infection in the bone marrow.[36] "This marrow deposit," Snow surmised, "leads to local tumor-formation or to fracture only in exceptional instances; far more often, it progresses insidiously, perhaps for several years, with comparatively inconspicuous local indications of its presence, but with a gradual and steady deterioration in the general health."

Snow argued that in the case of cancer in the breast this long latency had previously "favoured the constitutional theory."[37] Constitutionalism had provided a very plausible framework for understanding many of cancer's unique clinical features such as the appearance of cancer in multiple places in the body and the inexorable progression to exhaustion and death in many patients. Notions of reciprocity, sympathy, humors, constitution, action at a distance, and disease as an aggregate sum of a body's experience over time offered a set of convenient explanations for why disease might begin in the breast but appear elsewhere in the body later on in the same patient, and which in many cases led to exhaustion, cachexia, and ultimately death. But as the more materialist conception of cancer cells spreading throughout the body was understood and accepted, the constitutional explanation of metastasis and latency lost ground.

The new reductionist and mechanistic consensus on metastasis, like the older constitutional notions it replaced, posed a challenge to surgical extirpation of primary tumors. What good was surgery if tumors may have already spread throughout the body in a latent way? Late-nineteenth-century surgeons began to answer this challenge by asserting that there existed a discrete time interval in the natural history of cancer during which latent metastasis had not yet occurred. During this interval, cancer spread only by direct, local extension.

That cancer was a local disease before spreading throughout the body was to become a central dogma of the ascending model of cancer's natural history. It permitted a less pessimistic view of surgery, because cancer was presumably within the reach of the knife during this interval. Instead of the more traditional notion about cancer's malignancy that posited some transformative moment in which innocent tumors became malignant, this newer view of cancer's natural history implied that a tumor's malignancy or malignant potential might be fully formed with no need for a transformation, but existed for some period in a localized area before spreading throughout the body. Cancer was increasingly viewed as an orderly, mechanistic biological process whose potential for future harm depended on when in its natural history it was discovered and extirpated. This notion was implicit in the ideas and practices of earlier physicians, as in Physick's comment to Emlen that the wisdom of surgery would not be revealed until the "parts were laid open," but was not made into an optimistic credo for rationalizing surgery until the late nineteenth and early twentieth centuries in Anglo-American surgical practice. Then and now, however, this view of cancer's natural history was more asserted than proven, in part because it was and is impossible to prove that at any hypothesized "early" period in a cancer's natural history metastasis has not already occurred.

What Causes Cancer in the Breast?

Unlike the consensus about cancer's natural history, there was no late-nineteenth-century medical breakthrough or consensus about what causes cancer. This failure was especially disturbing because cancer rates were widely perceived to be increasing. There were no reliable clues to evasive action at either the individual or population level. Cancer seemed to strike at random and was feared more than in earlier eras.

Randomness was not well tolerated. American and British doctors in the latter half of the nineteenth century made halting attempts to bring some order to this disturbing area of uncertainty, reconfiguring older assumptions about cancer with the new reductionist style of explaining disease. The practice of Willard Parker (1800–1884), a busy New York surgeon, serves as an ideal place to explore this style of causal thinking and its relationship to clinical practice. Parker both published a text on cancer in the breast and recorded his day-to-day impressions about individual patients in a cancer casebook. He made some 457 brief entries in this book, almost exclusively about cancers of the breast, from 1852 to 1879. This large number of consultations, itself only a small part of a very diverse surgical and administrative career, is evidence of the increase in surgical consultations for breast tumors, cancer surgery, and cancer specialization in the latter half of the nineteenth century. The increasing number of breast cases Parker saw throughout this time reflects the calculus of market success in nineteenth-century urban specialization. "A surgeon will get a reputation as the only possible man to consult in cancer cases," one New York journalist ironically observed, "simply because he has cut off more breasts than any one else."[38] Parker and his son used this casebook as the basis for a posthumously published text on cancer in the breast.[39]

Parker, Agnew, and other American surgeons of the time were taught about the leading, largely German, theories of cancer's origins. Parker's casebook contained lecture notes from 1873 in which he recorded competing theories such as Rudolph Virchow's theory that cancer cells derived from connective tissue, Julius Cohnheim's theory that cancer originated in cells that retained the embryonic capacity for cell division and unrestrained growth, and other theories that stressed the role of various germs or parasites. Although cancer was evidently a cellular disease, Parker concluded in his text that it might also spread "by causing, through infection, a growth similar to itself in adjacent healthy cellular elements."[40] But these differing theories about cancer's tissue origins had little bearing on clinical practice and none was clearly superior to the others. "Among these various and conflicting doctrines, what one is to be accepted as the most plausible?" Agnew rhetorically asked after reviewing the different principal doctrines about the origins of cancer. "For it is doing no injustice to say that not one has been demonstrated to be true."[41]

One nineteenth-century insight into the tissue origins of cancer was generally accepted and at least held out some promise for a more fundamental insight into cancer's etiology: the notion that cell differentiation in embryonic development is essentially a one-way process, such that the large number of malignant tumors composed of epithelial tissues (the various carcinomas, as distinguished from sarcomas) all derived from cells that differentiated into epithelial tissues during fetal life.[42] Beyond bringing order to cancer classification or tracing earlier steps in a complex causal pathway, nineteenth-century histologists hoped that finding other general principles of embryonal development would ultimately explain – by error and deviation from normal differentiation – the formation of cancer. De Morgan, for example, believed that the same principles that determined how "one atom in the germinal membrane becomes muscle, another bone, another brain" would determine "what we call morbid growths."[43]

Parker initially recorded a few isolated demographic and clinical observations in his casebook. With time, he recorded more clinical information in a simple tabular system under the headings Name, Residence, Family (typically a notation of "taint" or "no taint"), Location (of breast problem), and Remarks. Under Remarks he typically included follow-up information as was available (especially decisions about surgery and their outcomes) as well as the chronology of discovery and medical attention, exciting causes (e.g., blows to the breast), and short details from the patient's life that might be relevant to cancer (mostly details about grief and other stresses and strains). These schematic notations became the basis for the tables that formed half of the posthumously published text.

Parker's system of classifying cases reflected the expectation that knowledge about causes might emerge from quantitative analysis and pathological–clinical correlation from the raw material of clinical practice. In his text, Parker put each case into one of nine categories, some based on the patient's age at cancer diagnosis (very young and very old), some on the disease's clinical behavior (rapid, slow, or benign for a long time before an abrupt shift to malignancy), some on constitutional criteria (from consumptive or cancer families), or on the physical appearance of the tumor (cystic or ordinary scirrhus). While each case was assigned to only one category, these demographic, physiological, familial, and physical criteria overlapped so much that a particular case might have been classified equally well under a few different headings. Parker's classification system thus reflected a faith in an ontological scheme in which each case could be categorized as a unique and discrete subtype of cancer in the breast, although he was not committed to the priority of any particular level of analysis (i.e., the pathological did not trump the clinical) and his placement of cases into particular categories seems in retrospect to be arbitrary.

However much faith Parker had in this empirical, bottom-up approach to causal inference, he nevertheless understood that the ultimate causes of cancer were going to be found elsewhere. He wrote that "we shall have to observe the habits of individuals, of communities, and of nation, and their surrounding circumstances."[44] Parker argued that medicine had come to rely too much on the "microscope as a means of arriving at ultimate causes, and the consequence is that there has not been as much advance in the etiology and *nature* of the disease."[45]

While Parker's tables demonstrated few new etiological clues, it typified the style of recording and analysis of aggregate data that many clinicians and others expected would soon yield results about the causes of cancer in the breast. Parker did draw some tentative conclusions from his quantitative analyses. As we discussed earlier, the cessation of menses had been linked to cancer in the breast since antiquity. Parker nevertheless found that in the 353 cases in which he had information on menstrual status, 189 developed cancer in the breast before menses ceased, 84 developed it at the time of the cessation of menses, and only 80 after menses had stopped.

Without having a specific statistical vocabulary, clinicians like Parker often evidenced a subtle grasp of the complexity of causal inference. In another instance, when his tabulations suggested counterintuitive results, Parker inferred an association as a probable instance of what would later be labeled as *confounding*. Parker dismissed the apparent "protective" effect of child bearing on cancer in the breast that he found in his tabulations – an association commonly appreciated as robust today – as resulting from a common cause that made women both barren and cancerous.[46]

Parker's speculations about the emotional and psychological etiology of cancer in the breast harkened back to traditional notions and served to bring some order to the apparent randomness of who developed cancer and when the disease appeared. They also rationalized actions that aimed to comfort patients and allay their fears. "Her husband had been sick a long time, and her care and anxiety had been very great," Parker wrote of one patient. "She had never conceived, and I believe these were sufficient traceable causes for the malignant epithelial growth."[47] Parker's casebook is filled with similar notations about patients – some having had surgery while others not – whom he observed to be suffering grief and sorrow and whose nervous constitution he had tried to calm. Only typical was the case of a woman who had a "nervous temperament" and whose mass Parker had removed under ether 2 years earlier (she had no axillary involvement at the time). She had "remained entirely well until May 18, 1862 when her husband died suddenly and she was in great grief and sorrow. She called on me in August and the disease is cancer had made [sic] its appearance in the old place ... I advised to keep her mind quiet by keeping it occupied."[48] More generally, Parker concluded that therapy "must seek to modify the patient's constitution so that it will be no longer prone to reproduce the disease; and then only may the surgeon be satisfied that he has done his duty."[49] Although localist ideas were ascendant among elite physicians considering the natural history of cancer, clinical practice was still strongly influenced by constitutional ones.

Parker evidenced a more mechanistic style of explaining the link between emotions and cancer than in earlier eras. He frequently evoked the mediating role played by the nervous system. Breast and other tissue development were "under the normal influence of the nervous system." Cancer resulted when there was a "tendency to pervert relations between proliferating cells and the terminal nerves," resulting in "retrograde development."[50] Paget had similarly suggested the traditional link between women's emotional life and subsequent development of cancer, adding a mediating somatic link in poor nutrition.[51]

Parker and other nineteenth-century clinicians frequently observed that physical trauma preceded cancer in the breast.[52] In 1841, a 23-year-old woman consulted Philadelphia physician George Washington Norris, presenting with a heavy and lobulated tumor that appeared a year after a "blow upon her right breast." In addition, Norris also recorded that her freely "secreted milk" from a previous pregnancy had been "dried up by her physician," thus combining trauma with older mechanico-humoral ideas such as that cancer in the breast derived from stagnation and obstruction of normal lactation.[53] Parker had concluded that there was a traumatic exciting cause in 229 cases. In one case he noted, "exciting cause – a blow from the handle of a pump about 2 years ago. She was hurt at the time and a tumor was soon discovered." In another case, he noted a woman whose husband 18 years previously had struck her breast "during nightmare. Later hit by gentleman who was lifting her up."[54]

Along with discrete physical blows, Parker and his contemporaries frequently emphasized "habitual" physical pressure. Parker meant habits such as "wearing tight stays and dresses."[55] Such speculation was in keeping with many other late-nineteenth-century clinical descriptions of chronic irritation. This idea, often associated with Virchow, remained prominent well into the twentieth century (as in the writings of prominent twentieth-century cancer pathologist James Ewing). Chronic irritation's appeal and tenacity probably reflects its focus on the physical interface between discrete bits of environment and parts of bodies. Snow's 1891 model of chronic irritation anticipated twentieth-century "two hit" theories of carcinogenesis with their emphasis on the processes of cancer initiation at the body's exterior surface and damaged repair mechanisms. Snow emphasized repeated insults to a "functionally healthy mucous membrane," where "repair is slow and tedious," so that the "door for initiation of the cancerous process is thrown widely open." In the case of alcohol as a chronic irritant, Snow combined specific and general causes, cellular mechanisms, and constitutional insults, by arguing that alcohol not only chronically irritated and thus disordered epithelial cells but it also lowered general vitality.[56]

Some late-nineteenth-century physicians were skeptical about the use of chronic irritation to explain everything and to support a localist view of cancer, while obscuring ignorance of the actual mechanisms of cellular change that produced cancer cells. Mr. Rivington, a skeptical surgeon at the London pathology conference remarked that "even if we could refer all cases of cancer to some source of local irritation, we should only be one step nearer an explanation; we should still require to know how it was that local irritations could cause an abnormal development of natural elements, since we know that this is not the ordinary effect of injury or irritation."[57]

In keeping with the more localist and mechanistic ideals of late-nineteenth-century medicine, elite clinicians did not generally place much emphasis on heredity. The physical, biological basis of hereditarian transmission remained obscure. There was also confusing aggregate data. While some clinicians believed that the familial clustering of cancer cases was self-evident in practice, a 1859 review of the experience at the Middlesex Hospital in London noted that only 8.75 percent of cancer patients recalled another close family member with cancer.[58] Heredity generally was evoked more as a vector of cancer than as a specific contribution to disease etiology. In the era before the rediscovery of Mendel, the work of Weissman, and the discovery of chromosomes, speculating on heredity, lacking in mechanisms and physicality, was often viewed as a scientific dead end. The method of inheritance, Paget wrote in 1887, is "so mysterious; it is so utterly impossible to conceive the form of the material in which the impregnated ovum contains that which will become or be made cancerous, that it cannot be safe or useful to think that we can deduce anything from the bare fact. We are apt to speak of potentiality, tendency and predisposition as if they were forces independent of matter or structure; but when we try to think of the very things on which they depend, we find ourselves in a cloud-land of mystery, where the difficulty of discovering truth is as great as the facility of guessing."[59]

Parker downplayed any strong deterministic role for heredity in the development of cancer in the breast, arguing that such a focus distracted women from avoiding the more well-accepted exciting causes such as tight lacing and too little or excessive breast feeding as well as unnecessarily stigmatizing and scaring women who had relatives with cancer. Parker and others preferred to associate cancer with different features of modern life. This association was plausible because there seemed to be a lot more cancer, especially from the vantage point of a surgeon specializing in cancer with a large clientele.[60] Framing cancer as a "disease of civilization" was also a standard way of explaining chronic diseases, especially those that primarily affected women.

Parker's conception of cancer as a disease of civilization was built on conventional assumptions about "primitive" culture and the transmission of acquired traits.[61] Parker observed that cancer was common in the American Negro while unheard of in native black populations of Africa. "Has the negro, by dwelling among the white race, acquired a constitutional predisposition, which is transmitted?"[62]

Inferences about modernity and civilization were frequently combined with assumptions about gender. More than was the case earlier in the century, clinicians and others understood and interpreted aggregate statistics and clinical observations about cancer and women in an increasingly authoritative, quantitative, and deterministic style. In this new style, women's biology, behavior, and changing roles were linked via specific, if speculative, somatic mechanisms to the genesis of cancer.

Snow's 1891 tract, *The Proclivity of Women to Cancerous Diseases*, made most of these connections explicit. For Snow, cancer was a women's disease because the two most prevalent sites for cancer – the uterus and the breast – occurred only in women (a few men did of course get cancer in the breast). Snow observed that "these are most prone to frequent modifications and changes, either in individual growth; or in relative arrangement" and that they "exhibit the most intimate subordination to the nervous system."[63] "Modifications and changes" in breast and uterine tissue referred to changes associated with menstruation and pregnancy. Italian public health official Rignoni-Stern similarly explained the proclivity of the breast and uterus to cancer as "due to the temporary execution of the natural functions of the uterus and breasts, or to the periodicity associated with these same functions, or even more importantly, it may be due to the great propensity these organs have to mechanical damage."[64]

The special vulnerability of these female organs was plausible because of the accepted etiological role of chronic irritation in cancer and because of older assumptions about the dangers of life cycle events – puberty, menstruation, lactation, and menopause – associated with these organs. The nervous system mediated the ways that the stresses and strains of modern life and civilization for women led to cancer in the breast. Snow and others used the fact that suckling stimulates lactation to argue that breasts were under direct and rich nervous control.

A crucial link in a model that connected modern life, women, nerves, and cancer was the role played by benign breast and uterine tumors. Snow wrote that these "benign tumor formations" were "a simple over-growth of normal tissue" as a result of "perverted development, the result of some factor which interferes with the local nutrition of the organs in question" and which only occurred among the "civilized races."[65] For Snow and others, these benign tumors were consequences of some unexplained factors in modern industrialized life. Benign tumors could and did turn into malignant cancers if women were exposed to worrisome exciting causes.

Snow also pointed to other specific mechanisms – habits, states of mind and body, such as constipation, overpressure at school, and abuse of neurotics (tea) – that might cause women to have increased amounts of cancer.[66] Like Parker and others, Snow was especially critical of the evil results of tight lacing in cancer in the breast, calling attention to the way that this "energetic application" was done to female children in their tender years.[67]

In cancer sites in which physicians observed a lower prevalence among women, Snow and others offered other types of explanations. Snow observed, for example, that women were more attentive to their appearance and used less alcohol and tobacco. Attentiveness to physical appearance thus protected women from the exciting causes of head, neck, mouth, and skin cancers. Exciting irritating conditions and warts, for example, would infrequently develop in a body well taken care of and monitored. Avoiding alcohol and tobacco reduced cancer among women because the routine use of these substances led to more functional derangements, which over a long period of time might produce cancer (it was an article of faith that "functional disorder or derangement is apt to generate organic disease").[68]

Self-evidently, the underlying cause for the attitudes, behaviors, and states of mind that linked women to cancer was modern civilization. Like Parker, Snow noted, "It is also found that carcinoma is almost absent in the savage; while rapidly increasing in prevalence among the civilized."[69] Snow and others explicitly connected cancer in the breast and elsewhere to neurasthenia, chlorosis, and other late-nineteenth-century medical ailments that particularly ailed women and whose ultimate causes lay in modernity.[70] The links among civilization, female stress, nerves, and cancer and other "nerve weaknesses" led Snow to "the practical conclusion" that we need to "aim at removing the causes which, among us, so conspicuously impede the female sexual organs in the due performance of their allotted functions. You will then succeed in hugely diminishing the prevalence, not only of cancer, but of every other specially female complaint; and will go far to remove that reproach of chronic invalidism under which the fairer half of our community now so needlessly rests."[71]

Although linked by Snow and others to nerve weakness, cancer in the breast and elsewhere was widely understood to be a much more somatically based affliction than neurasthenia and other sorts of chronic invalidism. Alice James, sister of Henry and William James, spent much of her life as a chronic invalid but was dramatically relieved of the stigma and psychological burden of this social role when a physician diagnosed a breast lump she had been living with as cancer in 1891:

> To him who waits, all things come! My aspirations may have been eccentric, but I cannot complain now, that they have now been brilliantly fulfilled. Ever since I have been ill, I have longed and longed for some palpable disease, no matter how conventionally dreadful a label it might have, but I was always driven back to stagger alone under the monstrous mass of subjective sensations, which that sympathetic being "the medical man" had no higher inspiration than to assure me I was personally responsible for. . . . [72]

Finally, the acceptance of the germ theory in the century's closing decades not only fed expectations of progress but also contributed to new frameworks for understanding cancer's causes and clinical course.

It did so in part by direct extension as there was considerable speculation about the parasitic origin of cancer as well as a more general hope
to find some small and localized "germ" of cancer. There were no credible reports of finding such a germ or well-accepted demonstrations of the
contagiousness of cancer. But given the rapid rate of progress in understanding infectious diseases, many believed that clinical and laboratory
correlation would soon uncover the specific germ of cancer.

Paget characterized the contemporary inability to find such a necessary
and sufficient agent (likely to be an infectious organism) as comparable to
the situation a generation earlier when hard evidence for specific germs
in infectious disease was lacking. "When I last lectured here on this subject," Paget said 1887, "if similar questions had been asked concerning
tuberculosis, leprosy, tetanus, or many other diseases now known to be
dependent on parasitic or other specific materials in the blood, they could
not have been answered; or, most probably, those which could then have
been answered 'No' would now be more correctly answered 'yes.'"[73]

The Problematic Diagnosis and Treatment
of Cancer in the Breast

Although ether had allowed longer and therefore more extensive operations, cancer surgery had not been technically transformed. "Excision of
the mammary gland is not an operation of any great difficulty," Agnew
wrote in 1881, "nor is it especially necessary that the patient should be
subjected to any protracted preparatory treatment." He taught that the
operation could be performed in a bed or on an operating table.

Agnew recommended either removing the tumor and gland and closing the wound with existing skin or performing a more extensive operation that included removing overlying skin. The latter was to be reserved
for extreme cases. If axillary disease was present, Agnew advised the oper-
ator to "enucleate" the disease in the armpit with the fingers because this
provided more "safety than the knife."[74] While he articulated a goal of
removing all visible tumor, Agnew did not call for a routine extensive
operation to remove cancer that could not be seen. Experimentation with
more "radical" surgery against such invisible disease was occurring much
more in Europe than in the United States.

Surgery, even if done more frequently and less painfully than earlier
in the century, was still risky. Lay persons could read in the newspapers

about fatal outcomes of breast amputations, such as an 1883 news report of a woman dying from erysipelas and lockjaw after "a cancer was recently removed from her breast."[75] Agnew pointed to a 10-percent mortality for the more extensive operations.[76] And there was also considerable morbidity, especially from arm swelling. In the era before surgery that routinely involved removal of the axillary lymph glands was common in the United States, the clinical syndrome we now call *lymphedema* was more commonly seen as a consequence of cancer in the breast than surgery. "Among the distressing complications which belong to the life history of the disease," Agnew wrote, "are the great swelling and pain of the arm which follow the venous obstruction due to the pressure of the indurated axillary glands."[77]

Although surgery for cancer in the breast was done more frequently and was less horrific, clinical diagnosis remained difficult. Even at the end of the nineteenth century, clinicians knew that they did not have the technical means to always divine the potential of a tumor to behave malignantly by examining gross or microscopic abnormalities. The operative and preoperative routines, which would later link surgery and pathology to clinical decision-making in the operating room, such as the use of interoperative biopsy with frozen sections, were not yet routinely deployed. Surgeons generally amputated breasts without pre- or perisurgical microscopic pathology. They could be reasonably sure in most cases that tumors were cancerous, but there remained great uncertainty in other cases.

Nor were tumors routinely examined under the microscope after surgery, even though this was technically possible and could have helped determine prognosis and assisted in future decisions (e.g., the lack of microscopic evidence of extensive cancer could presumably suggest a good prognosis). Surgeons (who until the twentieth century typically served as their own pathologist in the minority of cases that had postsurgical or postmortem analysis) generally believed that clinical diagnosis based on factors such as the patient's history and the look and feel of the tumor before surgery was superior to microscopic diagnosis done on surgical specimens. Pathological diagnosis was not a "gold standard" by which clinical diagnosis was confirmed or rejected. There were few revelatory moments where microscopic diagnosis brought clarity to obscure clinical signs.

In 1882, for example, Philadelphia surgeon Addinell Hewson recorded a case history of a patient that he had operated on years earlier whose amputated breast had been sent for pathological examination under the microscope. The specimen was judged not to contain cancer. But later events proved this judgment to be erroneous. Hewson observed that the disease had reappeared in the operative scar and in the opposite breast and the patient was now dying of exhaustion caused by cancer. This patient had undoubtedly been suffering from cancer at the time of her original surgery. Experiences such as these reinforced the idea that cancer was most reliably diagnosed based on what clinicians directly observed with their eyes and palpated with their hands. Hewson wrote the following terse and ironic note on the front and back of a photograph of his patient's large, ulcerating breast tumor: "Microscopically the mass was found to be composed of epithelial cells without any traces of cancer."[78]

For some surgeons, such as prominent nineteenth-century French surgeon and cancer authority Alfred-Armand Velpeau (1795–1867) the issue was not simply the greater accuracy of the surgeon's eyes and hands than the pathologist's microscope. Clinical diagnosis was necessary because cancer was not primarily a cellular disease but was caused by an elusive specific agent that could not be seen by the microscope.[79] But clinical diagnosis was also not easy or reliable and often considerable uncertainty remained about the nature of tumors. Despite the need to determine whether cancers had spread to the axilla, surgeons could not often make such judgments. "It is impossible, from any external signs," Agnew noted, "to determine the limits of this infiltration, a fact which must necessarily have great practical bearing on all operations for the removal of carcinomatous tumors."[80]

In addition to the fallibility of both clinical and pathological diagnosis, decision-making in cancer in the breast was difficult because of the highly idiosyncratic clinical course of the disease. "The clinical aspects of the disease are exceedingly varied," Agnew wrote in his text, "scarcely two cases being alike in their life history."[81]

When late-nineteenth-century American and British surgeons had confidence in their diagnosis, they believed, as did surgeons and physicians in earlier eras, that the prognosis was miserable, with or without surgery. In 1887, Paget wrote that surgery for cancer "does not do all we want; the disease returns after even complete removal of the diseased parts. All that is locally wrong may be removed, the local portion of the disease may be deemed cured, but something remains, or, after a time, is renewed, and similar disease reappears and, in some form or degree, is usually worse than the first, and always tending towards death."[82]

Agnew believed that although the prognosis was miserable, there was a rationale for surgery even if it did not cure cancer. "In general it may be said that the prognosis in carcinoma is most discouraging, if not hopeless," Agnew observed. "The great question to be determined in any case of mammary carcinoma at the present state of surgery, in my judgment, is not how best to cure or eradicate the disease, but what course will give the patient the longest lease on life. This question can only be determined by the comparison and analysis of a large number of cases treated by tentative and operative means."[83]

Agnew was aware that existing statistical analyses of treated and untreated patients did not really present a fair comparison of different approaches. Showing a remarkable understanding of the limitations of existing data, Agnew argued that such comparisons, while "strictly correct," did not "represent the real or bottom truth of this subject. There are more than mathematical processes involved in striking the averages between the two different lines of treating the same disease." Agnew went on to stress the many ways in which operated patients might have a better prognosis than those who did not have surgery ("the prudent surgeon will exercise some selective judgment in the cases of mammary carcinoma which he consigns to the knife, selecting the most favorable for operation and relegating the more hopeless ones to the mercy of nature"). "It will not do to place these two classes on opposite sides in the race of life," he argued, "and, when the death-goal is reached by each, to credit the difference of days or months to certain plans of treatment."[84]

Agnew was not nihilistic. He extrapolated from his own clinical experience and published data that there was a modest benefit from surgery in selected cases. He understood that local recurrences usually occurred within 3 and 12 months after surgery.[85] The benefit of surgery, however small, was only to be seen in terms of extended life and "comfort of the patient" and only in selected cases.[86] Cures would have to wait for future advances. "The blessed achievement will, I believe," Agnew wrote, "never be wrought by the knife of the surgeon. We may hope, however, for the discovery of some drug which, operating through the general system, will follow and destroy the vagrant cells and do for cancer what mercury and the iodide of potassium have done for syphilis."[87]

More quantitative evaluation of surgery and less subjective means of categorizing cancer resulted in more confident – if negative – judgments about the efficacy of existing therapeutics. Hence surgeons at the end of the nineteenth century were often as pessimistic about breast amputations as those at the beginning. While they carried out more surgery, they often did so with a similar reluctance and when there was no good way to avoid doing it.

Parker observed that more careful, quantitative follow-up of surgical patients and developments in histology in the latter part of the century had made the contemporary surgeon even more skeptical about the efficacy of breast amputations. "One reason for the unsettled state of opinion," Parker wrote in 1885 of earlier eras in which exaggerated claims of surgical efficacy and extreme skepticism coexisted "was the lack of subsequent histories of cases which had been operated on, and which were often wrongly reported as cures as soon as the patient had recovered from the operation. Another cause of erroneous opinion was the lack of that histological knowledge which now shows that in most cases of cancer there is, at an early period, a degree of infiltration of the cancerous elements beyond what was formerly suspected."[88]

In the 178 cases in which Parker could reliably judge the duration of life after the appearance of cancer, the average duration was 3.38 years. But there was little difference in this average duration among the 100 subjects who had surgery (3.54 years) and the 78 cases who did not (3.22 years).[89] Despite these pessimistic numbers, Parker believed that surgery was beneficial for some women without axillary swellings. Parker and others could draw some limited optimistic gleanings in part because his case series included 16 women who in 1882 were still living when last heard from.

The "propriety of amputation" for good prognosis cancer was an idea more assented to in medical texts and articles than enthusiastically embraced in practice. "Not the least important part of the work is that in which the view is sought to be maintained by an abundant array of facts," prominent Philadelphia surgeon Samuel Gross wrote in the introduction to his 1880 treatise of mammary tumors, "that carcinoma may be permanently relieved by thorough operations practiced in the early stage of its evolution."[90] Parker similarly wrote that "there is such a consensus of opinion as to the advisability of early removal of the growth, that a discussion of this subject would be useless."[91]

Yet there was a disjuncture between these espoused views and actual practice. In Parker's notebooks there are many examples of surgery done on women with bad prognostic signs and not offered to others who showed no evidence of axillary disease. In one revealing case, Parker was seemingly influenced by both a patient's young age and regret over an earlier decision not to operate, to perform surgery on a woman with bad prognostic signs. Mrs. T., was 35 years old when she consulted Parker in September 1862. She was "very fat" and in "good circumstances." Three and a half years earlier, Parker had noted a small tumor in her left breast during a pregnancy but had not operated. She had been well up until 6 months prior to the 1862 visit but the tumor "was now growing fast," extended to the axilla, and her nipple was retracted, tender, and hot. Parker noted that she was a "bad case for operation" but nevertheless operated on her in May 1863. Parker's last entry was, "The disease was extensive in axilla and involving the pectoral which I cut away. Died July 2, 1863."[92] Surgery was increasingly being done as a way of not giving up hope, sometimes called a "moral" rationale.

In many cases, an important criterion for operation was the patient's state of mind, in particular, how resigned women were to their cancer diagnosis. If they were resigned, then an ineffective and mutilating operation could be avoided. In 1863, a 54-year-old woman consulted Parker who had "accidentally discovered tumor 2.5 years ago in left breast above the nipple." Parker's decision to "sustain and palliate" rather than operate was based on clinical criteria such as the spread to the axilla, but also because "the mind is quiet."[93]

In Parker's practice and in others, surgery could be deferred because the tumor was too small and innocent, in which case the body might take care of it by itself, or too large in which case surgery would be futile.[94] Surgery was generally avoided or delayed unless the patient was young and healthy, demanded it, and had not had previous surgery, and there was clear evidence on gross examination that the cancer had not spread to the axillary area.[95]

Surgery was of course done for other reasons besides cure or moral purposes. Breast surgery, especially in the years after ether was introduced, was often done to remove an unpleasant mass more than for the rationale of cancer cure per se. Surgeons often expressed their disgust at the tumors they removed. For example, Gross wrote a colleague about a woman whose breast tumor was a tangled mass of ulcerations and growths. He had performed an autopsy and derisively concluded that she died of "sheer exhaustion from the stinking discharge."[96]

Whether to cure or to remove an unpleasant mass, surgeons would often do repeat surgery on patients as cancer frequently returned in the area of surgery.[97] One response to this situation was that elite American surgeons began to experiment with and advocate for more extensive operations. As a corollary, they began to deride less extensive operations. In one illustrative case, Parker mockingly referred to the actions of a "cancer doctor" who "applied caustic and removed a portion of the breast." About a year after this, the breast became the seat of a more rapid development, which Parker entirely removed.[98]

While only a minority of surgeons called for extensive surgery, those who did exhorted their peers to perform extensive cancer surgery on "early" cases. Gross in 1880 wrote that he was "aware that this general doctrine [surgical curability of early cancers] will not meet with general acceptance on the part of the purely mechanical surgeons." Gross's caricature of "purely mechanical surgeons" was part of a larger intraprofessional conflict brewing in American surgery in which more elite, academically oriented surgeons laid claim to more detailed, scientific, pathological knowledge such as the natural history of cancer and proclaimed it relevant for practice.[99] While there was a good deal of late-nineteenth-century clinical experimentation with more extensive surgery, especially in Europe, it would not be until the early twentieth century that American surgeons fully embraced the dogma of entirely removing cancer through increasingly "radical" operations, along with a model of cancer's natural history in which the time of clinical intervention was the crucial variable.

The Experience of Cancer in the Breast at the End of the Century

Mary Cope died from cancer in the breast in early 1888. Unlike Shipley, Cope underwent surgery despite having advanced disease. Unlike Emlen, who had lived for years with cancer in the breast, Cope died only a few months after her diagnosis. Thus she had neither enough time nor health to leave an extensive written record of her life with cancer.

Cope, an unmarried daughter of a prominent Philadelphia Quaker businessman, had turned 35 during the summer of 1887. By today's standards, Cope's death at 35 from breast cancer seems very early, but in the late nineteenth century, the average age of an American women dying from cancer in the breast was in the 40s.[100] We can partially reconstruct some events of that summer because her first cousin Rachel Cope Evans had left Philadelphia with her children for the cooler climate of Newport, Rhode Island, and received almost daily letters from her husband Jonathan Evans, who had stayed behind in Philadelphia to manage his business. Jonathan Evans's letters chronicled the illnesses and comings and goings of the tight knit Cope family and their friends, many of whom lived together during the year in a small Philadelphia [Germantown] Quaker compound called Awbury.

Jonathan Evans first noted Cope's poor health, which family members described simply as "not strong," on June 22, 1887.[101] The family had recently employed a nurse who did not think Cope's health was improving. Probably because of this lack of progress and because she felt "the heat very much," Cope soon left Philadelphia for Spring Lake and in early July moved down the road to Sea Girt, both New Jersey shore resorts. The change of climate may have had its desired effect for Cope was able to come "to the table to dinner and tea which is more than she has done at home for sometime."[102]

Cope's father, Thomas Pym Cope II (1823–1900), was also suffering some ill-defined ailment that summer. He and his wife Elizabeth joined their daughter and her nurse in Sea Girt in late July. Jonathan Evan's letters depicted Uncle Tom's concerns for his daughter's health and vice versa but did not make clear who was the sicker of the two nor did they give specific symptoms of either illness.[103] Cope's family worked to keep her at rest and to minimize social contacts, tactics not unlike those used in the mid-to-late nineteenth century to deal with chronic invalids and neurasthenics. Jonathan Evans's letters recounted so many neurasthenic-like illnesses that summer among the younger women in the family that it is not clear that he believed that anything much out of the ordinary was going on with either Cope or her father.

By early September, the weather was "so cool" in Philadelphia that Cope's brother Walter went down to Sea Girt to bring her back to

Awbury. Dr. Danach came to the Cope home and discovered that Cope had a breast tumor. Jonathan Evans was not sure when, or even if, Cope knew that she had breast troubles. At one point, Jonathan Evans wrote that Cope did not have "an idea of what it was until Dr. Danach examined it," but later added that Cope knew what was going on but had confided only in her nurse.[104] In a later letter, Jonathan Evans related "a curious thing" that occurred when Cope's sister Ellen had last visited. "Ellen caught cold and it settled in one of her breasts and it threatened to gather. One morning he [George Emlen, Ellen's husband] said Mary said to Ellen I have thought of this a great deal during the night for I have had a sympathetic pain in my left breast nearly all night. George seemed to think that altho' Mary noticed nothing more it was likely the commencement of the Cancer."[105] Cope's family's concern over the circumstances in which her breast tumor developed, that is, their speculation that Cope's "sympathy" with her sister's chest cold was the start of her cancer, reflected the fact that many lay persons still held traditional notions about cancer and the holistic, idiosyncratic, and contingent nature of cancer and illness generally at a period when elite medical men were often in the grip of a more reductionist temper.

On or about September 19, D. Hayes Agnew amputated Cope's left breast, probably in her Awbury home. We do not know the extent of her cancer, but it is highly probable from subsequent events that her poor prognosis was evident to Agnew. Agnew might have rationalized surgery in terms of a very modest increase in the length of her life or for moral purposes, especially in a young woman from a very concerned family.

"There seems little doubt of its being a cancer," Jonathan Evans wrote after the surgery.[106] Throughout this ordeal, Cope's aunt Hetty, writing to her sister-in-law, marveled at Cope's "composure, wh' was unbroken from the first time I saw her, on her return from Sea Girt, till the ether was administered not a symptom of nervousness was manifested from first to last, nor has there been since; she is uniformly cheerful and submissive, of course she has pain but nothing has been referred to except incidentally."[107] Family members in this period were much more likely to find hope and comfort in patients' courage in the face of progressive disease and painful treatment, rather than in their spiritual reckoning.

The relative ease and safety with which surgery could be carried out made cancer surgery less feared and momentous.[108] Operations were not only carried out more frequently on women whose physicians believed they could not cure, as Agnew in all likelihood viewed Cope's life chances, but the substance and style of decision-making had changed. Cope and her family members appeared to agonize much less about whether to consent to surgery and made this decision much more quickly than was the case with Emlen 70 years earlier.

Most of Jonathan Evan's and Aunt Hetty's references to Cope in the immediate aftermath of the operation concerned efforts to conceal news of Cope's tumor and operation from her parents. "It seems to me a *fearful* responsibility for them [Cope, her nurse, relatives in the know like Aunt Hetty] to take," Jonathan Evans wrote 3 days after Cope's surgery, "Don't it all seem very very sad. Please don't say a word of all this ... until they [Cope's parents] hears it from other quarters for I donts want it to come from me."[109] Aunt Hetty wrote, "Mary was so desirous that her parents should not know she was to have an operation performed that we were obliged to keep the matter very quiet lest something might reach them thro letters." Aunt Hetty herself felt "intensely for brother and sister [Cope's parents] tho' it has been an immense relief to them to be spared the suspense that preceded the operation, and the anxiety that followed, tho' the doctor assured us no serious consequences would follow the operation."[110] Cope's parents ultimately learned about the operation a week later. They felt "entirely satisfied with what had been done" and planned to stay away from Awbury "as long as was thought best." Jonathan Evans was relieved that there were no more family secrets to keep.[111]

Cope's and her family's efforts to protect her parents from news of the cancer operation were part of a more general attempt to soften the grim realities of dangerous and mutilating surgery done with little expectation of cure. While concerned about shielding Cope's parents from worry about her surgery, Jonathan Evans had no problem uttering the word cancer in letters to his wife. There appeared to be no special shame over the cancer diagnosis.

Agnew and another doctor came to the Cope home 5 days after the surgery to change dressings. "They both pronounced her doing remarkably well," Aunt Hetty wrote, "but had hardly left the house when she was taken with a violent dyspepsia, causing distressing moans, the inflated condition of the stomach pressed upon the wound increased the pain there, and about the breast, so that it was 4 hours before she was relieved."[112] In the weeks following the operation, Cope had repeated severe attacks of abdominal pain, which her doctors attributed to colic but which her relatives understood in terms of cancer in the abdomen. "I am afraid the disease may have affected her stomach," Jonathan Evans wrote his wife on September 29. "The developments of the place in her breast was so rapid that it seems to me it may have even this short time made its appearance elsewhere. But thee knows I am naturally very anxious and inclined to look on the dark side of things."[113] Cope's sister Margaret similarly understood that despite the fact that the "doctor does not discourage us however and says the wound is healing very well" and that she "don't like to think of discouragement after being so very hopeful as we have been," she was nevertheless "anxious" and "discouraged" because of Cope's continued pain and inability to eat.[114]

Compared to the beginning of the century, there was a greater gap between physician and patient in communication and knowledge about cancer, reflected in Cope's physicians' optimistic comments and their darker interpretation by her close relations. While care remained in the home, there was less intimacy and personal attention given by Agnew and Danach compared to what Physick and colleagues had provided Emlen 70 years earlier. Cope's family experienced a wide gulf between the episodic care and perspective provided by doctors (whose home visits by today's standards seem so attentive) and their own continuous witnessing at home of postsurgical problems and the progressive symptoms of cancer.

Cope's doctors' optimistic comments did not prevent the family from inferring that Cope's cancer "may have even this short time made its appearance elsewhere." Cope's family members understood that her physicians were offering overly optimistic assessments and had little trouble apprehending the grim reality of Cope's situation. Truth telling in cancer diagnosis and prognosis was not yet routinely avoided, but it was being modified by medical intervention despite lack of hope for cure, increased medical certainty about the dismal future of patients with cancer, and the less intimate and more sporadic relationship between doctors, especially infrequently consulted specialists, and families.

Over the next few months, Cope was cared for by a nurse and a small group of family members. They described efforts to keep Cope at rest in her home and not to disturb her with visitors. They found a few optimistic things to say about her nerves ("much stronger than they were a month ago") and her doctors predicted Cope's recovery "would be more rapid because of her remarkable equanimity."[115] But with the end of the summer separations, letters dwindled, and the only further indication of Cope's fate was an announcement in a Philadelphia Quaker newspaper: "Mary S. Cope, daughter of Thomas P. and Elizabeth W. Cope, died in the 35th year of her age, at the residence of her parents, Germantown, Philadelphia, on Fourth-day evening, 1/4/88."[116] Neither Cope's surgery under ether, new ideas such as the ascending localist consensus about breast cancer, nor the new scientific medicine seemed to have much impact on the rapid, destructive course of her breast cancer.

Promise and Pessimism at the End of the Century

Due to both clinical experience and widely held beliefs, most late-nineteenth-century surgeons remained deeply pessimistic about the efficacy of existing means to control cancer in the breast or elsewhere. This pessimism about cancer was brought into bold relief by comparison to medical progress against the many nineteenth-century fevers and symptom complexes that had been dramatically refashioned as specific infectious diseases. In infectious disease, progress was apparent not just in medical knowledge but also in terms of morbidity and mortality. By the latter decades of the nineteenth century the so-called epidemiological transition was in full force. A broad range of American society not only experienced and perceived major improvements in infant mortality, life span, and general health, but also attributed them to clinical and public health practices directed at specific diseases.

In contrast, Americans did not generally perceive that there were attitudinal, behavioral, intellectual, or technological changes that resulted in significant improvements in the ways people lived or died with cancer. Throughout the nineteenth century, physicians and patients continued to feel impotent in the face of cancer in the breast and other sites. Surgeons performed more and more cancer surgery as the century progressed, but did so as or more reluctantly than in earlier periods. Cancer surgery was still feared by patients, if more for the resulting mutilation than because of pain and its inherent dangers. Moreover, the mortality and morbidity from cancer seemed to increase rather than decrease as the nineteenth century progressed. Partly, this was a matter of the epidemiological transition itself – more people were alive and alive at later ages who would then suffer and die from chronic diseases such as cancer. But some contemporary observers and many today also attributed a definite etiological role to different aspects of modern life in the apparent increase in cancer, especially cancer in the breast.

Yet, to American medical observers at the end of the nineteenth century, the significance of the contrasting developments in cancer and infectious disease was not that the direction of scientific thought and clinical innovation in cancer was wrong. The bets waged by contemporary medical men and scientists about cancer were not dissimilar in substance or style to those strategies and ideas that came to be seen as prescient, useful, and having had major, real, biological impact in infectious disease. They just needed more time to work. Given the achievements in medical science generally and the many other technological achievements of the nineteenth century, many physicians, surgeons, and lay people at the end of the nineteenth century expected that significant progress in cancer control and understanding was just around the corner.

A few American and British surgeons began to articulate the idea that if diagnosed and operated on at an early stage, "cancer would surely cease to be what it has so long been termed, the 'opprobrium of surgery.'"[117] This promise has its clearest expression in Thomas Eakins' *The Agnew Clinic*, arguably the most famous heroic painting of late-nineteenth-century American medicine and surgery, which has found its way into the covers of numerous medical books and which hangs today at the University of Pennsylvania in a grand passageway between a building erected in the late nineteenth century for pathological research and medical education and an even more palatial one recently built to house research into the molecular basis of health and disease (see Figure 3.1).

The bloodless surgical scene depicted by Eakins is very different from Agnew's actual bloody mastectomies that were carried on women such as Cope. To the modern eye, the classical and idealized scene depicts dangerous surgical practices, which would soon be changed such as ungloved hands, unmasked faces, and open surgical amphitheaters. Agnew's assistant in the painting, Dr. White, had called the operation "the present opprobrium" and like Agnew and most nineteenth-century American surgeons was well aware of the high operative mortality and near impossibility of surgical cure.[118] "I should hesitate, with my present experience" Agnew had written pessimistically, "to claim a single case of absolute

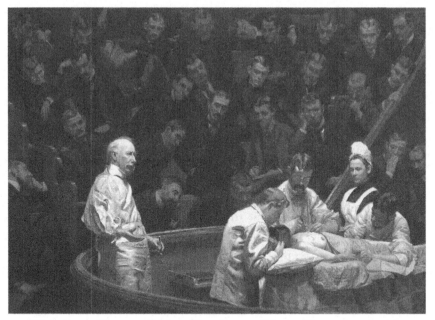

Figure 3.1. Thomas Eakins: The Agnew Clinic. (Reproduced with permission of the University of Pennsylvania Art Collection.)

cure where the diagnosis of carcinoma had been verified by microscopic examination."[119]

Yet Eakins' heroic scene does accurately capture the faith that many doctors, patients, and other Americans had by the end of the nineteenth century in the future of scientific surgery and its potential to deliver health benefits. The value placed on this potential, and its contrast to the realities on the ground only makes sense when we take stock of hope and confidence in future rewards. In earlier eras as well as our own, physicians and patients have often made fundamental decisions, such as whether or not to consult a doctor for a breast lump or choose one type of therapy over another because of the vision of the future with which they most closely identify.

At the end of the nineteenth century, there was thus a widespread and profound ambivalence about progress against cancer in the breast and at other sites. Age-old pessimism and fears about surgical or other cures became, if anything, more severe and pervasive and yet coexisted with heightened expectations about progress that was about to happen. This profound ambivalence would shape later events. Twentieth-century

American surgeons turned their frustrations about current practice and their expectations about the promise of scientific developments into a new dogma whose elements included a localist and orderly model of cancer's natural history, "early" and "complete" surgical eradication, and a public health campaign that promoted these ideas and more "positive" attitudes about cancer. The very lack of optimism by some skeptical physicians and the larger public was imagined to be the enemy and thus the target of their educational campaigns.

FOUR

Taking Responsibility for Cancer

Dr. William S. Halsted (1852–1922) is the American surgeon frequently credited with establishing extensive, radical surgery as the standard treatment for breast cancer. At Johns Hopkins, where he was the first Professor of Surgery and founder of an innovative surgical residency, he trained a generation of surgeons who spread his practices, ideas, and reputation throughout the country and beyond.

Halsted's innovative role in breast cancer surgery has been told from different vantage points for various purposes. Scholars have taken stock of Halsted's many unique contributions to operative practice,[1] examined the role of breast surgery in relation to Halsted's other contributions to surgery and surgical training,[2] and analyzed the many social dimensions of Halsted's practice such as gender, the status of medical authority, nationalistic attitudes, and economic competition among professionals.[3] The context for much of this attention in recent decades has been the controversy over radical cancer surgery. In contrast to hagiographies by former trainees, breast cancer activists in recent decades have often vilified Halsted and the "Halsted mastectomy," which has been depicted as a mutilating operation imposed on women by patronizing and insensitive male surgeons. Reaction and counterreaction have followed.

But Halsted is not just an icon in the history of surgery or breast cancer or a lightning rod for controversy. He was a busy, practicing doctor to many women with breast cancer. He carried on an extensive correspondence with women and their families, general practitioners, and surgeons throughout the country, perplexed over what to do about breast lumps and breast cancer in a time of great change and rising expectations. I will consider Halsted mostly in these clinical and consultative roles in this and the next chapter. Sometimes this means using Halsted as a mere fly on the wall to sample the concerns and aspirations of a large group of geographically spread out patients and physicians.

It is of course problematic to generalize from the life and correspondence of perhaps the most prominent U.S. surgeon to American attitudes and practices about cancer. Yet many of the problems with which Halsted and his correspondents wrestled would soon become the common experience of a much larger group of patients, their families, and their doctors. Halsted's many physician correspondents also represent a very diverse group of practitioners and styles of practice. His breast cancer patients, while largely drawn from the middle and upper classes, came from around the country and had many different medical problems.

Much of Halsted's correspondence exists because of his interest in the "end results" of surgery. On the anniversary of patients' surgery, Halsted had one of his assistants send out a short letter asking patients about their general condition and specifically about their arm mobility. Halsted's patients often understood these letters as a sign of his personal interest and responded with personal details and questions, prompting a response from Halsted, and so on. Another common reason for letters was that general practitioners and patients often needed to determine in advance whether a long-distance consultation was worthwhile and if so, fees had to be negotiated.

This chapter focuses on medical practice, especially cancer surgery, while the next focuses on doctor–patient relations, the breast cancer experience, and decision-making. A central question is how and why breast cancer surgery changed from the "opprobrium of medicine" to something perceived as new, scientific, and effective. While this change has often been understood as a direct consequence of technical innovations in operative procedure that allowed for better results, Halsted's and other surgeons' promotion of new *attitudes* toward cancer, surgery, and the cancer patient may have been the more profound and lasting explanation. The central attitudinal change was a heightened sense of surgical responsibility for cancer. This heightened responsibility is key to understanding many other developments, such as Halsted's career-long attempt to see the complications of breast surgery as being caused by something and somebody else besides surgery and surgeons. This heightened responsibility would soon envelop cancer patients' understanding of their own disease and their relations with their doctors.

Halsted and the Complete Operation

While ether anesthesia and other mid- to late-nineteenth-century technological innovations were necessary conditions for extending the reach of cancer surgery, the push to do so followed from the miserable outcomes of more limited surgery and the centuries-old belief that these poor outcomes resulted from a failure to remove cancer's "invisible roots." Extending the reach of cancer surgery was also common sense, finding its parallel in mundane aspects of nonmedical life, such as removing wide, visibly normal margins when cutting away rotten fruit or termite-infested wood.

Halsted was one among a number of mostly European surgeons who experimented with extending the scope of breast amputations in the late-nineteenth century.[4] He is generally credited with extending breast cancer surgery in the 1880s and early 1890s to include not only the pectoralis minor but also the pectoralis major muscles (chest wall muscles that rotate arms and raise ribs). Joseph Bloodgood, a prominent pupil and later a surgical and pathological colleague of Halsted at Hopkins, recalled that in 1886 other American surgeons such as Dr. Nicholas Senn in Milwaukee routinely performed "complete operations" for cancer in the breast but they did not remove pectoral muscles as Halsted was doing at that time.[5] Halsted advocated removing these muscles, the axillary lymph glands, and the entire breast "en bloc," in one piece (see Figure 4.1). Although Halsted frequently advocated and performed more extensive surgery, such as exploring and removing lymph nodes above the collarbone and along the neck, this was not part of the canonized "Halsted mastectomy."

Through the efforts of Halsted and his trainees in the first decades of the twentieth century, the complete operation rapidly became the standard approach to breast cancer patients. Its ascendency represented much more than the successful diffusion of an effective, innovative technology. It also signified a change in attitudes about cancer treatment that partly constituted and set in motion fundamental changes in how surgeons and women with breast lumps understood and experienced cancer. Unlike surgical responses to cancer of the breast throughout most of the nineteenth century, which were characterized by a chaotic mix of traditional therapeutics and limited surgery, typically done for "moral" reasons and suffused with pessimism, the complete operation as performed at Johns Hopkins by the first years of the twentieth century was done with expectation that it "worked," that it should be offered to all women

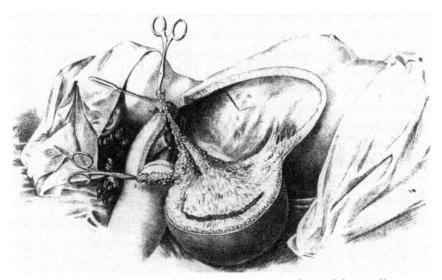

Figure 4.1. The Complete Operation as performed by William Halsted. (From W. S. Halsted, "The result of operations for the cure of cancer of the breast performed at the Johns Hopkins Hospital from June 1889 to January 1894," *Johns Hopkins Hospital Bulletin*, 4 (1894–1895): 297.)

with breast lumps thought cancerous, and that it be performed in a uniform way.

Some of Halsted's contemporaries objected to the false promise implied by terms such as complete and radical.[6] "The words constantly used to qualify the operation of the day as "complete" and "radical" are anatomical misnomers," surgeon Rudolph Matas pointedly observed in 1898, "which serve only to indicate evolutionary phases in the surgical technique, and are illusory if used in the sense that they root out the evil with any degree of certainty."[7]

A few months before he died, Halsted wrote his colleague William Welch about his own place in a long line of surgical innovation in breast amputations. While others recommended stripping the fascia and the superficial fibers of the pectoralis major muscle, Halsted wrote that he was the first to recommend its complete excision. Halsted also credited Willy Meyer with independently and simultaneously recommending removal of the pectoralis minor muscle. Revealingly, Halsted took major credit not so much for these extensions of the operation but for a set of proper surgical attitudes such as meticulousness in cleaning out cancer from the axillary area, a respect for the dangers of cutting into tissues for biopsy (because this itself might spread cancer), and the surgeons' privileged position as cancer diagnostician. He claimed that he was "one of the first surgeons in this country able macroscopically to make the diagnosis of the common tumors."[8] I would add to Halsted's list his important role in changing the character of decision-making and prognostication in breast cancer from one based on the physician's assessment of the patient's individual constitution, attitudes, and social circumstance to a more uniform surgical approach based on purely clinical findings. Halsted helped make operative practice fit the more specific, uniform, localized, surgical disease *breast cancer* that had emerged from earlier notions of *cancer in the breast*.

While the shift to heightened medical responsibility for breast and other cancers during the first few decades of the twentieth century was dramatic and extensive, Halsted's complete operation did not become received practice everywhere. Among the generation of surgeons who practiced in the years immediately following Halsted's death, there was a good deal of skepticism about the need for radical breast surgery. D. A. Power's historical account of breast amputations written in 1934 (which depicted Halsted as an innovator on a par with many others, especially Halsted's contemporary Mitchell Banks whose obscurity Power attributed to the "force of circumstances and his surroundings") depicted, for example, a general English skepticism. "He (Halsted) went perhaps a little too far, and the pendulum is swinging back to less extensive operations than he carried out."[9]

The shift to heightened medical authority and responsibility for cancer also did not mean that nineteenth-century therapeutic pessimism was discarded. In 1932, Hopkins medical historian Henry Sigerist wrote the following assessment of cancer therapeutics, which could easily have been voiced 75 years earlier – or later: "The history of the therapy of cancer is very dull. The principles we are following today, namely, the elimination of the tumor as radically as possible, were discovered in far remote antiquity. Our operative methods are much more efficient than theirs were, and besides the knife we have x-rays and radium to destroy the tumor cells, but we have not found any new principle yet."[10]

The Perceived Efficacy of the Complete Operation

One reason that early-twentieth-century surgeons perceived the complete operation to be superior to less extensive operations was that women were much less likely to have recurrences in the operated breast and surrounding tissues (which were generally called "local recurrences" although the boundaries separating local, regional, and distal disease were in-flux and contested) and thus need second and third operations. As was the case with Emlen and many of Parker's patients, local recurrences after surgery were common in the nineteenth century. Charles P. Childe, as part of his 1905 cancer education book, which stressed the virtues of modern, extensive surgery for "early cancer," recalled a case of a woman who had three successive surgeries between 1876 and 1879, all "due to cancer cells left behind at the time of the first operation.... But there can be no doubt, looking at the case through modern glasses, that these recurrences were due to an imperfect operation. In the operation as done today, the cancer cells giving rise to them, would have been removed at the first sitting, and the patient would have been cured, ab initio."[11]

Halsted similarly attributed recurrent, local disease and the need for repeat operations to "less-than-complete" initial operations. Many surgeons wrote Halsted with stories of repeated limited surgery in patients who had not had complete operations as their initial treatment.[12] Dr. Frank Small from York, Pennsylvania, wrote Halsted in 1897 about how he had removed a mass the size of a hen's egg from a 25-year-old patient. A few months later, the patient returned with an "indurated gland" below the operative scar, which was removed in a second surgery. A few months after the second surgery, the patient returned with an "angry" looking scar and some new glandular enlargement in that breast. "I rather urged the advisability and necessity of more radical procedure for the entire removal of the diseased tissues," Small wrote Halsted belatedly.[13]

One reason that the efficacy of more extensive surgery in reducing local recurrences was so readily apparent was that women were still typically presenting to doctors with very advanced disease. In Halsted's era, as in Physick's and Agnew's, clinicians (like Dr. Small) generally estimated the size of women's breast tumors on their initial visit as being the size of one or another bird egg.[14] The great majority of women prior to the early twentieth century also presented with clinical evidence of swelling in the armpit, long known to be a sign of poor prognosis. In such cases, the chance of local recurrence after less-than-radical surgery was high. Halsted had tabulated local recurrence rates of greater than 60 percent among other leading nineteenth-century surgeons who practiced different degrees of less extensive surgery.[15]

Halsted's own notion of the superiority of the complete operation over more limited surgery was much more closely tied to claims about reducing local recurrence rates than saving women's lives. Halsted did claim, however, in at least one publication that women who underwent complete operations were cured more often than women who had more limited surgery.[16] Like other surgeons and observers throughout the nineteenth and most of the twentieth centuries, Halsted compared the survival experience of women who did or did not have surgery.[17] While such claims would be skeptically received today because of selection biases, uncertain pathological diagnoses, and unsubstantiated historical comparisons, many of Halsted's contemporaries accepted these survival data at face value and attributed the prolonged survival of some of their own patients to complete operations. At the same time, some contemporaries as well as observers in earlier eras, such as Agnew, were well aware of the limitations of these comparisons.

Halsted's associate Joseph Bloodgood, not surprisingly, introduced his recollection of Halsted's breast surgery with a photograph of the (then) "oldest living patient [82, had surgery 38 years earlier] operated upon by Dr. Halsted for cancer in the breast" both to illustrate the successful operative technique (the "perfect" use of the arm and the absence of pectoral muscles) and the apparent effectiveness of surgery given the woman's advanced age.[18] Surgeons in earlier periods had frequently observed the long survival of some patients with breast cancer, and sometimes claimed that surgery as then practiced was responsible. But as we have seen, their predominant view was that cancer surgery produced few cures and the idiosyncrasy of cancer in the breast, including that some women lived with breast cancer for decades or more, was well accepted.

THE STATUS OF EXTENSIVE CANCER SURGERY AS PRESTIGIOUS, SCIENtific, and more effective was also buoyed by the seriousness of its task – the cure of cancer – relative to the goals of other surgical procedures promoted in this era. In contrast to the growing surgical and popular enthusiasm for hysterectomies, tonsillectomies, oophorectomies, and so forth, cancer surgery was distinguished by its goal of evading a painful and certain death. "What consistency, I ask," surgeon W. L. Rodman rhetorically questioned in 1908, "is there in advising a woman with a small ovarian cyst or myoma of the uterus – neither of which has a tendency per se to shorten, much less to terminate, life – to travel hundreds of miles so that the specialist may do a laparotomy, and the same day, perhaps, admonish her sister or friend with a mammary tumor that she must calmly and resignedly await a lingering, painful and loathsome death, rather than submit to a less dangerous operation curing permanently all benign growths and at least one-third of the malignant ones?"[19]

Surgeons believed so strongly in the efficacy of radical cancer surgery that it was sometimes done on women who were known to have newly described benign conditions that were classified and understood as having some increased probability of later developing into cancer. In 1923, Rodman argued that "20% of chronic mastitis will unquestionably become cancer. But if we must make a mistake and, being human, we will make them, I prefer doing a radical operation and leaving only a scar, thus doing too much rather than too little and having the patient die a hopeless cancer death."[20] Giving the label "chronic mastitis" to a noncancerous breast condition and offering a precise, quantitative probability of this entity turning into breast cancer lowered the threshold for performing extensive operations and increased their use – a pattern that would be repeated throughout the twentieth century.

The technical intricacies of the more extensive operation also buoyed its status. Harvey Cushing, one of Halsted's early trainees who would later become a leading American neurosurgeon, recalled his surprise when first experiencing Halsted's more intricate approach to breast surgery. In Boston, where Cushing had trained earlier, "amputation of the breast was usually accomplished in 19 minutes flat." So when a patient from Cushing's ward at Hopkins was away in the operating room for over 4 hours (typical for Halsted's extensive operation), Cushing assumed something dreadful had happened and prepared to treat the patient for shock. "To his [Cushing's] amazement, when the patient arrived after her four hour ordeal, her pulse was 80 and she was not in shock at all."[21]

A Disease for the Complete Operation – Halsted's Breast Cancer

Halsted's writings on cancer in the breast were remarkably different from those of his immediate American predecessors such as Parker or Agnew. Halsted almost never noted hereditary taint, predisposing factors (such as chronic irritations or trauma), or other individual characteristics in his published clinical descriptions nor in his correspondence with patients and other doctors. Halsted did not engage in etiological speculation nor was he a participant in the early-twentieth-century public health and

education campaigns that focused on early patient recognition of dangerous cancer signs. While Halsted acknowledged individual variation and
the importance of finding the causes of cancer, he acted as if a rational,
scientific understanding of cancer's etiology was not possible in his era or
at least not germane to the surgeon's task. Although the titles of Halsted's
major papers continue to refer to "cancer of the breast," he frequently
referred to the disease as "mammary cancer" in their texts. This usage
emphasized that the disease was not so much a site for a more generalized
cancerous process, but was autonomous and had its own unique clinical
and pathological identity. For Halsted and others, "mammary cancer" or
the increasingly used "breast cancer" was a specific, ontological category
that demanded a uniform clinical response.

Halsted was a chief exponent of the late-nineteenth-century synthesis
that cancer spread in an orderly, slow, and localized manner, contigu-
ous with its site of origin, along physical planes that separated tissues.
Unlike Agnew, Paget, and others, he put little emphasis on metastatic
spread via the lymphatic and blood systems. Halsted approvingly cited
the ideas of British surgeon W. Sampson Handley (1872–1962) who
had dismissed the idea that cancer spread by metastasis, which Handley
defined as cancer's random spread to distant sites via the blood system.[22]
"We believed with Handley," Halsted wrote in 1907, "that cancer of the
breast in spreading centrifugally preserves in the main continuity with
the original growth, and before involving the viscera may become widely
diffused along surface planes."[23] In his 1907 surgical case series, Halsted
reproduced Handley's figures, which showed the spread of breast cancer
in the body. These figures depicted how breast cancer spared the distal
extremities and were offered as evidence that cancer spread in very specific, nonrandom, ways. If cancer appeared in some organs and places
and not others, the argument went, then it did not spread willy-nilly via
the blood system.[24] But despite the assertion of agreement with Handley,
Halsted's qualification "in the main" as well as his acknowledgment that
routes to the viscera were another matter makes clear that Halsted did
not reject the reality of blood-borne, less-than-orderly metastasis so much
as sought to de-emphasize it.

Halsted's commitment to cancer's localized spread led him to posit
pathways of direct extension which seem fanciful in retrospect and
extreme in their surgical implications. Halsted wrote in 1907 that breast
cancer might very well travel by direct extension to the humerus, so

that "amputation of the shoulder joint plus a proper removal of the soft parts might eradicate the disease.... So, too, it is conceivable that ultimately, when our knowledge of the lymphatics traversed in cases of femur involvement becomes sufficiently exact, amputation at the hip joint may seem indicated."[25]

According to Halsted's and Handley's theory of cancer spread, early and extensive surgery might catch cancer before it spread too distally and in too many directions. But surgeons such as Halsted and Handley at the same time had to accommodate a set of observations about cancer that potentially undermined a strictly localized conception of its spread. For example, clinicians had long observed that cancer spread to internal organs and other distant sites in some women who had only limited local disease.[26] In other cases, women who had no clinical or pathological spread of cancer at the time of surgery would soon succumb to cancer. Part of this accommodation, which in Halsted's case was more evident in his communication with individual patients than in his scientific writings, was the idea that breast cancer was in effect two diseases, localized and metastatic cancer. Halsted recognized that complete operations were ineffective against the latter and thus bracketed off and largely ignored metastatic disease in his rationale for the complete operation. Most often – in publications and in his dealings with patients – he was silent or even evasive on the subject.

By pushing metastasis to the margins of his clinical gaze, Halsted defined breast cancer as the right disease for the complete operation. Breast cancer's local destructiveness was understood as having an independent life from cancer's potential for metastatic devastation. "The efficiency of an operation is measured truer in terms of local recurrence than of ultimate cure," Halsted wrote in 1899. "For some lives are rescued only by repeated operations for local recurrence, and others, free from local recurrence, are lost from internal metastases."[27] By positing the distinct and separate clinical course of local disease and metastatic disease, Halsted rationalized his emphasis on measuring the success of the complete operation by the absence of local recurrences rather than saving his patients' lives.[28]

In Halsted's view, preventing local recurrences was thus the best, if limited, measure of cancer surgery's effectiveness.[29] As a corollary, surgeons should not be held *responsible* for the spread of metastases that ultimately would account for fatalities from breast cancer. "When operating for cancer of the breast, we cannot be responsible for undiscoverable metastases in the skin," he asserted. Halsted's many case reports in his early papers did not hide this restricted (and, from the patient's standpoint, myopic) definition of success. Like the early nineteenth-century testaments of the efficacy of compression therapy, many of Halsted's "successes" are patients who succumbed to cancer but did so without having local recurrences. In one case, Halsted reported that a 60-year-old woman with evident axillary disease at the time of the complete operation "died in two years and seven months of internal metastasis. Letter from friends does not mention local return."[30]

Halsted was so intent on proving his operation a success that a letter from his patients' friends that did not mention local return was sufficient for him to categorize the case as having no recurrence of local disease. Halsted's determination to adhere to this standard of success was so strong that in many instances he accompanied a condolence note with a query about whether the loved one or patient died with or without such local recurrence. It is unclear how these queries were received by their recipients, but many seem tactless in retrospect.

It is striking that Halsted, unlike surgeons before him (such as Parker), almost never turned away patients as having disease too advanced for surgery. According to the logic of the complete operation, even terminal patients might benefit from surgery because they would suffer less from the recurrence of local disease. While Halsted did not turn away patients as inoperable, he did report in his 1907 paper that he carried out limited surgery on 65 women for what he called "moral purposes." Having promoted surgery as efficacious, Halsted may have felt the need to at least do limited surgery to preserve hope. These cases were excluded from survival statistics because the complete operation was not performed.

Halsted's 1907 paper was the one place where he reported cure rates in addition to recurrence statistics; indeed he highlighted them in the paper's title, "The results of radical operations for the cure of carcinoma of the breast." The oft-quoted major result was that of the 64 women thought to be without "glandular involvement," 45 were "tabulated as cured," by which Halsted meant they had survived for more than 3 years after surgery.[31] Despite the high cure rate for women without axillary involvement, Halsted was careful to stress that curing patients was not the sole or even the main goal of surgery.[32] "It is interesting to note how late the metastasis occurred in these cases with undetected axillary involvement"; Halsted wrote in this paper, "another argument for wide operating."[33] For Halsted, preventing local recurrence or delaying metastasis was a compelling rationale for surgery, even for the great majority of patients who could not be cured by the surgery. In his other papers and in his dealings with patients and colleagues throughout his career, Halsted did not explicitly invoke the curative goal of the complete operation.

One reason for Halsted's reluctance to tout cancer cures from surgery was that only a small proportion of women who presented to him had prognostic signs that predicted a possible surgical cure. Halsted did *not* want to conclude that the complete operation be reserved for this small minority of patients.

Halsted had tailored a breast cancer that was the effective complement to the new operation – a specific disease whose potential for local extension and destruction was placed in the foreground while its metastatic mischief was bracketed and largely ignored. Success was defined as what the complete operation could possibly accomplish (dramatically reduced local recurrences), rather than the survival or cure that patients desperately hoped for and surgeons wished they could deliver. In future years, the gap between Halsted's and others' use of ambivalent definitions of success and the expectations of patients and other physicians would become increasingly problematic, widening the divide between the perceived success of medical and public health interventions and their impact on breast cancer's deadliness.

Making Breast Cancer the Surgeon's Diagnosis and Disease

Halsted vigorously objected to any prior or concurrent exploratory incision for diagnosis. He feared that cutting into the cancerous tissue could cause cancer cells to spread throughout the body, just as some older surgical practices had exposed the blood system to germs.[34] Throughout his career, Halsted had worked to reduce surgical risk of infection. He had changed the scope and techniques of different operations to eliminate "dead space" in which germs might multiply.[35] His vigilance about practices that might increase the danger of cancer "infection" was consistent with and an extension of this work, as well as reflecting the seriousness of the surgeon's responsibility to adhere to these effective principles and practices. "I believe that we should never cut through cancerous tissues," Halsted preached, leaving little room for deviation. "The division of one lymphatic vessel and the liberation of one cell may be enough to start a new cancer."[36]

In addition to seeing biopsy as a dangerous operative practice, Halsted did not believe that microscopic examination of tumors was the right way to diagnose cancer. While cancer was evidently a disease of disordered cells and tissues, Halsted emphasized that cancer should be diagnosed by the surgeon based on what he saw and felt in the examining and operating rooms. Cancer was a macroscopic disease – and the diagnostic property of the surgeon rather than the pathologist.

Halsted's belief that the surgeon's macroscopic diagnosis was superior to the pathologist's microscopic one was more than a reassertion of nineteenth-century suspicion of pathological inaccuracy; it was also integral to Halsted's vision of cancer as a surgical disease and surgery as a scientific practice. He understood that surgical diagnosis was extremely difficult and required knowledge of pathology as well as lots of clinical and operating experience. "The naked eye diagnosis of the surgeon should count for nothing unless he is a sound pathologist and the macroscopic findings are specifically detailed," Halsted acknowledged.[37] William Welch, Halsted's contemporary and Hopkins pathologist, recalled that in cases where the pathologist and a surgeon of Halsted's caliber disagreed about the cancer diagnosis, "the experienced surgeons were always right."[38]

As discussed earlier, pathologists' mistakes in cancer diagnosis were part of the surgeon's stock in trade throughout the nineteenth century. Many of Halsted's twentieth-century surgical correspondents similarly characterized pathology as a false siren, luring them from trusting their own clinical judgment, leading to dangerous repeat surgeries and worse outcomes for patients. H. B. Walter wrote Halsted about "a very worthy young woman under my care has had a rapid growth of the breast. I at once removed it – our pathologist reported it as negative. It recurred at once. I did a larger operation, and insisted that it was malignant. Then I was told it was."[39] Another surgeon wrote Halsted in 1908 about a woman whose small tumor was incorrectly diagnosed by pathologists: "I removed it, but seeing it was not a lipoma sent it to another pathologist, who pronounced it probably an adenoma. . . . Upon seeing the breast the real nature of the growth was apparent, and I advised her to put herself under your treatment at once."[40]

Halsted believed that surgeons were better at cancer diagnosis than pathologists because of their intimate knowledge of physical examination and the clinical course of cancer. "There is a gap between the surgeon and the pathologist which can be filled only by the surgeon," Halsted wrote in 1898. "The pathologist seldom has the opportunity to see the diseased conditions as the surgeon sees them. A tumour on a plate and a tumour in the breast of a patient, how different! Its blood, its colour, its form, its freshness, its consistency are more or less lost when the tumour has been removed."[41] While Halsted posited an almost mystical quality to the surgeon's familiarity with cancer, structural factors such as the poor quality and limited availability of pathologists and their technologies in many hospitals were also important arguments for making the surgeon responsible for cancer diagnosis. Halsted also believed that surgeons should be in charge of cancer diagnosis for moral reasons. Surgeons, not pathologists, were ultimately responsible for their patients' surgical outcomes.

Bloodgood recalled that Halsted "was not as interested in the immediate observations of microscopic pathology, as up until 1915 it was of no particular value in the operating room, and was just as useful to him in the form of a report."[42] In general, Halsted felt that the pathological classification of breast cancers had "not been very successful" and "for the physician, as well as the layman, a cancer of the breast is a cancer of the breast."[43] Halsted ridiculed contemporary pathologists' efforts to give more and more microscopic detail divorced from the clinical perspective. "I have read long and careful descriptions of the minute appearances of tumors which might be interpreted to mean almost anything," Halsted wrote. "If drawings were to be made by several individuals based on some of these descriptions, I doubt if any two of them would depict the same thing."[44]

Halsted's belief in the surgeon as supreme cancer diagnostician led him to use a system of cancer classification that was largely based on what he observed at preoperative examination, during surgery, and by gross dissection and examination of tumors immediately after excision. Halsted's 1907 surgical case series contained 210 cases, 147 of which were classified as a type of scirrhus carcinoma (by then an almost anachronistic term for hard rather than ulcerating tumors) based on macroscopic features.[45]

Many surgeons who referred their patients to Halsted assumed that he relied on exploratory surgery and pathology to determine if their patients really had cancer. In one typical case, Halsted offered only a dismissive silence to the queries of a general practitioner who requested that his patient undergo an exploratory incision prior to considering the complete operation. In 1907, Dr. William Ely, a Rochester physician, referred a woman with an enlarged breast to Halsted, having told the patient's husband, Dr. Roe, "that you [Halsted] could begin the operation for the removal of the indurated mass, and could determine its nature so speedily as to decide at once whether it would be necessary to amputate the breast."[46] Despite Dr. Ely's plea for an interoperative or preoperative diagnosis, Halsted made the clinical diagnosis of cancer and performed a complete operation in one step without other pathological determination. After the operation Dr. Ely wrote Halsted that he "regretted very much that the necessity for the removal of her breast was so apparent. When the examination of the specimen has been completed, please let me hear again about the final diagnosis of the trouble."[47] Dr. Ely did not understand Halsted's modus operandi. The gold standard for cancer diagnosis was the surgeon's clinical judgment – there would be no "final diagnosis" from the pathologist's microscopic examination.

While Halsted acknowledged that macroscopic diagnosis of cancer was often extremely difficult, he did not seem to worry that his standards were too high for others. It is not clear how much of American surgery outside Halsted and his circle upheld the principle of surgeons' preeminence in cancer diagnosis and definition, but it was far from being the contemporary norm.

In 1916, Dr. Biggs, a Crescent City, Florida, surgeon, wrote Halsted about a case that exemplified the problematic state of the clinical diagnosis of breast cancer among less than elite surgeons. Biggs wanted advice and help in the diagnosis and treatment of a 36-year-old female patient, Mrs. Crumb.[48] Crumb had come to Biggs 2 years earlier with a breast tumor. Biggs removed the tumor, which he believed was benign for a number of reasons, especially that Crumb told him that it had been "in the same spot and of the same size for six or seven years." Biggs had kept the tumor in alcohol but had never sent it for pathological examination, in part because Crumb had told Biggs that she "did not see any necessity."

Crumb had recently returned with a new "glandular enlargement" in the same breast. Biggs sent the specimen from 2 years earlier to a New York Skin and Cancer Hospital pathologist, who reported by telegram that the tumor was a scirrhus carcinoma.[49] Biggs then removed the new growth, and sent it to New York and soon received news that it too, unsurprisingly, was cancerous. Biggs was now sending Crumb to Halsted for more extensive surgery.[50] Halsted agreed to take care of Crumb but feared "from what you tell me that the disease must already be generally disseminated, but possibly a local cure can be obtained."[51] Halsted was probably especially pessimistic about cure because Crumb had lived with cancer for at least 6 years and because her two previous surgeries put her at added danger.

Biggs' letter to Halsted evokes the complexity of cancer diagnosis and how concerns about responsibility and competence cast long shadows on surgeons who were caught between the limitations of their own training, knowledge, and resources and the high expectations of the "Halstedian" ideal. Biggs worked far away from the university-affiliated surgeons who were promoting new techniques and knowledge. It was one thing for Halsted to pontificate on the centrality of surgical diagnostic acumen, but a general surgeon from Crescent City, Florida, did not necessarily have enough clinical skill, experience, and knowledge to suspect that an innocent seeming tumor that had not grown for 6 or 7 years in a 34-year-old woman was cancerous. Biggs also did not have access to either local pathological laboratories or clinical expertise in gross or microscopic diagnosis of cancer.

Biggs' suggestion that he did not initially send Crumb's tumor to a pathologist because she had not requested it seems like a graceless attempt to shift responsibility for botched diagnosis onto someone besides himself. Such shifts were part of an ineluctable slide from surgical and medical guilt and responsibility to patient responsibility, as evidenced by Biggs' later telling Crumb "not to delay any longer" and consult Halsted, as if she were in some way responsible for the previous delay in diagnosis and treatment.[52]

Crumb had the complete operation at Hopkins, immediately after which Halsted and colleagues cut into the excised breast and "were quite sure that we found a spot in the old scar which was either carcinoma or a spot over-rich in parenchyma."[53] This judgment was not contradicted by Bloodgood's later inability to find any evidence of cancer on microscopic, pathological examination of Crumb's tumor after the operation. In Crumb's case and almost all others, microscopic pathology remained for Halsted a less reliable, post hoc commentary on clinical decision-making.

Many other of Halsted's surgical correspondents were more familiar with Halsted's diagnostic ideals and elite beliefs than Biggs was and frequently voiced criticisms of older ways of diagnosing and treating breast cancer. But structural realities often resulted in their suspension between traditional practices and newer ideals.

In 1900, Dr. J. C. Wysor, the "surgeon in charge" of the Chesapeake and Ohio Hospital in Clifton Forge, Virginia, wrote a letter to Halsted that was accompanied by "a section of mammary gland and also some lymphatics from axilla of my brother's wife." Wysor told the sad story of his sister-in-law's nearly 2-year saga. After she had noted a breast hardness while nursing her youngest child, she was treated with topical treatments (such as a poultice, similar to Susan Emlen's initial treatment a 100 years earlier) and was directed to change her nursing routine.[54] Despite these treatments, Wysor's sister-in-law felt that her breast "was never quite right since that time" but did not consult another physician until over a year later when she noted that her breast seemed larger.

Wysor did not hesitate to operate on his sister-in-law after another physician noted an induration in her breast. His decision to operate was also informed by his knowledge that his sister-in-law's aunt had died of "cancer of breast." Although Wysor "removed breast with glands in axilla" he did not do the complete operation with its en bloc resection of pectoral muscles. Wysor implied that he knew his approach was wanting and wrote Halsted that "I should like very much to run over and see you do this operation *as you do it*." At the same time, both his lack of clinical experience and the absence of reliable, on-site pathological expertise at his hospital, made him wonder if the operation had been justified – that is, had he removed a cancerous or a normal breast? He noted that the removed breast contained "a little hard nodule," which "makes me think that the operation was very justifiable and performed none too soon."[55]

Unlike Halsted and his steadfast self-confidence, Wysor had worried whether his operation was justified. Such doubts about the diagnosis of cancer frequently bedeviled general practitioners and general surgeons who could not reasonably emulate Halsted's skill and self-confidence. The number of women presenting to physicians with breast lumps was rapidly increasing in the early decades of the twentieth century, and this led to an increased demand for surgeons competent in cancer diagnosis and surgery. And with the increasing prestige and rising expectations of what medicine and surgery could deliver, there were more incentives for early-twentieth-century American general surgeons practicing far from University hospitals to take up cancer surgery.

These shifts exacerbated the already untenable tensions in diagnosis and treatment and undoubtedly contributed to the eventual ascendency and diffusion of more objective means of diagnosis such as the microscopic, pathological diagnosis of breast cancer. This process was slow and halting. In 1927, Bloodgood wrote to surgeons and pathologists throughout the United States about their current practice of tissue diagnosis in the operating room and whether and how they used frozen section technology. The replies suggested that tissue diagnosis in the operating room was still rare and that reliable pathological expertise was available only at the leading hospitals.[56]

After Halsted's death, the microscopic diagnosis of cancer became the gold standard even among Halsted's students and colleagues at Johns Hopkins. Bloodgood believed that this shift was largely explained by the different spectrum of disease facing the surgeon and pathologist, since "the enlightened individual, due to modern educational methods, comes under observation in a much earlier stage of the disease." At this earlier stage in which lumps were small, surgeons had more difficulty distinguishing cancerous from benign tumors and became more reliant on the microscope. There were also so many more patients presenting for evaluation.[57] "Cancer has become a microscopic disease," Bloodgood wrote in 1934.[58]

Cancer became a microscopic disease by the 1930s in part due to pathologists retrofitting the frozen section, a technology for fixing, freezing, and cutting tissue that allowed microscopic pathological examination immediately after excision. Frozen section technology had been in sporadic use since the 1890s so its emergence as an intraoperative aide to surgical decision-making in the 1920s was not simply a consequence of technological improvements.[59] In the first decades of the twentieth century, frozen section technology was sporadically used – like most pathological techniques – as a more immediate but still after-the-fact way of evaluating surgical decision-making. Bloodgood recalled that in 1886, when he was a medical student, he had been dining with a prominent pathologist who earlier in the day had been sent a specimen from a complete operation. After dinner, they returned to the laboratory and made a frozen section from the morning's operation that confirmed their earlier, gross impression of cancer. "Frozen sections were not made in the operating room," Bloodgood recalled. Bloodgood related a later incident in which William Welch, prominent Hopkins pathologist and close Halsted colleague, had once examined an operative specimen using frozen section techniques immediately after Halsted had removed a small portion of a tumor that Halsted suspected was benign (which, as we have seen, was a highly unusual procedure for Halsted). Welch rushed to the operating room to tell Halsted not to proceed with the complete operation but Halsted had already made that "correct" determination on his own on gross criteria and without Welch's frozen section diagnosis. The evident moral of this story was that Halsted did not want or need this kind of confirmation.[60]

Neither Halsted nor many of his contemporaries gave serious thought to using frozen sections as they would later be used.[61] The reasons were numerous: intraoperative cancer diagnosis by frozen section was not necessary to distinguish cancer from noncancer given the advanced stage at which cancer was presenting; physicians believed there were blurred boundaries between benign and malignant disease and in any event they generally lacked faith in the reliability of microscopic pathology; surgeons believed that cutting through live tissue might spread cancer through the body; pathologists had no recognized role in clinical decision-making; and few hospitals had the infrastructure to provide pathological expertise and technology.

Halsted ultimately and posthumously lost the battle to make the surgeon the arbiter of the cancer diagnosis based on the look and feel of cancer. Along with the use of the frozen section intraoperatively, a new specialty emerged, surgical pathology, whose practitioners had a definite, if consulting, role in clinical decision-making.[62] Frozen sections and surgical pathology were responses to the surgeon's problem of deciding whether or not to carry out a severe, mutilating operation on the basis of increasingly difficult-to-interpret clinical clues. But despite losing the battle for control over the diagnosis, Halsted's commitment to the surgeon's clinical diagnosis of cancer, disdain for exploratory operations, and low threshold for operation had succeeded in bringing order and standardization to the chaotic and arbitrary decision-making that was evidenced in Parker's and others' practices.

Elephantiasis Chirurgica: Was the Disease or the Operator Responsible?

Along with the rising expectations that the new, extensive surgery worked and the promotion of the surgeon as in charge of cancer diagnosis came a heightened sense of the surgeon's responsibility for clinical decisions and surgical outcomes. In Halsted's case, this led to a lifelong attempt to find causes besides surgery for some of the complications experienced by his patients.

In 1914, in response to Halsted's first anniversary query, which included questions about general health as well as specific ones about arm swelling and mobility, Hilda Martin sent measurements of her arms: her left arm (side of complete operation) measured 11.5 inches in circumference while the right measured 10 inches. She described that a "noticeable restriction in the use of the arm occurs when someone tries to help me from a lower to a higher level by taking my left hand – as in stepping up from a boat. Also, in arranging my hair, my left arm tires easily, and perhaps has to be rested, although I can accomplish the result." When Halsted asked for photographs of the limits of her ability to raise her arms, Mrs. Martin dutifully complied (see Figure 4.2 that shows a mild restriction in her ability to raise her swollen left arm).[63] In a subsequent letter, Mrs. Martin wrote that the "effect" of the swelling was "larger" than the photos indicated and that the swelling was hard. Halsted personally thanked her for the photos, "they help me, I am sure, to improve the operation in which we are so much interested."[64]

Throughout his long surgical career, Halsted both in private correspondence and in published writings disputed the conventional wisdom that the arm swelling and restriction of motion following the complete operation was "an inevitable consequence of the removal of the axillary glands."[65] Halsted's argument was multifaceted. As we saw earlier, arm swelling was a common clinical finding in nineteenth-century patients who presented "late" and did not have surgery (as was the case with Mary Shipley). When the patient did undergo surgery, swelling often began years after the operation and had clinical characteristics that suggested causes other than obstruction from surgery such as the repeated, episodic nature of attacks, redness and warmth, and constitutional disturbances. Halsted also noted that experimental obstruction of axillary lymphatics in dogs did not produce arm swelling.

Halsted's competing conception of what we would now call lymphedema granted only a small potential facilitative role for surgery as an occasional part of a more complex causal chain. Other factors, most notably infection, "played a conspicuous part in the determination of the amount of the swelling and the time of its manifestation." Halsted's evidence for the role of infection was based on clinical observation of the circumstances surrounding bouts of swelling, but in his 1921 paper he

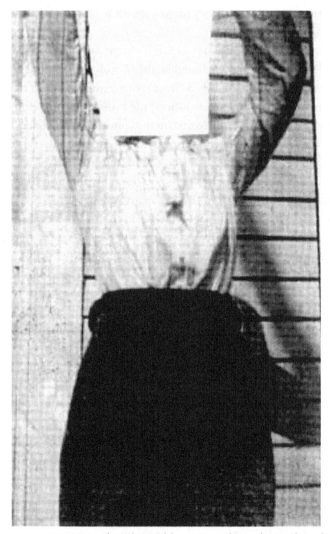

Figure 4.2. Pictures taken by Hilde Martin (pseudonym) and sent to Halsted showing her limited ability to raise her left arm. (Reproduced with permission of The Alan Mason Chesney Medical Archives, the Johns Hopkins Medical Institutions.)

acknowledged that he was not yet prepared to "submit figures" and the "infection may quite conceivably be so mild in degree as to escape the observation even of those intently on the lookout for it." He drew an analogy to the swelling caused by the filaria parasite that caused a tropical disease known as elephantiasis. Trying to make the point and perhaps move conventional wisdom in his direction in one rhetorical stroke, Halsted proposed a new name for the condition that would evoke an infectious etiology, "Elephantiasis chirurgica" (surgical elephantiasis).[66]

Halsted claimed in a 1921 article that "swollen arms of dimensions sufficient to distress or annoy the patient were no longer observed" after he had modified 11 years earlier the way the skin was incised and the wound closed.[67] While lymphedema was ultimately caused by something other than surgery, Halsted believed that changes in operative routine could reduce the chances of it occurring. Halsted also claimed that even prior to this modification in 1910, no patient was "herself sufficiently incommoded by the restriction of movement" to consent to a repeat operation aimed at providing more mobility.[68] These assertions are hard to reconcile, however, with the many examples in Halsted's correspondence of patient complaints and worries about their arm swelling and restricted movements before and after 1910.

Halsted was so passionately committed to the complete operation and so concerned over the possible threat to its acceptance posed by this operative complication that it colored the way he observed, recorded, and published his clinical experience. It is also highly probable, as in Martin's case, that it was easy to dismiss the functional impairments caused by arm swelling because of the deferential style female patients assumed with Halsted and because patient impairments were often depicted as affecting strictly female functions such as being helped out of a boat or "arranging" one's hair. Halsted also minimized side effects of a lifesaving (although more accurately, local recurrence sparing) operation in women who were already past their prime. "Furthermore, these patients are old," Halsted wrote in 1899. "Their average age is nearly 55 years. They are no longer very active members of society. We should, perhaps, sacrifice many lives if we were to consider the disability which might result from removing a little more tissue here and there."[69]

Halsted sincerely believed the claims he made about the dramatic improvements in arm swelling following changes in his operative practice in 1910. He sounded the same notes in his correspondence with patients and colleagues as he did in print. Halsted's extraordinary efforts to get data on arm complications in his follow-up studies were similarly not actions of someone trying to hide bad results. They were an effort to identify and prove an infectious or other nonoperative etiology for lymphedema.

In a letter to prominent Philadelphian surgeon John B. Deaver in 1922, Halsted recalled that prior to his "present style of operating, which to my surprise practically eliminated the swollen arms, it did not occur to me that surgeons were responsible for this distressing complication." Given that so many other doctors had deduced a connection between breast amputations and arm swelling, statements like this suggest some measure of denial on Halsted's part. In the same letter, Halsted went on to say he had received a letter from Sir Almroth Wright "which happily strengthens me in the belief that infection is responsible. Our experimental work briefly referred to in my paper seems to indicate that the removal of the axillary contents does not alone suffice to produce the swelling."[70]

While current wisdom and many of Halsted's contemporaries' common sense more directly implicated surgical practice as the "cause" of arm complications, Halsted supported his more complex infectious/multifactorial theory with a series of clinical observations and arguments by analogy to other clinical entities. Nevertheless, it is clear that Halsted's passionate commitment (evidenced in his publications and years of clinical research) to promoting a more complicated, multifactorial view of arm complications in which the complete operation was a bit player was motivated by his desire to remove a threat to the widespread acceptance of the radical operation. This is not only a plausible reconstruction of the way Halsted conducted his follow-up studies and his seeming blind-sightedness to contrary data. Halsted also acknowledged this motivation in print, citing with evident disapproval the links others had made between arm swelling after extensive cancer surgery and calls to restrict the extent of the operation.[71]

Halsted's fixation on the problem of arm complications colored a great deal of his correspondence with other doctors and patients. His passionate interest in discovering and promoting an infectious etiology for his patients' arm swelling led him frequently to query patients about the timing of infectious illnesses and arm swelling. He not only persistently asked questions about the character and circumstances surrounding arm swelling but relentlessly focused on this concern to the exclusion of more serious issues or those of greater concern to patients and colleagues.[72]

Although Halsted worked hard to avoid blaming arm swelling on his "complete operation," he harshly judged the arm swelling in *other* surgeons' patients to be due to mechanical obstruction and infection caused by their unnecessary mucking about in the axilla. "There may be a little swelling but if so this might, I think, be attributed to the operation of the Jersey City surgeon, whose second performance was followed by very great swelling of the arm."[73]

Arm complications following surgery were Halsted's Achilles heel, more so than mortality from cancer, because Halsted believed he was personally responsible in a way that he was not for the late effects of the cancer itself on the body. As we shall see in later chapters, the avoidance and management of responsibility for cancer, often more than the avoidance of cancer itself, would become one of the most powerful influences on cancer prevention and treatment throughout the twentieth century.[74]

Heightened Responsibility in Surgical Practice

The rise and acceptance of the "complete operation" was both a consequence of, and contributed to, a heightened responsibility for clinical decisions and surgical outcomes. One aspect was higher expectations of proper surgical conduct and procedure. Another was less tolerance of practice diversity. In one sense, this heightened responsibility was a logical consequence of the increased status and extensiveness of cancer surgery. To the degree that surgeons and patients increasingly believed that new surgical procedures were effective, there was more at stake in distinguishing good from bad surgical practices. As the amount and scope of cancer surgery greatly expanded, surgeons also felt increasingly responsible for evaluating and justifying the greater amount of surgical morbidity. And as a largely unregulated profession with many diverse groups competing in the marketplace, early-twentieth-century surgeons often engaged in rhetorical battles with one another, which focused on correct practice, blame, and responsibility.

This heightened responsibility was not confined to cancer and cancer surgery. Some early-twentieth-century American surgeons, for example, agitated for systems to evaluate operative "end results" while others waged highly visible campaigns that highlighted the high prevalence of diagnostic error (as compared to autopsy) in clinical practice.[75] But the increasing use and extensiveness of cancer surgery, as well as cancer's devastating impact on individuals, made it an intense focus of this crusade.

One specific way Halsted's and others' surgical innovations contributed to this intensity was by increasing the gap between idealized and routine surgical practice. Halsted's efforts to make difficult-to-achieve competencies, such as the diagnosis of cancer on gross anatomical grounds, the norms for surgical practice, led to problems for surgeons who could not meet these high standards. There was little awareness of the distinction made by today's policy makers between the efficacy of practices and their benefit under ideal conditions, and their effectiveness and benefit under the conditions in which they were actually likely to be performed. Halsted and other elite practitioners neither acknowledged nor explicitly accommodated the paradox of promoting difficult-to-achieve practices as the desired norms for surgical behavior. The ensuing tensions were inevitable.[76]

The very words most often used to describe extensive breast amputations, *the complete operation*, implied that operations less extensive were by definition "incomplete" and wanting. Similarly, the other common term *radical* not only acknowledged the extensive mutilation but connoted, via its political meaning, a zealotry and "leave no prisoners" extremism toward cancer.[77] Bloodgood made these assumptions explicit in 1904 when he wrote, "In regards to tumors...lynch law is by far the better procedure than 'due process.'" As well as summary justice, cancer's evil nature required the surgeon's constant vigilance. "To be able to assert with any degree of positiveness that the axilla and neck are negative involves *infinite toil*," Halsted wrote in 1907.[78]

When Bloodgood recalled that Halsted did not "risk" limited operations, he was capturing some of the moralistic force behind the precepts about carrying out complete operations.[79] In those rare times when Halsted decided against operating because he thought that a breast tumor was benign on the basis of physical examination, Halsted remarked on the "heavy responsibility" of not operating because of the remote possibility of cancer. He recalled that early in his career he operated "because I did not dare do otherwise." While he dared otherwise more frequently with the passage of time and greater experience, Halsted noted that those (untreated) cases "still keep me apprehensive." "Although not uneasy," Halsted wrote in 1915 to the husband of a patient whom he offered to visit at home, "I shall be apprehensive until I can assure myself that Mrs. B. is not mistaken in the conviction that her swelling is diminishing."[80]

In accepting the heightened responsibility of the cancer diagnosis and commitment to extensive surgery, surgeons were also establishing their increased authority in the medical and larger social worlds, reinforced and recapitulated by the asymmetrical relationship between male surgeon and female cancer patient. At the same time, surgeons remained dependent on women to recognize breast problems and seek medical attention. "As I read over my records again and again, the remarkable fact stands out that we have rarely palpated a distinct lump which the patient had not felt," Bloodgood noted in 1923, remarking on the surgeon's ultimate dependence on the patient to initiate cancer diagnosis and treatment.[81]

Although this heightened responsibility pervaded almost every aspect of elite surgical practice surrounding cancer, Halsted did not in his dealings with patients, letters to other physicians, or published writings about cancer bemoan or blame patients who had come to his attention too late. He certainly believed, like most physicians concerned with cancer in the early twentieth century, that patients should not delay medical care for suspicious cancer signs, but he was steadfast in seeing the physician's role as relieving, where possible, the guilt and anxieties of patients. It also helped that Halsted understood that for the great majority of breast cancer patients, coming to medical attention sooner from the point at which they recognized a lump would not have altered the disease's deadliness.

"It's Not Entirely My Fault": A Case Study of Surgical Responsibility for Diagnosis and Management

While most of Halsted's referring surgeons believed in the efficacy of the extensive and technically complex complete operation, they often practiced far away from elite medical institutions like Hopkins and under very different conditions. They had less direct experience with breast cancer and the complete operation and had less confidence that they practiced the right way. Many surgeons were suspended between belief in the promise of new surgical management and older styles of managing women with breast lumps. This suspension only increased the concern with blame and responsibility, especially when patients fared poorly.

A few letters from a Kansas City surgeon, Dr. W. W. Duke, to Halsted about his patient, Mrs. J. L. Buxton, illustrate the nature and implications of the gap between old and new surgical practices and ideals. Buxton first consulted Duke in August 1912, was definitively diagnosed and operated on in November, and died in April 1913. This rapid course exacerbated

Duke's awkward attempts to apportion blame and guilt among himself, Buxton, and her disease.

Duke wrote Halsted that Buxton had first consulted him "on account of pain in her left breast. At the time, there was no lump to be felt where the cancer is at present." Duke did see some redness and felt a small moveable mass in her breast, which he believed was a subpectoral lymph gland. "For want of a better diagnosis, I called it Neuritis and told her to return in a month for further examination."

Buxton returned 3 months later with a large mass with the overlying skin dimpled – sure signs of cancer. Duke wrote to Halsted that he "told her husband that it was Carcinoma but said I hoped it would prove Tuberculosis or an infection of some kind." Duke wanted to send Buxton to Baltimore and asked if Halsted could do an exploratory incision before the complete operation, unless he felt "absolutely convinced it is Carcinoma." While Duke's request for an exploratory incision was consistent with his equivocation to Buxton's husband that he "hoped it would prove Tuberculosis," it went against Halsted's teachings and was at odds with Duke's straightforward description of the process as cancer elsewhere in the letter. After observing that Buxton had "a tender cord reaching from the tumor mass to the axilla," Duke wrote more straightforwardly about his fears for Buxton and his own responsibility for her situation: "This makes me fear that the prognosis is rather bad, but hope you will be able to clean it all out. I feel badly for having let a Carcinoma progress so far, but console myself by thinking it was not entirely my fault."[82]

With some medical hindsight, it seems highly probable that Duke failed to notice or appreciate the malignant potential of the "small moveable mass" in Buxton's breast at the initial visit. Duke's awareness of his mistake and perhaps his regret over his dismissive attitude revealed in the "neuritis" diagnosis colored his retelling of events and his half admission and half deflection of responsibility, "it's not entirely my fault" (responsibility for the delayed diagnosis could presumably be shared with Buxton, as it was her fault for returning in 3 months rather than 1). The public education campaign to get women to recognize cancer warning signs and to seek care without delay that was just beginning in these years would only exacerbate physicians' concerns about the delayed diagnosis from initially attributing a patient's complaint to a functional disorder.

A note scribbled on Duke's first letter indicated that Halsted performed a complete operation on November 30, 1912. In February 1913, Duke wrote with evident concern about a recent visit from Buxton, now back in Kansas City, during which Duke palpated some hard glands in her neck. In this letter, Duke communicated both a grim assessment of probable cancer and hope for a nonmalignant explanation. "I have been trying to attribute this condition so far to a chronic pharyngitis from which she has been suffering, but cannot help fearing that it is a metastatic condition starting in the neck." Duke wondered if removing these glands would prolong Buxton's life. "I hate to send the patient back again [to Baltimore] for she is as nervous as she can be about the condition now, but will gladly do so if you advise it."[83] As in the initial visit, Duke actively worked to place Buxton's signs and symptoms in a functional, noncancer framework even as his suspicions of cancer recurrence grew.[84] The difficult balancing act of hope and despair was sometimes as much as an intrapsychic negotiation for physicians as one between physician and patient, both exacerbated by clinical uncertainty and insecurity.

Only 11 days later, Duke wrote Halsted that "everything seems to be going pretty well" and again struggled to place Buxton's signs and symptoms in a stereotyped, neurotic (female) sick role. "She is troubled some with cough and pain in the chest, but I am inclined to believe that it is more of a neurotic affair than metastatic carcinoma." Similarly, Duke noted some small white areas over the scar but was not sure if they were "metastatic carcinoma" or a "hair follicle or sebaceous gland developing." He concluded the letter asking, "if it would be a good idea to have them treated first with an x-ray as a precautionary measure."[85] Buxton's proposed "precautionary" x-ray treatments were made possible by recent technological innovations. X-ray treatments, as we will see in Chapter 5, were one of a few legitimate treatments for cancer recurrence after complete operations. Such postsurgical treatments were partly a response to greater physician responsibility for the course of the disease after surgery.

Duke wrote Halsted again on March 6, 1913, "I am afraid that the outlook in Mrs. Buxton's case is at present pretty bad."[86] Duke's avoidance of the cancer diagnosis had also made treatment difficult (see discussion on truthful diagnosis in the next chapter). "I hate to let her know that there is a recurrence and I am afraid if we used the cautery she would be sure of it. At present, she is unable to come downtown and I suppose that even the x-ray treatment will have to be given up and the case regarded as hopeless." Duke wrote Halsted that he was "sorry the case had advanced so far before it got into your hands. It seems to have made all of your elegant work of little avail." ("Elegant work" is also in striking contrast to Duke's earlier hope that Halsted will be able to "clean it all out," which while literally true and descriptive, had winked at the crude mechanical nature of the complete operation.) "I have learned a good lesson myself and will hereafter advise exploratory incision if there is a faintest suggestion of cancer," Duke concluded in this letter, drawing a lesson to do exploratory incisions that Halsted vigorously opposed.[87] At the same time, the lesson Duke drew hinted at a vigilance for increased surveillance and early surgery whose momentum would build in coming decades, rooted in the increased sense of responsibility experienced by doctors and patients.

Duke's last letter to Halsted, dated April 16, 1913, related news of Buxton's death on April 11. Duke had performed an autopsy and was able to give Halsted a precise anatomical description of her cancer's extension. Buxton's autopsy showed "internal metastasis of lung, pleura, spine, and ribs. Hydrothorax and pulmonary oedema were the immediate causes of death. She had a few small local recurrences in the scar and also a small metastatic growth in the right breast."[88] Buxton's disease had defeated Halsted in his own terms of success, preventing local recurrence, while its extensiveness might have mitigated – but did not – Duke's burden of guilt for initial misdiagnosis and delay. Duke's style of personalized, functional diagnosis and watchful waiting were a poor fit with the ascending belief in the efficacy of extensive cancer surgery done in a uniform way without delay.

FIVE

Living at Risk

"Living With Such a Terrible Threat Hanging Over Her Head"

Halsted's patient Elizabeth Smith was diagnosed with breast cancer in 1914 and died in 1921. Her experience was in many ways closer to that of an early–twenty-first-century breast cancer patient than to Mary Cope's less than three decades earlier. Smith and her husband General John Watts Smith first consulted Halsted in the fall of 1914. Smith was 40 years old at the time. It is not clear from the correspondence how Smith, who lived with her husband, a former general in the New Jersey National Guard, on a mountaintop outside of Charlottesville, Virginia, came to consult Halsted but many women of means with breast lumps from throughout the eastern half of the United States were referred to him or, less commonly, sought him out on their own. We do know that she discovered a lump in her right breast in June 1914 and that the lump was at first misdiagnosed as a benign tumor.[1]

The correspondence with Halsted began shortly after Smith underwent the complete operation sometime in November 1914. General Smith first wrote Halsted to inquire about his wife's prognosis. Unlike the home surgery and aftercare provided to Susan Emlen and Mary Cope, Smith's surgery and prolonged recovery occurred at an elite medical institution, Johns Hopkins Hospital, far from home and without the attendance and oversight of General Smith or other family members. General Smith necessarily had to inquire by post because he had not been present during her 6-week stay at the hospital. General Smith described his mental state as the "most disordered uncertainty" and as desperate for information about his wife's life after the "terrible cataclysm," which was her surgery.

General Smith had learned from his wife that the "chances of her cure were only 75 percent, – not the chance of life of a soldier going into battle," and had a difficult time accepting these odds. He was also shocked by the extensiveness of the operation and drew the inference that this signaled a poor prognosis. He asked Halsted whether the operation merely prolonged his wife's life "or whether she is reasonably exempt from further trouble." "What and how much she has learned from you of her condition I do not know," General Smith wrote, "for she is absolutely reticent on the subject."[2] It is not clear how much of General Smith's anguished ignorance was due to the ambiguity of the situation, Halsted's evasiveness about his wife's poor prognosis that was revealed in subsequent letters, the norms of marital communication surrounding mutilating surgery and a feared disease among people of means in this period, or the idiosyncrasies of the Smith marriage.

Halsted was much more explicit about Smith's prognosis in his reply to her husband's queries than he would ever be to Smith herself. Halsted wrote General Smith that although Smith's disease was "quite advanced," he hoped that there would be "no local recurrence." This formulation, which reflected Halsted's view of breast cancer and the goals of surgery but which was almost certainly obscure to patients and their families, allowed Halsted to signal an accurate, and in this case dismal, prognosis while at the same time communicating a tincture of hope. The message's ambiguity depended on the growing gulf between medical and lay knowledge about body and health generally and cancer in particular. Halsted could say "no local recurrence" and the patient and family could think "cure." Halsted knew, however, that patients like Smith, whose disease had spread to the axillary nodes, would almost certainly die of metastatic disease although they would probably not suffer recurrences in the surgical scar, chest wall, or armpit. Since physicians could not perfectly predict developments in any one patient, Halsted further cushioned despair by writing General Smith that "what the ultimate results will be so far as metastases to distant organs we cannot foresee."

Halsted wrote General Smith that he did not tell his wife the nature of her tumor, "but I think she probably knows." It had become routine to avoid explicitly offering the cancer diagnosis to patients, yet Halsted's acknowledgment that Smith probably understood her situation demonstrates that many patients and doctors nevertheless indirectly communicated important and frightening information. One part of this indirect communication was the very circumstances that brought doctors and patients together. Many women could easily infer that such extreme means as the complete operation were being done to prevent or cure something worse, that is, cancer. Whatever Smith could infer from indirect codes or context, Halsted had strong beliefs about what patients should be explicitly told. Halsted wrote General Smith without equivocation that he thought that Smith "should not be told that there is a possibility ultimately of a recurrence of the disease in some other part of the body."[3] Halsted did not want to increase women's fears of cancer spreading in their bodies, especially since he believed that there were no effective interventions against metastatic disease.

General Smith's response acknowledged Halsted's indirectness and its goal of softening a harsh reality. But he persisted in asking for more complete and unhedged information. "Your reply is very satisfactory – satisfactory in the sense that it is frank," General Smith wrote. "Your opinion, however, is stated with such delicacy and tact, that some reading between the lines is necessary to its full understanding." After repeating the details of his wife's disfigurement and its effects on her life, General Smith judged that "her present condition of safety ... more than compensates for her bodily mutilation and the consequent humiliation growing out of it." And revealing the heightened sense of personal danger women and their families experienced, General Smith wrote that "we have still hope left, and for that we must rely in the future. It is hard though to think of such a young and seemingly healthy person as Mrs. Smith living with such a terrible threat hanging over her head."[4]

Enclosing a check to Halsted in a subsequent letter, General Smith rehashed the troubling calculus of the greatest mutilation in exchange for best chances of survival that Fanny Burney and many women since then have articulated. He hoped "that such favorable results will ensue that will more than compensate for all the moral and physical agony through which she has gone." General Smith offered more detail about the emotional and physical consequences of the surgery for his wife, noting that "her moral attitude is still one of depression. She has practically no use of her arm, and there is still one wound unhealed – the one under the arm."[5]

Although surgery had moved into the hospital, much of the after-care remained home-based in this period, especially among Halsted's far-flung clientele. The Smiths had employed a nurse, Mary Thomas, who also corresponded with Halsted about Smith's healing wounds, points of break down, and the local treatments she was applying under Halsted's direction.[6] Almost to the point of obsession, Halsted continuously sought from Thomas, General Smith, and Smith herself details of the physical consequences of arm swelling and motion limitations in order to attribute responsibility to something other than the physical obstruction caused by the complete operation.

Sometime around May 1915, Smith herself began to write Halsted. Her stimulus to begin this correspondence and what would sustain it afterward were her fears of cancer recurrence. While such fears motivated some of the consultations of Susan Emlen and other women in the nineteenth century, Smith appeared to survey her body more intensively and had more faith that recognizing changes would lead to either effective medical interventions or specific reassurances from her doctor. Perhaps her own earlier misdiagnosis and the ensuing wasted time motivated Smith as well. Smith had been "made slightly apprehensive" by something that appeared in the incisional wound, which she thought might be a stitch or something more worrisome. She made a crude drawing (see Figure 5.1) of the location of the problem ("I made (?) this diagram showing the position of scab and slight redness thinking it may give you a better idea, it is *between* the *ribs*") and wanted some "assurance" since the "slightest change in my conditions fills me with alarm."[7] She arranged to come down to Baltimore for another examination at which time Halsted excised the worrisome red swelling. Halsted wrote Smith afterwards that the "little tumor is not of bad nature; it is what we call an infectious granuloma," probably arising from a stitch. He had, he said, already told Mrs. Smith, but he feared that she "was not sufficiently recovered from the gas when I left to recall what I said."[8]

More problems soon ensued. Smith wrote Halsted in August 1915 that she was "a little apprehensive of troubles beginning in my left breast – it is slightly tender and the left arm and shoulder joint are weak – I can find no lump in the breast tissue such as I discovered last June in the right breast, which made known to me first my troubles. Can you reassure me at all as to this being only a false alarm due to slight rheumatism or tell me of some slight tests by which I may make sure of this being a similar trouble or not, of course I being alarmed at the least condition that it is not normal – if it were not for my previous trouble I do not think I would even have noticed these symptoms which do not annoy or inconvenience me."[9]

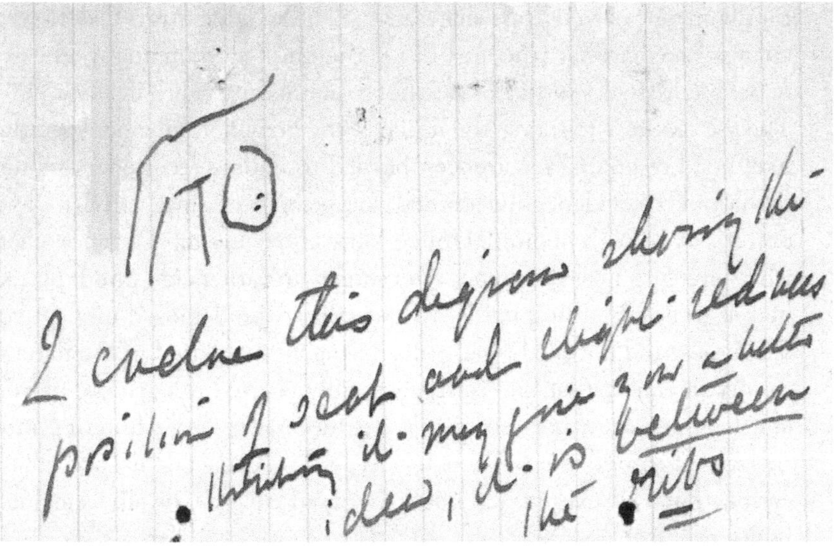

Figure 5.1. Drawing made by Elizabeth Smith (pseudonym) and sent to Halsted showing her worrisome problem in the area of her surgical incision. (Reproduced with permission of The Alan Mason Chesney Medical Archives, the Johns Hopkins Medical Institutions.)

Like so many women after her and qualitatively different from the experiences of women in earlier eras, Smith had entered a lifetime of "little" apprehensions and need for reassurance and "slight tests." She wrote Halsted in September 1915 that she had another red spot in the same place as the "infectious granuloma" which Halsted removed the previous spring.[10] Halsted reassured her by letter that the spot was likely to be benign. In subsequent letters, Smith wrote Halsted that this spot appeared less worrisome and that Halsted could wait until her planned visit to Baltimore later in the fall to observe these changes. She wrote Halsted that she was "perfectly well as far as I can judge, and only stop in Baltimore to see you as a precaution."[11] However well she felt, Smith, like many other twentieth-century women, understood that her ability to detect cancer recurrence was limited, necessitating precautionary visits to physicians.

After being examined in early November of 1915, Halsted presumably believed Smith had recurrent cancer because he referred her to his Hopkins colleague and prominent obstetrician/gynecologist Howard Kelly for radium treatments of her neck and axillary region. Curtis

Burnham, one of Kelly's associates, wrote Halsted that x-rays had showed enlarged mediastinal (the area inside the chest surrounding the heart) nodes but he took "particular care not to alarm Mrs. Smith in any way."[12] The use of x-rays to survey the inside of the body not only increased the likelihood of finding recurrences, but led to finding recurrences sooner than would be evident clinically and gave greater certainty, authority, and objectivity to such findings. Unlike Mary Cope and most other women who suffered cancer recurrence after surgery in earlier eras, Smith placed herself in a web of hospital-based specialists who deployed innovative, dangerous, and untested treatments during a time period in the natural history of cancer that had earlier generally elicited resignation, prayer, and measures aimed at restoring constitutional balance. Entering into this web also often removed whatever vestige of cancer denial and obfuscation that still existed, although the word *cancer* typically remained unuttered.

While Halsted had little hope for curing his patient, Smith took an increasingly more active and visible role in her treatment decisions and negotiations. After requesting additional radium treatments for new spots on her surgical scar, she wrote Halsted presciently in December 1915 that "it looks as though you will never be quite rid of me as a patient."[13] Halsted then helped arrange the additional radium treatments but in a follow-up visit in early May 1916 he suspected that her cancer was not responding to these treatments. The next day Smith wrote Halsted about how her reaction to this bad news "was so disturbing to me that I fear I did not show the proper appreciation and gratitude yesterday," echoing a century of hopelessness and despair upon learning of cancer's advance and the way female patients often felt the need to apologize for such expressions or in some other way make sure that their physicians did not perceive them as ungrateful or questioning of their competence.[14]

With Dr. Kelly's treatments apparently not working, Halsted suggested that Smith consult Dr. James Murphy at the Rockefeller Institute in New York City for a different type of radiation treatment. Murphy (1884–1950) had been developing a theory and a technique for irradiating white blood cells, believing that such irradiated cells would then attack cancer.[15] "I should be very pleased if you care to take her in charge and stimulate her lymphatic system with the x-ray – provided that you would be interested to do so," Halsted wrote Murphy in November 1916.[16]

Thus in response to rising expectations about medical interventions and greater numbers of women aware of recurrences and aided by technological innovations (such as radium and therapeutic x-rays) and improvements in communication and transportation, Halsted and his colleagues had established at this early date technologies, networks, and routines with which they could provide both hope and what would later in the century be called "salvage treatments" for patients whose cancers persisted or recurred after cancer surgery.

During this same period, Halsted described Smith to Murphy as a case "in which there were certainly lymphatic metastasis beyond the field of operation. She does not know the seriousness or the extent of her disease." Yet Smith's initial communication of seriousness to her husband, her vigilance toward her body, her depression after hearing bad news, and her continued partnership in the ever increasing amount, type, and distance of treatments undermined Halsted's claim that she "does not know." As we saw in her earlier apology for communicating her despair at the news that Kelley's treatments were not working, Smith worked hard to present a face to Halsted that was stoical and upbeat. The mutual evasion of the cancer diagnosis and explicit prognosis was a key supporting prop in maintaining this facade. Revealing Smith's and Halsted's collaborative efforts at evasion, Halsted wrote to Murphy in this same introductory letter that Smith was "particularly anxious that no one should know or suspect that she has had an operation performed."[17]

Evasion of patients' diagnosis and miserable prognosis reinforced medical authority and alleviated some patient fears and physician anxiety. It also made for less-than-honest doctor–patient communication and patient self-understanding. Halsted would never deliver the details of Smith's prognosis as explicitly and candidly to Smith as he had done to Murphy and other physician members of his network or even to her husband. Having felt a new if tiny lymph gland high in Smith's neck earlier in the week, Halsted wrote Murphy, "I am quite confident that we have never cured a case of breast carcinoma so advanced as Mrs. Smith's." Halsted also wrote Murphy that he had previously "told General Smith that the chances for ultimate cure were about nil."[18] What he had actually written General Smith 2 years earlier was that Smith's disease was "quite advanced," that he hoped there would be no local recurrence, but "what the ultimate results will be so far as metastases to distant organs we cannot foresee." Halsted nearly always took pains to sustain some hope in his communications with patients and their families.

Smith wrote Halsted that her "experience [with Murphy] was not as unpleasant as I had feared – I had only one treatment which took all together about an hour then three times a week I had blood tests – I did not stay in the hospital and I found Dr. Murphy altogether very agreeable and considerate. He detained me only two weeks – which was a surprise."[19] Some of Smith's surprise over the short treatment and frequent blood tests reflected another contemporary ambiguity – the conflation of treatment and clinical experimentation (which required blood tests). Many of Halsted's patients, for example, seem to have misunderstood Halsted's requests for follow-up information as part of their own personal clinical care rather than as research.[20] Halsted's described Murphy to Smith as "one of the most original and brilliant men in the Rockefeller Institute," terms more appropriate for a researcher than a clinician.[21]

Halsted wrote Murphy in June of 1917, "Mrs. Smith called to see me the other day. It will soon be three years since her operation. She seems to be perfectly well, although I considered her case incurable."[22] To Halsted's surprise but consistent with the idiosyncratic and unpredictable nature of breast cancer, Smith would survive, intact and without further recurrences, for yet another 4 years. But although "perfectly well," Smith lived in a state of heightened concern and fear, continuing to write Halsted for reassurance about possible cancer signs and advice about the need for physician surveillance. In April 1918, she wrote Halsted for advice about a pain in her ear, which although "not unbearable," was "alarming, as I am always apprehensive of the older trouble in new form."[23] Smith later wrote Halsted that the "pain of which I wrote you has entirely disappeared. I presume it was a slight neuralgia so my alarm is relieved."[24] As cancer recurrence had become the focus of their long-standing relationship, Smith's worry about the "older trouble in a new form" rather than "cancer recurrence" seems a thin euphemism serving shared social ends, that is, it reflected a taboo against uttering the term rather than an evasion of the cancer reality.

Three years after her mastectomy, Smith's fears continued to run deep and included fears of cancer contagion. She asked Halsted in July 1917 "another very vital question – will you tell me frankly – what the danger of communication is to my child – in using the same table service, or occupying adjoining rooms – should things be disinfected? This question worries me more than almost anything else – the danger to others."[25] This fear was not shared by Halsted or most contemporary physicians. It was just one element in the growing gap between the lay understanding of cancer and the increasing complex and specific medical understandings of the disease.

From the time of Smith's treatments at the Rockefeller Institute in 1917 until 1920 there were no definite signs of recurrence. What had happened in these intervening years? Had Murphy's treatments worked? In June 1919, Smith expressed to Halsted both her relief and concern at her disengagement with her doctors during this period, writing him that "as far as I can judge I am quite well, perhaps it is not necessary to see you at all in which case I need not to worry you with making an appointment in these difficult times – Dr. Murphy seems to have abandoned me as well – perhaps he has gone to France. I have heard nothing from anyone at the Institute since my last treatment."[26]

But in February 1920 Smith wrote Halsted that she had "just discovered a smaller knob in the gland of my throat and of course it alarms me greatly. Can it be the return of my trouble after *five* years of perfect health?...The knot seems about the size of a pea and is not visible but I am always anticipating trouble – Could it be from any other cause?"[27] Smith soon went to Baltimore and saw Halsted's colleagues Drs. Boggs and Follis. Follis diagnosed several cancerous glands in the right supra-clavicular triangle (an area just below the neck) and slight ptosis (drooping of the eyelid, often due to cancer).[28] Follis told Smith that "an operation will be quite useless."[29]

Unlike the quick demise of Mary Cope in her home or the spiritual acceptance reached for by Susan Emlen at the end of her life, Smith sought and received more treatment at Hopkins. Follis wrote Halsted that Dr. Kelly was giving her more radium.[30] Halsted wrote Follis thanking him for the news of Smith, adding only "it is too sad that there is no hope for her but we have had none from the beginning."[31] If we take Halsted at his word ("no hope ... from the beginning") then his earlier statements offering some hope or at least uncertainty to the Smiths were patently false. But the situation was less cut and dried. Halsted and other physicians had their own personal motivations (e.g., sympathy for patients and reducing the cognitive dissonance surrounding their own therapies and other efforts) and clinical reasons (the uncertainties of the diagnosis, the idiosyncrasies of disease, and the limitations of extant medical knowledge) to have at least partly believed their own early optimistic pronouncements.

Compared to previous eras, Halsted and colleagues seemed to be more darkly pessimistic than their predecessors in their private medical communication while being more evasive in the acts of diagnosis and prognosis. The new, more powerful salvage therapies signaled that there was still some hope and that patients would not be abandoned. In this way, the Hopkins doctors continued to treat Smith with whatever was available and attempted to relieve fear if not inspire hope until she finally succumbed to cancer. The final correspondence was a letter from General Smith to Halsted, whose voice had been missing from the time his wife took charge of her disease a few months after her complete operation. "Dear Doctor, assured of your sympathy, I write to let you know that Elizabeth Smith died on the morning of May 31st last. Apparently she passed away without a struggle, but I fear that in her heroic efforts to spare us all the sorrow she could, she suffered more than we knew. Mrs. Smith had the greatest confidence in you, and I know that she felt that you did for her all that human power was capable of."[32]

Heightened Fears and Greater Demand for Surveillance and Intervention: "Could Anything Be Wrong Without My Knowing It, as Must Have Been the Case Before?"

The 7 years between Smith's surgery and her death were in some ways an historically new stage of disease. Unlike most breast cancer patients in earlier periods, Smith and many other women who underwent complete operations generally lived and died without experiencing recurrences in the remaining breast tissue and the immediate surroundings. Patients had lost some of the usual signposts that signaled disease stability or progression. Breast cancer had in effect been driven "deeper" and further away by extensive surgery, making the cancer experience similar to that of people suffering cancers whose sites of origin were in internal organs such as the stomach or lung. Women after surgery also knew that cancer could be progressing in their bodies in the absence of any signs or symptoms.

As they struggled with the side effects of surgery, women like Smith worried about the meaning of rashes, pains, lumps, and other signs and symptoms arising in different parts of their bodies. Compared to earlier eras, they seemed to survey their bodies more frequently and want precautionary medical examinations. Partly, this was a response to the educational campaign for women to recognize "early" cancer signs and seek medical attention that was beginning to be promulgated in the early twentieth century (next chapter). The earlier experience of accidentally detecting a breast lump (which many women understood as potentially lifesaving) suggested to many women that further cancer progression might be invisible to them and only discoverable via a medical examination. Given the apparent efficacy of the complete operation and the growing prestige of modern therapeutics, breast cancer patients often placed more faith in medicine to both find and treat recurrences.

In Halsted's practice, the annual follow-up queries contributed to patients' self-surveillance and also to their desire for Halsted to examine them.[33] In addition to sending Halsted pictures and descriptions of her arm movements (see Chapter 4), Hilda Martin responded to Halsted's annual query with some questions of her own. "Could anything be wrong without knowing it?" she wrote Halsted. She wondered if she might benefit from precautionary radium treatments that she had heard were sometimes given to other patients. Martin also wondered if there was a possibility of "not knowing of the existence of anything wrong, because that was the case before I came to you, the discovery being accidental. It occurred to me that perhaps I ought not to feel so sure and ought to have an examination occasionally."[34]

Halsted wrote Martin back that he did not think she should be examined or get preventive radium treatments because "I am sure that nothing remains to be cured, and second, because even if there were traces of the disease anywhere in the body, neither radium nor the x-ray could find them."[35] This ambiguous formulation was typical of Halsted's response to requests for preventive examinations and treatments. Halsted's only advice was that patients live out their lives as if they did not have cancer. The complete operation was effective at reducing the rate of local recurrences. There was nothing more doctors or individuals could do against the possible development of metastatic disease. Halsted was probably aware that most patients did not fully understand the nature of this limited liability and were the better for that partial ignorance. Martin responded that Halsted had completely reassured her, that she was "absolutely at ease in regard to that."[36] But despite her protests, it is plausible that Martin remained only partially reassured.

Halsted's uniform and technically accurate response to his patients' cancer fears and requests for surveillance and preventive treatment were different from that of many of his peers. Unlike Halsted, many of his physician correspondents dealt with their patients' fears of cancer recurrence and requests for surveillance by attributing them to female nervous constitution and propensity toward excessive worry. "Mrs. Short is still suffering from her breast," Dr. Warwick Evans wrote Halsted about a patient Halsted did not think had recurrent cancer, "and yet I think her pain much magnified by a very nervous temperament – she is of scrofular diathesis and some years since had enlarged cervical glands removed. If she continues to suffer this acute pain as she alleges she does would it not be best to have the breast removed at once?"[37] Dr. Evans believed that surgery was an appropriate response to "alleged" pains and fears of cancer recurrence.

Halsted's response to the state of heightened risk was the antithesis of traditional styles of managing chronic disease that stressed actions individuals might do to "support the system." Halsted saw cancer as a specific, localized disease of unclear etiology. He therefore did not suggest to patients how they should live their lives; rarely if ever offering advice about what patients should eat, what they might avoid, or what they might do to prevent cancer recurrence. His response to patients was tailored to his understanding of cancer's natural history, not the life history of individual patients.

As in his dealings with Martin and Smith, Halsted expected and encouraged women to have "brave and sensible" attitudes toward the future. Women so implored often had to find indirect means to express their fears and worries about cancer and cancer recurrence. Typical of this indirection was Florence Miller's attempts to explain her fears about an upcoming surgery and to communicate her awareness of the emotional gulf that separated her from Halsted and other doctors. Miller wrote that she wished her surgical interventions "were all over, as little a job as you think it is, it makes me nervous. However, I am not going to worry over it."[38] In a letter to Halsted after her surgery, prompted in part by news that Halsted had been ill, Miller again communicated her nervous and depressed emotional state while trying not to be dismissed as a nervous woman. She also signaled her acceptance of women's subordinate political status. "I am feeling pretty well," Miller began, "but get powerfully blue sometimes, because I can't do as much as I used to be able to do. I look fine, so everyone says, and am surely glad to be alive and well ... This evening we go to register for you see I have a vote up here in New York State. Ha! Ha! Whether shall take advantage of it or not I don't know yet. I have my hands full enough with my household duties without attempting more ... Now, be good, mind your nurse and doctors, like I was compelled to do, and get well soon."[39]

As in Smith's case, Halsted never initiated precautionary checkups nor cautioned patients to survey their bodies for signs of cancer recurrence. Halsted was not a member or enthusiast of the American Society for the Control of Cancer, an organization that, as we shall see in Chapter 6, urged men and women to survey their bodies for cancer signs and symptoms (Halsted's protégée Joseph Bloodgood was an instrumental member of the inner circle of this organization). Halsted argued in print that physicians should avoid exacerbating patients' fears and uncertainties about events out of their own and their physicians' control by giving "expert advice," and offering "useless examinations."[40]

Not Naming Cancer: "The Necessity of Her Knowing It Are of Course Matters for You to Decide"

Unlike Physick's or Agnew's typical style of communication, Halsted routinely avoided telling patients that they had cancer. Halsted's behavior was normative for his medical generation.[41] This was of course related to the way Halsted and others avoided any detailed discussion of individual prognosis and the mention of possible future cancer recurrence, as it was difficult if not impossible to offer detailed prognoses when the cancer diagnosis was unacknowledged or left implicit.

It is striking that only a few of Halsted's patients (but many husbands and family members) ever directly asked "what do I have?" or "do I have cancer?" Halsted must have communicated that this question was off limits. He did not typically substitute benign, provisional, euphemistic, or misleading diagnoses for cancer. Rather, the whole subject was actively and consciously avoided, as we saw in Halsted's instructions to General Smith.

In many instances, family members implored Halsted to not give the cancer diagnosis to the patient while asking Halsted to tell them the uncensored truth. Ruth Francis, the sister of Halsted's patient Helen Francis, wrote Halsted in 1915 that her sister's prior New York physician, Dr. Cannon, had not told her sister of the possibility of cancer, nor did she, "knowing that plucky as she is it would add one more thing to worry about and she is a person who does worry underneath."[42] After Francis's surgery, Ruth asked Halsted about her sister's prognosis. Halsted's response balanced clinical realities with his own sense of what relatives were able and wanted to hear. He first mentioned that the hardness in her sister's breast was the result of previous operations, not cancer, but also that her sister's "axillary glands showed signs of beginning malignant changes so it is well that they have been removed...I hope that in Miss Francis's case the disease will prove to be relatively benign."[43] To his Hopkins colleague Dr. Burnham, who was assisting Howard Kelly in giving radiation treatments to Francis, Halsted was much more pessimistic and direct. "There has been no local recurrence but the axillary glands were macroscopically involved up the apex of the cervical axilla. I feel that the case is hopeless from a surgical standpoint."[44]

A few months later, Ruth Francis tried again to get clearer and more specific information about her sister's prognosis from Halsted. Her request was couched in terms of the family's practical needs. Ruth Francis explained that her sister had given "much of her time" to caring for their 86-year-old mother and so she needed to know "what is going to be best for my sister. Is she responding to the treatments in such a way that there is a possibility even, of a cure?" Would she be able to care for their mother? Another doctor in New York had given her "definite word" (which she was glad to get "so frankly") that the probabilities were from "two to five years of active life, if the progress of the disease should be as slow in the future as it was in the past."[45] Halsted's response to this query was to paraphrase what he had told the patient herself. Halsted emphasized the disease's varied course, "that one could never be sure that the disease might not return, even as late as twenty years, and advised her to lead her usual normal life because we know of nothing which can hasten the progress of the disease."[46] By referring to breast cancer's idiosyncratic course (just as Physick had done 100 years earlier), Halsted was able to communicate some hope for prolonged survival while being medically accurate.

The very fact that physicians and family members often had to make special pleas to avoid the cancer diagnosis and sometimes gave detailed instructions about who should be told suggests that the norms of truth telling were neither absolute nor uniformly applied. For example, Dr. A. Peskind of Cleveland, Ohio, wrote Halsted in 1908 about his patient Mrs. H. Schwartz. Peskind had told Schwartz that she probably needed a radical operation but had "no apprehension of anything serious." Peskind asked Halsted to "kindly spare her feelings as much as possible but let her husband be informed of your candid opinion. If possible furnish me with a statement of your diagnosis."[47]

As was the case with Smith, patients could of course infer that they had cancer from the very fact that they had a tumor or underwent radical surgery, from family members who were more accurately informed, and from other indirect means. Such inferences and indirection could be adaptive, allowing patients to apprehend the reality of their situation to the extent they wanted and at their own pace while relieving their doctors of the uncomfortable task of delivering harsh prognoses.[48]

Mrs. W. A. (Ida) Price, the wife of a prominent Chicago engineer, underwent the complete operation in December 1921. At the physician-to-physician level, there was direct communication about the suspicion of cancer. Price's physician, James G. Kiernan had been watching a breast mass for 3 years that he considered to be a "nervous adenoma" but which had later developed into something more suspicious. Kiernan had referred Price to Halsted for an evaluation.[49] After examining Price, Halsted sent a telegram to Kiernan saying that he was "confident that the tumor of breast is malignant. Do you wish me to operate?"[50] Kiernan assented and Halsted carried out the operation. Afterward, Halsted wrote Kiernan that "the tumor was a typical carcinoma."[51]

Price's husband sheepishly asked Halsted about the diagnosis and prognosis of her "problems." "If it is proper for me to know," he asked, "I would very much appreciate it if you would advise me ... whether or not you are of the opinion that the operation will permanently eliminate Mrs. Price's problems."[52] Halsted's response to Price's husband was much more detailed, accurate, and medical than he would ever tell a patient directly, but as usual he stressed the goal of no local recurrence and drew something positive from the operative findings: "The wound has healed ideally, and I believe there will be no disability as the result of the operation. Nor do I think she will ever have a local recurrence. Some of the lymphatic glands in the axilla were cancerous, but those nearest the chest (highest in the axilla) were normal; hence I am in hopes that the disease may not have gone to other parts of the body, but of this I cannot be sure."[53]

Ida Price herself wrote to Halsted describing many small details of her wound, arm movements, and postoperative functioning. While she did not utter the word *cancer*, Price made it clear to Halsted that she understood not only her diagnosis, but the fact that she might never be free of the danger of cancer recurrence. "I intend to have examinations made as often as you think necessary until danger of recurrence is over if there ever is such a time."[54]

Patients not only made it clear that they understood they had cancer but sometimes themselves evaded or obfuscated medical details for their own purposes. In 1914, Mrs. Judith Wheaton wrote Halsted about her sister-in-law Ruth Green's medical situation. Wheaton asked Halsted to hide the diagnosis of cancer from Green because she was nervous and frail. "Because of several recent sorrows and her nervous condition the doctors have thought it best for her not to know that it is malignant, though they tell me that there is very little doubt in their minds," Wheaton wrote Halsted. "Whether it is malignant or not and the necessity for her knowing it are of course matters for you to decide when you see her. She has definitely decided on operation and feels that every day is so much time lost."[55]

After Green had radical surgery (without being told the diagnosis), she herself wrote Halsted about her own attempts to avoid telling her friends the true nature of her surgery. "My friends all say, 'how well you look since your rest cure at the Hopkins' – so I haven't said a word about my operation." Green's friends assumed she experienced a more stereotypical female ailment and treatment (the rest cure was a treatment for neurasthenia and kindred conditions), which allowed her to maintain a wanted privacy about her cancer diagnosis and treatment. Green also wrote that the operation had caused her "just a little trouble," probably minimizing its effects in order to please her surgeon who had so much riding on the success of the operation.[56]

A year after her complete operation, Green developed breast cancer in the remaining breast and in her bones. Halsted believed that further surgery would be futile, an assessment that was taken as "a great blow to her [Mrs. Green's] father."[57] Halsted then asked prominent New York cancer specialist James Ewing about the possibility that Mrs. Green might try an unspecified promising therapy that Ewing was developing. Halsted chose to mention in his letter to Ewing that Green "is a genteel young woman from Georgia who has sufficient means to pay for a private room and nurse."[58]

Ewing did not think the new treatment was appropriate for Green. Halsted graciously accepted Ewing's judgment, noting that Green was in any event too weak to travel from Georgia to New York. Consistent with his practice of shielding patients from the burden of regret, Halsted wrote Ewing that he had "not told her [Mrs. Green] of the new treatment at the Memorial Hospital."[59] To Green's sister-in-law, Halsted was more honest. He wrote that the "situation is indeed most distressing and it is mortifying to be so helpless in the presence of this dreadful disease. There is, of course, nothing to do for Mrs. Green except to try to relieve her pain."[60]

Why was there a more literal evasion of the cancer diagnosis and more reluctance to offer specific and individualized prognoses than in earlier periods? Some historical accounts have understood such behavior as indicative of a more paternalistic doctor–patient relationship, sustained by medical and popular conceptions of the female body as weak and inferior.[61] While such macrolevel shifts in the doctor–patient relationship and medical and popular ideas about the female body undoubtedly influenced how breast cancer was understood and responded to, these shifts seem less important and the extent of change in the doctor–patient relationship less great, when we factor in the changed clinical context surrounding the act of cancer diagnosis and prognosis.

The physician's diagnosis of cancer often had a radically different meaning in Halsted's time than in Physick's. In the early nineteenth century, physicians' diagnosis of cancer did not completely determine patients' hopes and fears. As we saw with Emlen's cancer recurrence in England, the diagnosis was often contingent and shifting. Emlen's first English physicians may have suspected cancer but their initial and provisional diagnosis of nonspecific glandular involvement or a scirrhus-like tumor permitted Emlen to hope for survival. Not only did patients and families, much more than physicians, direct the flow of information, there was much less of a gap between physician knowledge about cancer and that of an educated lay person. Physicians had less to conceal from patients. There were thus fewer opportunities for either dramatic truth telling or literal evasion.

By the late nineteenth century, cancer had become a more specific and objective entity. Cancer had become a cellular, microscopic disease that could often be diagnosed by clinicians on the basis of reliable clinical or objective microscopic or radiological criteria, not a tumor diagnosed retrospectively because it was relentless and did not respond to therapy. Smith's chest recurrence, diagnosed by x-rays at Hopkins, while perhaps not totally unambiguous was an objective sign of cancer recurrence. For many early-twentieth-century doctors, the act of cancer diagnosis was potentially imbued with a different, more deterministic meaning than in the period when cancer was more of a gestalt clinical diagnosis, revealed ultimately and retrospectively by its destructive course.

Breast cancer was by the early twentieth century a similar disease in all women and followed a destructive natural history. Of course, breast cancer's idiosyncrasy was still apparent and acknowledged and could and was used to hedge a hopeless prognosis. But both patient and doctor believed that this idiosyncrasy largely reflected a contingent medical ignorance much more than an individual's ability to influence and evade subsequent developments. Physicians felt more self-confident (certainly Halsted did) about the accuracy and meaning of their diagnosis, and patients were cognizant of this greater certainty. There was thus much more to potentially fear in receiving the diagnosis than in the past.

As a result of these changes, the physicians' diagnosis of cancer was transformed into a potential revelatory moment in which hope might be instantaneously lost. In order to sustain hope for survival, a seemingly timeless goal at least in the early period of disease, there was a greater need to more literally evade the diagnosis. So, looked at in terms of underlying function, there may be more continuity in active patient and physician collusion to avoid despair and hopelessness than any historical progression to greater dishonesty from Physick's to Halsted's era.

The complete operation itself often served as a gesture of hope. By the early twentieth century "inoperable cancer" had become synonymous with hopeless cancer. Halsted rarely, if ever, deemed patients as inoperable. Halsted's silence about diagnosis and his reticence to discuss prognosis maintained the symbolic, hope-giving nature of the operation, which could only be deflated by a clear understanding of its limited reach. Halsted and other early-twentieth-century doctors also did not want to offer patients like Smith detailed prognostic information after surgery that would exacerbate their already primed fears of cancer recurrence when they believed that there was nothing more to be done.

The often close familiarity of doctor and patient and the locus of surgery and care in the home sustained a different pattern of diagnosis and prognosis in the early nineteenth century than 100 years later. Unlike Burney and Emlen who were close intimates of their surgeons, Smith did not know Halsted until her breast problems developed. Halsted's efforts to avoid telling Smith her hopeless prognosis may have been helped by their more strictly professional relationship, the geographical distance between them, and the location of their episodic encounters in hospitals rather than in the Smiths' home.

The pattern of evading diagnosis and prognosis that Halsted and other doctors followed had consequences. Halsted's begrudging, limited, yet technically honest prognostication, which stressed that breast cancer's natural history after surgery was autonomous from individual action and medical attention, was unsettling to many patients and family members. Some of Halsted's patients experienced a reduced sense of control over their future and therefore felt a greater need for medical and self-surveillance. Evasions were also often in conflict with other needs and goals. In a number of Halsted's cases, patients' treatment was complicated because they had never been told that they had cancer. For example, Dr. J. Peebles Proctor of Athens, Georgia, wrote Halsted in 1912 about the care of Mrs. Blake, a patient on whom Halsted had previously operated. Proctor observed that Blake's general condition was worse and wanted her to consult Halsted again "but neither she nor her husband approve of it yet. I do not insist because I do not wish Mrs. Blake to get the idea that her condition is not favorable. It might be well for you to write me a letter which I can show to them, requesting that she be sent back to you."[62]

Evasion of the diagnosis and the possibility of recurrent disease was also sometimes in conflict with Halsted's "end results" research program. Halsted's annual queries about postoperative complications and general health prompted some women to examine themselves and worry more about disease progression. Florence Miller received a follow-up query on the third anniversary of her complete operation. Miller's husband wrote Halsted that his wife had discovered a worrisome spot on her arm and was close to a "complete nervous breakdown. I recall that at the time of the operation the exact nature of the her trouble was concealed, thanks to your kind consideration, and while she is apparently still ignorant of the real cause of trouble, she suspects its nature, due to the suggestion contained in blank sent her. And this, of course, is not helping matters."[63]

Treatments Other Than the Knife

Smith's highly intervened-in life after her breast amputation foreshadowed the experiences of many American women with breast cancer later in the century. Smith and other Halsted patients with recurrent disease after surgery often entered into a web of specialists who deployed novel, powerful salvage treatments whose use in specific contexts Halsted and others considered appropriate.

Early-twentieth-century modalities of "salvage" therapy shared features with some nineteenth-century innovations like Emlen's compression therapy. Compression therapy was similarly intensive, of long duration, applied by physicians, produced (or was perceived to produce) observable changes in the breast, caused significant side effects, and was understood as new and experimental. But there were also important differences. The early-twentieth-century salvage therapies such as radiation therapy or radium were more directly the result of technological innovation and scientific experiment. They had more powerful and visible effects on the body. They sustained medical and surgical commitment to patients who had braved extensive, mutilating surgery but were not cured. Doctors and patients had high expectations that these nonsurgical treatments might be effective, although doctors understood that they controlled rather than eliminated cancer. Perhaps most profoundly, these treatments were fundamental parts of a halting and incomplete yet very real shift from a patient-centered, spiritual reckoning at the end of life to a more crowded, secular, and medicalized last rite of breast cancer.

While Halsted directed the traffic to specialists and sometimes their fees, he did not administer these second-line, nonsurgical treatments himself. Each therapy had its own specialist. The two salvage treatments that Smith experienced – radium treatments administered by Halsted's Hopkins colleague Howard Kelly and the experimental radiation treatments by Rockefeller Institute researcher James Murphy – were the ones that Halsted most consistently urged on his "complete operation" patients with local, regional, or distal disease that might be reached by them. As described earlier, Murphy's "treatments" were an extension of his animal research. Patients such as Smith and Francis appeared not to understand that they were in part research subjects, writing Halsted about their surprise over their individual attention and free "care."

Along with Halsted, William Osler, and William Welch, Howard Kelly (1858–1943) was one of the four pillars of the Hopkins medical faculty. In addition to leading gynecological surgery at Hopkins, Kelly had become a pioneer in radium treatment of cancers, especially gynecological malignancies. The deployment of radium, discovered by the Curies in 1898, into human cancer therapeutics was swift but was limited by its worldwide scarcity. Kelly had been instrumental in arranging for the U.S. Bureau of Mines in 1913 to extract radium from the Colorado plateau and for a period he was in control of the small amount of radium (7 g) available for medical use in the United States at his private clinic in Baltimore. With his close colleague Curtis Burnham, Kelly implanted radium into deep-seated, gynecological tumors and had observed dramatic cures in some cases.

There was a lot of variation in how radium and x-rays were used and rationalized, even among elite surgeons who did extensive cancer surgery and shared similar beliefs. Halsted's closest surgical counterpart in Great Britain was W. Sampson Handley, whose skepticism about cancer metastasis was discussed earlier. Despite their many shared views, Handley used radiation and radium in a very different fashion than Halsted. Handley irradiated benign conditions such as chronic mastitis, borderline diagnostic cases, as well as tumors that he believed could not be cured by surgery. He also pioneered the implantation of radium-filled tubes into the chests of patients at the time of their initial breast cancer surgery in the hope that chest wall recurrences from occult metastases could be prevented.[64]

In contrast to Handley, Halsted deplored the use of radiation for initial treatment instead of, or with, surgery. Halsted worried that such initial x-ray treatment could compromise the benefits of a complete operation. In the case of Helen Francis, for example, Halsted had initially declined to perform the complete operation, whose uniform use in breast cancer he espoused, because she had already had a course of x-ray treatments.[65] Unlike the herbs, salves, opium, bark, and wine offered by Benjamin Rush to Mary Washington in the eighteenth century or the compression treatments used by Susan Emlen in the early nineteenth century, radium and radiation produced more visible and profound changes in the body – sometimes the literal burning away of tumors – and were capable of inducing more serious side effects. These side effects required elucidation and management by experienced, specialized physicians who saw enough patients to recognize patterns and modify treatments.

For example, Murphy and Halsted corresponded in 1917 about how to recognize and manage the side effects of radium and radiation treatment. Murphy wrote Halsted that these treatments sometimes produced a generalized sickness in addition to the more evident and visible localized burns to the body. "Miss Francis, after a recent treatment with radium," Murphy wrote Halsted, "had a very severe general reaction, with nausea, loss of appetite, and slight elevation of temperature. This lasted over several weeks. We put her on forced fluids, that is, a glass of water at least every hour, and her symptoms cleared up almost immediately. This, however, of course does not effect the local burn. The only treatment given locally was an occasional moistening of the tissues with alcohol."[66]

Having sought out Halsted's expertise, many patients and their families wanted their after-treatment to be managed by elite specialists as well. Helen Francis's sister wrote Halsted that she preferred that any further radiation treatment be given by Hopkins' specialists. "While I have no doubt that it [x-ray] has been as well given by our family physician as it can be by any one who is doing it only for an occasional patient, I cannot help feeling that the best results must be more likely to be attained by a man who has the experience that can come only when one is doing it constantly."[67] The very fact that Francis' initial radiation treatment was given by her family physician serves as a reminder that the dominance of specialist cancer therapeutics was not preordained but resulted from a more gradual jockeying about for control and influence. Halsted eventually referred Francis to Kelly and Burnham.

In Smith's case and others, there was often a significant gap between what the patient hoped and expected and what Halsted and the purveyors of these salvage treatments believed about their efficacy. Throughout Smith's illness, Halsted sounded pessimistic notes about her prognosis to Kelly and Murphy. Like Smith, most patients have hoped for cure of their recurrent disease, while their physicians often understood these experimental salvage treatments in narrower, less hopeful ways. Murphy understood that his radiation treatment of Smith and other patients would not cure their cancer but their use might advance scientific knowledge, palliate pain, remove a visible and disturbing reminder of disease, and sustain hope, especially in the aftermath of devastating surgery.

Halsted gave his patients much more control over the course of salvage therapy than he did over the initial "choice" of the complete operation. Salvage therapy arose from the need to offer something medical, with the trappings of efficacy to be sure, to patients whom Halsted had failed to cure but who retained faith in the efficacy of modern medical approaches to cancer. The initiation of salvage treatment was typically done at the patient's urging. Patients also had a degree of responsibility for transmitting information throughout the web of specialists.

Halsted also did not imbue salvage treatments like radium or radiation therapy with the same heavy dose of individual responsibility that surrounded the complete operation. Knowing that these salvage treatments were often experimental and of unproven value, for example, Halsted often attempted to relieve his patients of any guilt or regret that ensued from not choosing or not being able to afford treatment.

The case of Miss Janet Fleming, a Halsted breast cancer patient who was offered but did not end up getting salvage treatments, demonstrated the different moral territory these treatments generally inhabited. In response to the annual follow-up query, Fleming wrote Halsted from Culpeper County, Virginia, in 1915 that she had a new "tea cup" size lump on her left breast and was in poor health 11 years after her complete operation. "I shrink from another operation and from the long months of suffering before me," she pessimistically summarized the bad options before her.[68]

Halsted wrote back to offer both sympathy and reassurance that a decision not to operate was reasonable.[69] It was not until December 1915, 8 months after learning about problems in the second breast, that Halsted tentatively offered up radium treatment to Fleming. It may be that this delay followed from Halsted's knowledge of Fleming's modest economic means or that he was responding to cues in the earlier letter that Fleming was not enthusiastic about further treatment. In this and many other cases after cancer recurred, Halsted tailored his assessment of different treatment options so as to make the patient feel that she had made the right decision. "Quite remarkable results have been obtained," Halsted wrote, "particularly during the last year, in the treatment of cases like yours with radium. Very large amounts have to be employed, and I know of no one in this country excepting Dr. Kelly who has a sufficient quantity. If you care to come to Baltimore to give the radium a trial I shall take pleasure in arranging with Dr. Kelly for the treatment."[70] Fleming thanked Halsted for his interest but she did not have the money to come to Baltimore and communicated her resignation about her disease.[71]

"I am sorry that you cannot arrange to come to Baltimore," Halsted replied, aiming to make her miserable reality more bearable by not adding any guilt or regret that lack of money had prevented Mrs. Fleming from receiving treatment that could help her. "Although I am not sure that it would be worthwhile for you to make a great sacrifice to do so. Only a rather small percentage of the cases suffering with your trouble are relieved by the radium treatment, but in some instances the good effects are remarkable. Dr. Kelly is indeed most generous to patients who require the radium treatment."[72] In this and in many other situations, Halsted signaled not only that significant financial accommodations could be made but also took it upon himself to ease patients' anxiety about making or having to make wrong decisions in that sphere of therapy that was not part of the received canon of treatments, like the complete operation, which in Halsted's terms truly worked.

As we saw with Smith, Halsted was genuinely heartened when patients undergoing Kelley's x-ray and/or Murphy's radium treatments survived longer and with better than expected quality of life. In a brief letter to Murphy touching on the treatment of both Smith and Francis, Halsted expressed cautious optimism that they were both doing well, especially Francis, whose "prognosis seemed to me almost absolutely bad."[73]

It was not inevitable that Halsted, other elite physicians, and some patients considered these salvage treatments on a different, more legitimate plane than the many other nonsurgical cancer treatments promoted by a wide variety of practitioners. Radium's and x-rays' biological activity was apparent in the melting away of superficial tumors as well as highly visible side effects such as radiation burns and generalized sickness. Radium's prestige was also buoyed by its scarcity and the international attention given to the Curies' discovery. But the credibility of the promoters of radium and therapeutic x-rays was also very important. Kelley was Halsted's colleague and Murphy his former trainee. Kelley worked at Hopkins and Murphy at the prestigious Rockefeller Institute. In contrast to his close collaboration with Kelley and Murphy, Halsted strenuously objected to the x-ray treatments initially given to Helen Francis by an unfamiliar general practitioner working in a community setting. "Have you any fear that prolonged treatment with the x-ray might be attended with the risk of stimulating epithelial growth?" Halsted asked Francis's New York doctor in an uncharacteristically confrontational manner.[74]

One other type of cancer salvage treatment that Halsted used was surgery for relief of pain. In 1915, Halsted became extremely agitated over the case of Mrs. Dattwyler, in large measure because there was a specific, surgical option for the relief of her pain that was not being used.[75] In keeping with the heightened responsibility surrounding the complete operation, the fact that Halsted believed there was an effective and specific surgical response to a devastating medical problem created its own imperative to utilize it.

Dattwyler was apparently unable to travel from Alabama to Baltimore to undergo an operation that Halsted had proposed to relieve her excruciating arm pain that was not controlled by narcotics. Halsted implored Mrs. Dattwyler's daughter Rosalie that "there is only one relief for the pains and that is to divide the nerves in the neck ... It is a shame that your mother should suffer so when it is unnecessary. In the meantime I would give her large hypodermics of morphia."[76] Rosalie replied that it was impossible for her to get up to Baltimore at that time so she would give her mother opium. If opium did not work she would try to bring her mother to Baltimore in a few months.[77] But Halsted remained so concerned about this "unnecessary" suffering that he dispatched his assistant Hugh Young to also write Rosalie, having previously asked another assistant (Heuer) to write her. "A few days ago Heuer also had a letter from Mrs. Dattwyler stating that morphia no longer relieves her pain, and regretting that it is impossible for her to come to Baltimore," Halsted wrote Young. "It occurs to me that perhaps a line from you would influence them."[78] This degree of coordinated pressure not only reflected a compassionate interest in the patient, but a heightened sense of responsibility to deploy those select surgical techniques believed to "work," regardless of whether they were curative or not.

Negotiating Treatment at the Border of Quackery

Halsted's gradual and grudging acceptance of a questionable treatment for a patient whose disease was too advanced even for the salvage treatments he generally used provides a window into how the credibility of treatments and their purveyors was constructed. Halsted's assistant Dr. Follis first examined Mrs. W. E. Burgess in the summer of 1914, when she was just 33. Follis had found cancer in the axilla and neck, in part by doing an exploratory incision and biopsy, violating Halsted's operative principles (Halsted was away for the summer). Because her cancer had spread to the neck, Follis told Mrs. Burgess and her husband William that "it was hopeless" and that further surgery would only "shorten her life." Halsted's assistant Harvey Cushing created a sling to support the heavy left breast out of whose nipple there was a "slight discharge of pus." Mr. Burgess wrote Halsted that "it is almost impossible for me to believe that

Mrs. Burgess is to die very soon from her trouble for her general health is good and she looks fine." Because Mr. Burgess was in his own words "old fashioned and simple" in my beliefs, he still hoped, "the Almighty will direct things better than I have been told to expect." He wanted to know if Halsted was "able to direct us to help the trouble in some way, though I am afraid it is too much to ask anyone that is human in the present state of knowledge on the subject."[79]

A few days later, Halsted responded to Mr. Burgess that he agreed with Follis that an operation would not help and cautiously proposed radium treatment. Halsted offered to arrange for Mrs. Burgess to meet Kelly and get radium. But Halsted also added that "Coley's serum is also to be considered ... It is only occasionally that the Coley serum is efficient. Under the circumstances it should perhaps be tried, although I have not much hope of its efficacy."[80] William Coley was a New York physician who had experimented with provoking immune reactions against cancer by injecting patients with heat-killed bacteria.[81] Halsted had just a few days earlier received three physician testaments to the efficacy of Coley's toxins and also had some experience using this treatment with his sarcoma patients.

Mr. Burgess wrote Halsted back about their especially difficult situation. Follis had already made the referral for Kelly's radiation treatments, Halsted's typical first line of salvage therapy, but Kelly's assistant Dr. Burnham believed that "the trouble had spread over too large an area to make it advisable to do anything" and that radium treatments would only damage tissues and hasten death. As even the normal salvage routines were not appropriate, Mr. Burgess asked Halsted, mixing desperation and acceptance of the impending doom, "if there is anything you would do doctor if Mrs. Burgess was your own wife that I would like to do for her, but on the other hand there are cases where nature is best left alone to take her own course and we just have to submit to the results."[82]

Halsted replied somberly, "I regret that there is nothing for me to suggest for the relief of Mrs. Burgess. The Coley serum gives results in such a very small percentage of cases and its administration is attended with such great and distressing reaction that I do not feel like urging its employment. The day must come when cancer will be controlled by other than surgical means."[83] Perhaps Mr. Burgess's seeming acceptance of his wife's eventual death allowed Halsted to more directly communicate the hopelessness that he typically communicated only with other physicians. Halsted had gingerly raised and then tentatively withdrawn the suggestion of using Coley serum based on his changing assessment of the Burgesss' desperation and acceptance of the inevitable bad results.

In spite of what Halsted advised and his flip-flopping about Coley's serum, Mr. Burgess took the initiative and contacted Coley in New York. Coley then wrote Halsted to convince him of the possible benefits of his serum for Mrs. Burgess. Coley began by acknowledging that Halsted and others in Baltimore strongly advised Mr. Burgess "not to try the treatment." To overcome Halsted's presumed skepticism, Coley related the story of a woman with extensive and inoperable breast cancer who had an apparent cure from the administration of toxins. Almost apologetically, Coley wrote that "the toxins were used rather against my advice, to please the family, and the treatment was carried out by the local physician under my direction."[84] Coley intended to convince Halsted of the efficacy of his toxins both on the basis of the testaments of other physicians (one of whom was a Hopkins graduate – scribbled in by Coley on the letter) and by Coley's appropriately detached stand toward these toxins. Speaking of what transpired with the Burgesses, Coley wrote that he could not give any advice without examining Mrs. Burgess himself and that he very likely would advise against treatment since most of the successes were with sarcomas not carcinomas. And if he did treat her, he would do so without charge.[85]

In his reply to Coley, Halsted backpedaled from his prior negative message about Coley's toxins to Mr. Burgess and tried not to offend a senior clinical researcher from another prestigious research institution. He wrote Coley that Mr. Burgess "must have misquoted me . . . I should be sorry to have a misunderstanding for I have advocated the use of your toxins for many years. For two or three years we tried it systematically in practically every inoperable case of sarcoma, but without definite result. You will perhaps recall that from time to time I have sent you cases. I made use of the term "serum" to Mr. Burgess because "toxins" sounds a little dangerous to the layman."[86]

In a subsequent letter, Coley reiterated to Halsted that he had not pushed the toxins on the Burgesses and gave further details vouching to the credibility of toxin treatments. Parke Davis and Company were producing the toxins and doing so with the support of the Huntington Cancer Research Fund. They were being supplied free of charge to hospitals.[87] After Coley's appeals to proper credentials and motives, Halsted further changed his tune and wrote Mr. Burgess that "on further consultation with Dr. Coley and after due consideration I have concluded that it would be well for you to consult Dr. Coley, and should he advise the trial of his toxins, to place Mrs. Burgess in his hands."[88] In other words, Coley had made the right social attestations of credibility about his treatment, including the absence of profit motive, testaments of physicians from the right institutions, and appropriate modesty in his claims. These trappings of credibility and legitimacy, much more than testaments of efficacy or other "data," were the active ingredients in the successful negotiations to frame Coley's toxins as a legitimate salvage treatment rather than as quack therapy.

In addition, there was probably a more personal and social aspect to Coley's limited ability to gain some plausibility for his experimental work and for clinicians like Halsted to try it on some patients. In 1931, eminent Hopkins pathologist William Welch asked Murphy to have a personal conference with Coley to discuss claims Coley had made about the efficacy of his toxins among patients at the Hospital for Ruptured and Crippled and to "give Coley advice, criticism and help." In this letter, Welch noted that he liked Coley personally ("he is sincere, enthusiastic, and well meaning"), and he has "always tried to be sympathetic" and moreover "he [Coley] is close to Mr. Rockefeller" (the ultimate benefactor of the Rockefeller Institute in which Murphy worked). At the same time, Welch distanced himself from Coley's claims of efficacy, writing that "if half of what he claims is in fact true, the experimental results are revolutionary, but I need not tell you that I am skeptical."[89] Skepticism toward claims of cancer efficacy was and continues to be a safe bet.

Life at Risk

As a result of the complete operation, salvage treatments, and changes in the way patients' fears and hopes were managed, many of Halsted's patients experienced a "life at risk" after surgery that was qualitatively different from the experiences of Emlen, Cope, and other women in earlier periods. Radical surgery and salvage treatments had more powerful effects on women's bodies than less extensive surgery and older ways of treating recurrent disease. Women's lives were increasingly framed by side effects of treatment, like arm swelling and limited mobility. These side effects were considered acceptable because women and their doctors had greater faith in the scientific basis and efficacy of cancer treatments and practices. At the same time, Halsted understood that even his highly valued complete operation in almost all cases did little against the metastatic disease that ultimately killed most women with breast cancer.

The sword of Damocles hung over affected women's heads more intensely. The new natural history of breast cancer – beginning as a localized, slow growing, and (if caught "early") treatable disease that nevertheless almost always turns malignant and incurable – and Halsted's reticent style of managing patients' fears after surgery led many patients to crave some means with which to reassert control over this feared disease. Many patients demanded more medical guidance and surveillance and more closely attended to their own bodies for clues of cancer recurrence.

As the complete operation and associated beliefs and practices were widely adopted by other surgeons throughout the United States in the 1920s and 1930s, this "life at risk" became an increasingly common experience of breast cancer patients. Some aspects of this "life at risk," especially the fear of cancer and the demand for some means of control, were also to spread widely throughout the society. Other historical accounts have speculated about how popular fears of cancer grew in the early decades of the twentieth century, in part because some cancers (e.g., lung cancer) were becoming more prevalent and the declining overall mortality experience in the population itself increased the relative danger and visibility of cancer. Economic and social improvements may also have led to more people having a greater interest in avoiding cancer.[90] In the next chapter, I will trace the way the promotion of public health messages about cancer's dangers and the importance of seeking "early" medical attention for suspicious cancer signs helped make some aspects of this "life at risk" – fear of cancer, reduced sense of control, faith in medical surveillance and interventions – the experience of many unaffected men and women.

SIX

"Do Not Delay"

The War Against Time

Beware the beginnings for an after treatment comes often too late.

Thomas Aquinas[1]

At the same time as Halsted's complete operation was rapidly becoming the standard approach to breast cancer, other surgeons and gynecologists were starting a mass educational campaign to change cancer-related beliefs and behavior. The campaign's central message was that cancer surgery was effective if individuals would only "not delay" seeking medical help for any one of a number of suspicious cancer signs or symptoms. Spreading this educational message was the raison d'être for the establishment of the American Society for the Control of Cancer (ASCC) in 1913, the organization that would become the American Cancer Society in the 1940s.[2]

While Halsted promoted a single right surgical approach to cancer, he did not blame patients for seeking medical attention too late. It is unclear whether he believed that time was not a crucial variable in his patients' outcomes or whether he had ethical or other reasons for not adding to his patients' burdens. In contrast, the organizers of the early-twentieth-century cancer educational campaigns made delay and individual responsibility the central element in their message. Time was also central to twentieth-century research and clinical efforts to refashion the natural history of cancer. In effect, two parallel, interacting, yet distinct quests gained momentum in the early twentieth century: a medical and societal one to find women earlier in their own personal history of cancer and a scientific one to identify and understand earlier stages in the natural history of the disease.

In this chapter, I will first analyze the obstacles to the campaign's success, namely lay and medical fears of radical cancer surgery and skepticism about its efficacy, and the processes by which these obstacles were overcome and the campaign succeeded. While the resources deployed to start the campaign were considerable and the logic of "delay" timeless, the main engine for the campaign's remarkable success and endurance was an autocatalytic-like interaction between changed cancer beliefs and health-care-seeking behavior, on the one hand, and widespread perceptions of surgery's efficacy at the aggregate level, on the other. In effect, the campaign's products – especially increased visits to physicians with cancer signs and the resulting improved survival statistics – encouraged even greater compliance with the campaign, resulting in a cascade effect. Although delay in seeking care for breast lumps or a change in the nipple and overlying skin was the main target of the campaign, the campaign was built on attention to cancer signs and symptoms in general (including those that might indicate stomach cancer, uterine cancer, and oral cancer). As a result, my analysis will switch back and forth from changing beliefs, routines, and aggregate perceptions of both breast cancer and cancer in general.

The British surgeon Charles P. Childe, in the first edition of his *Control of a Scourge* (1906), a book read on both sides of the Atlantic in many different editions, laid out the basic "delay" story line and its many supporting subplots. "Cancer itself is not incurable," Childe wrote. "It becomes incurable from the simple fact that its unfortunate victims harbour and nurse their cancers till it is too late." According to Childe, people delayed seeking medical attention for a variety of reasons: the paralyzing fear of surgery, the temporizing habits of some general practitioners, the pessimism of surgeons, visits to quacks, the use of home remedies, and the stigma of cancer for both individuals and families (due to unfounded – according to Childe – constitutional and hereditarian notions). Women particularly delayed seeking medical help for breast cancer because they mistakenly believed that lumps due to breast cancer should be painful and because they were "falsely" and inappropriately modest about their breasts.

Childe, like so many proponents of public campaigns after him, sounded an ambivalent note about fear of cancer. Fear was both a cause of delay and a necessary and justifiable means to motivate ordinary people to seek medical care for troubling signs and symptoms. Not to employ fear was to allow the public to commit "involuntary suicide." Childe understood that the audience for the "delay" message was the educated middle classes but argued that there would be an inevitable trickle down effect to less fortunate members of society.[3]

There has been a remarkable stability to this core "delay" message. One of the most stable parts has been the list of six or seven (and on occasion, more or less) danger signs of cancer in the educational material of the ASCC and later, the American Cancer Society (ACS), dating from the late teens until the 1970s.[4] These danger signs have always prominently featured breast lumps among the many vague and common signs and symptoms, such as "a sore that doesn't heal" and "chronic indigestion," about which to be vigilant. These danger signs appeared in countless posters, post cards, trinkets (such as faux cosmetic cases), pamphlets, books, movies, and lectures, varying only slightly in format, number, and emphasis.[5]

While the core "delay" message has been remarkably stable, its style and pitch have varied by era, audience, media, and promoter. A 1930s narrative published in a cancer prevention journal published by the New York City Cancer Committee, for example, told the story of a young (and newly rich) bride who avoids seeking medical care for a suspicious chest lump. Her husband suspects the problem but cannot get his newlywed to see the family doctor, who happens also to be a personal friend. Upon hearing about the situation from the husband, the family doctor invites himself over for dinner. The doctor confronts the newlywed in the living room, tells her to take off her blouse, pays "no attention to her hysterical attitudes," examines her, and sends her by taxi to the hospital where she immediately has an operation. The pathologist reports that evening that the biopsy result was benign, the wife's worries disappear, and her promising life can now really begin.[6] The appeals to a good life that was almost lost, the ideal of the paternalistic family doctor, and the expectations of hysterical yet submissive young wives give a Depression-era twist to the core "delay" message.

It is by no means obvious why the "delay" message played such a central role in medical and lay responses to breast (and other) cancers for so many years. One might imagine that there was epidemiologic or other data proving that a woman's delay in seeking medical attention for a lump was a significant factor in the harm and loss of life caused by breast cancer.

This was not the case and, in any event, it has not been until recent decades that medical evidence in the form of observational studies and clinical trials has served as the agreed upon rationale for specific clinical and public health practices and ideas. Whether there is good evidence proving that delay is harmful in breast cancer is still debated, demonstrating both continued interest in the "delay" message and our own era's commitment, at least rhetorically, to evidence-based clinical practice. A 1999 systematic review (meta-analysis) of existing studies, for example, concluded that "delays of 3–6 months are associated with lower survival."[7] While this conclusion is problematic because of the quality of the data under review, the relevant historical observation is that during the heyday of the "delay" message such robust data were rarely offered and hardly ever sought.[8]

The fact that there was demand for a twentieth-century American public health campaign against cancer is not in itself surprising – cancer was a rising and significant cause of mortality and there were many other progressive-era health campaigns from which to draw motivation, resources, and guidance. The gynecologists, surgeons, and actuaries who launched the public campaign against cancer did not explicitly rationalize why they chose "delay" as the central cancer control message. In private and public, the rationale seemed self-evident on the basis of a set of commonly held assumptions about cancer and the state of public ignorance. Yet it is worth asking why this message and not another (e.g., to avoid chronic irritations or get annual cancer checkups) if only to begin to discern the less-than-inevitable aspects of the history of breast cancer.

One way to understand the choice of "delay" is that cancer activists faced the problem of justifying a public health campaign against a disease that was not contagious. Unlike people with tuberculosis, for example, people with cancer suffered but were not the vectors of the disease. Voluntary organizations such as the ASCC needed to find a compelling rationale for mass intervention against a disease that, at one level, was only an individual problem. The "delay" message allowed cancer activists to justify their public campaign by analogy to more traditional ones against infectious disease. Instead of blocking the transmission of germs, cancer activists could block the transmission of disease-causing assumptions and behavioral norms.

Clearly, the centrality and durability of the "delay" message followed from widely held assumptions about the natural history of cancer, a public health activism borne out of frustration over the lack of other effective prevention practices and treatments, and a medical and cultural reflex to make individuals, especially women, responsible for their disease (in contrast to stressing the limitations of medical knowledge and treatment or just not concerning ourselves with the question of responsibility). The centrality of the individual responsibility for detecting cancer was parallel to and perhaps encouraged by the increased medical and surgical responsibility for outcomes promoted by Halsted and others. But merely evoking these beliefs and values does not adequately explain why the "delay" message played such a prominent role in clinical and public health practices and in the everyday lives of women throughout much of the twentieth century. A more adequate – if still incomplete – explanation emerges by focusing on the interactions among these beliefs and values and the routines of women, doctors, researchers, public health activists, and other actors in this struggle to make sense of, and respond to, breast and other cancers.

More than just an appealing idea, the "delay" message contributed to changes in the routines of ordinary women, women with breast lumps, pathologists, surgeons, and cancer activists. These actions led to a perception of progress in the war against breast cancer, which in turn reinforced the apparent efficacy of the public messages about cancer – sustaining and encouraging further actions and beliefs.

"So Utterly Opposed": The Skepticism and Actions of Ordinary Women and Their Doctors

To understand how the American campaign worked, it is first necessary to understand who needed to be persuaded and what obstacles needed to be overcome. The "delay" campaign was aimed at overcoming women's fear of surgery and their own and their general practitioners' skepticism about its efficacy. Lay skepticism about cancer surgery's efficacy was widely shared by most doctors outside of the "delay" message's core constituency of elite surgeons and gynecologists. Most women were skeptical of surgery's efficacy because they were unlikely to have known other women who survived the disease with or without surgery.

What women feared and believed about efficacy mattered profoundly because, as contemporary physicians with extensive breast cancer experience in the era before mammography repeatedly observed, nearly all breast cancers were first detected by women rather than physicians.[9] Evidence that women generally avoided surgeons and surgery up until the first few decades of the twentieth century comes from surgeons' descriptions of women's delay, clinicians' reports of the large size and late stage of breast cancers in the early decades of the century as compared to later eras, and the many descriptions of women seeking out "quacks" instead of surgeons.

As we saw with Emlen in the early nineteenth century, women frequently resisted advice of their husbands and others to consult surgeons and actively sought out nonsurgical alternatives as first responses to the discovery of breast lumps. Although by the early twentieth century radical cancer surgery was touted as being more efficacious, patients feared the ensuing greater mutilation. One Halsted patient expressed her anger and depression when she read about supposedly curative nonsurgical procedures, which if true should "by law the process exposed" since she would, as a result of her own complete operation, "never again feel comfortable as long as I live."[10]

Many of Halsted and other surgeons' patients were "utterly opposed" to the idea of radical surgery.[11] In 1927, Ernst Daland described the experience of 100 women who had not had surgery for breast cancer and who were residents of two hospitals that cared for "incurables." Twenty-three of these women had been advised to have surgery but had refused (the rest were "inoperable" at the time of diagnosis). Such "refusers" constitute evidence that many women in the early decades of the century not only feared but probably doubted the utility of surgery for breast cancer.[12]

There is a good deal of evidence that most general practitioners remained far less enthusiastic about surgical cures for breast and other cancers than the general and gynecological surgeons who established the ASCC and led the campaign that stressed the surgical curability of cancer "taken in time." In 1921, a general practitioner wrote Halsted about a patient with "a growth in the breast. Some three years ago it had the characteristics of a nervous adenoma. In the last six months it presents other peculiarities which require attention from a surgeon. I have referred her to you knowing your well marked conservatism."[13] This general practitioner's initial decision not to refer a woman who had "a growth in her breast," instead labeling it with a functional diagnosis and observing her for 3 years, seems to conform to the stereotype of the ignorant, procrastinating general practitioner that was painted by cancer activists of this period. But his later decision to refer the woman to Halsted, his unapologetic rationale for delay, as well as his appeal to Halsted's "well marked conservatism," all suggest that he was confident that not rushing to surgery for all breast lumps was a defensible course of action. This was a norm that was about to change.

Cancer activists and cancer surgeons not only frequently portrayed general practitioners as procrastinating and overly pessimistic about cancer in their cancer control writings but also traded stories with each other about patients whose cancer symptoms were initially dismissed by general practitioners. One of Halsted's surgeon correspondents in 1897, for example, wrote indignantly of a patient whose general practitioner, a "female doctor" no less, had told her that her breast lump was harmless, resulting in a dangerous delay of surgery.[14]

Frederick Hoffman, a Prudential Insurance actuary/epidemiologist and ASCC activist, clipped the following exchange between a patient/reader and an advice-giving general practitioner/journalist, which appeared in a 1913 St. Louis newspaper, probably because it demonstrated the problem that cancer control activists saw in the practices and beliefs of general practitioners. "The lump on my breast, of which I wrote," began a women reader, "has been growing about a year. It does not pain me generally but occasionally I suffer from it. I have been told that kerosene rubbed on it was good for it, and I have tried that but it has hurt me very much . . . I am very much worried." The general practitioner responded that "you probably used kerosene when you had irritated the skin by intense rubbing. Bathe the spot thoroughly and apply a pad of antiphlogistan."[15] For Hoffman and other ASCC activists, the lack of surgical attention and physical examination, the local remedies, the temporizing, and the failure to consider the cancer diagnosis often placed the general practitioner, along with the much ridiculed quack, on the dark side of the struggle against cancer.

In discussing the fate of a woman who presented with advanced cancer, another of Halsted's correspondents wrote in 1912, "Poor thing. She is another victim of the quacks."[16] Despite the real antipathy toward "quacks" and the furious ASCC and AMA campaigns against them, one wonders if some of this venom was displaced from conflicts between specialists and general practitioners, in which debates about authority and legitimacy had to be conducted with more overt civility. As evidence for this, many of the tirades attacked both quacks and general practitioners in the same breath, for example: "Notwithstanding our ignorance of the cause, and despite the pessimistic utterances of the former type of family doctor (who didn't bother to make unpleasant examinations for trivial complaints), despite the blatant mockery of the unhuman sharks who declare in flaring advertisements that the knife is useless, the truth is this: Cancer Is Curable If Taken in Time."[17]

In the conflict between cancer specialist and general practitioner, each side accused the other of acting out of greed rather than for the best interest of the patient. The conflict was not only over temporizing, the value of surgery, clinical skill, and access to patients – the explicit terms of the debates – but also over what might be considered a style of practice. The "delay" message justified and promoted a style of practice that accentuated acute, fast paced, diagnosis-driven care as opposed to a more familiar, life-long, slower paced, person-oriented one.

A 1913 newspaper article told women who experienced out-of-the-ordinary uterine bleeding to insist that "your family doctor conduct you at once to an expert gynecologist. It can do no harm other than a slight fee, which the specialist, in spite of a popular notion to the contrary, can very well do without and doesn't care a hang about."[18] Writing in the early twentieth century, the prominent Philadelphia surgeon John B. Deaver argued that the main problem with early detection was the public's lack of confidence in the specialist class.[19] This lack of confidence arose from suspicions that specialists were motivated to perform unnecessary procedures to enrich themselves. And specialist attention was expensive, for example, Halsted's standard – but highly variable – operating fee for a mastectomy was $500. General practitioners frequently described the patient's "means" and pleaded for special financial accommodations in their referring letters to surgeons.

In the early decades of the twentieth century, general practitioners' and ordinary women's fear and skepticism was also reinforced by the low threshold that many surgeons set for surgery. Many elite surgeons believed that the mere suspicion of cancer was an indication for a radical operation. In effect, surgeons often held onto two parallel and mutually reinforcing idealizations – that women should seek medical attention for any lump or vague symptom that could be construed as a cancer danger sign and that surgeons should err on the side of radical cancer surgery if there was the slightest suspicion of cancer. But this "take no prisoners" surgical approach may have kept women away from surgeons in order to avoid unnecessary operations. This could and did lead to a vicious cycle.

The desire to find, label, and respond aggressively to "earlier" stages in cancer's natural history, a corollary medico-scientific effort to telling women to come in earlier in their personal history of disease, may have had the paradoxical effect of increasing skepticism about cancer surgery by further lowering the apparent threshold for surgery. Even before pathologists had "discovered," defined, and reached consensus about precancers, some surgeons imagined their existence and exhorted their peers to define such stages and perform complete operations on those diagnosed.[20] In 1927, New York physician Henry C. Coe wrote to Joseph Bloodgood that he was "beginning to believe that the 'cure' of cancer by surgery in the future will depend upon our increasing ability to recognize a well-defined 'precancerous stage' – how, I do not know. My own clinical observations and experience with three members of my own family, in which a small 'lump' in the breast was promptly recognized and radical operation done, lead me to be even more radical than you. Why should not every accessible 'lump' be widely excised?"[21]

Bloodgood wrote in 1922 that, up until then, the Halstedian dictum "if you suspect cancer, better to do a complete operation" was upheld by himself and others.[22] This attitude could exacerbate widely held fears of mutilating cancer surgery, especially when many general practitioners and patients were not convinced that surgery would lead to cure.

The Apparent Efficacy of Surgery When Cancer Is "Taken in Time"

"Delay" supporters overcame these obstacles by stressing the efficacy of cancer surgery and increasing fear of cancer rather than reducing women's fear of surgery. This strategy was understandable given the real and unavoidable devastation produced by the complete operation and other radical cancer surgery. Skepticism about cancer surgery was not going to be overcome by spreading Halsted's notion that surgery only controlled local disease and had little effect on metastatic disease. Not surprisingly, in the years after he died, Halsted's narrow definition of the efficacy of cancer surgery gave way to claims about curing patients. Surgeons and others offered aggregate data from their own and others' clinical experience to demonstrate that women whose cancers were "taken in time," that is, removed surgically without delay, not only had reduced local recurrences but improved survival over women who presented later in the natural history of their disease. In many ways, however, these data were subject to the same sorts of limitations as studies done in the nineteenth century.

According to the English physician and public health official Janet Lane-Claypon, whose sophisticated and prescient epidemiological studies of breast cancer in the 1920s probably represented the highest quality data of that time, "it can hardly be doubted that an operation in the precancerous stage would rob cancer of the breast of most of its dangers, and the percentage of cures be greatly increased." At one level, such statements merely reflected clinical common sense – surgery would cure cancer if the disease was caught "early" in its natural history. Yet some observers questioned whether existing surgical practices actually removed cancer at an early enough stage to save lives.

Lane-Claypon attempted to answer such doubts by compiling statistics on breast cancer survival, carrying out a kind of crude meta-analysis of clinical observations, case series, and case reports in the published surgical literature from the early nineteenth century to the early 1920s. Her historical review of older surgeons' attitudes stressed their contempt for nonsurgical treatment rather than the more prevalent deeply rooted pessimism about surgery. "By much the larger portion of patients received into the cancer ward of the Middlesex Hospital have spent their last penny, and, what is worse, they have lost that precious time in which they might have been cured," Lane-Claypon quoted early-nineteenth-century surgeon Sir Charles Bell on medical men who did not recommend surgery as "the most unfeeling wretches that ever disgraced a country."

Lane-Claypon's more quantitative conclusion was that the mean duration of survival of breast cancer patients who underwent surgery was 5.7 years as compared with 3.6 years for those who did not. She also determined that survival was increased in women who presented at earlier stages of their cancer. In addition to these survival statistics (which were subject to selection and other biases noted by Agnew and others in the nineteenth century), Lane-Claypon determined that 43.1 percent of breast cancer patients in the pre-1924 literature had waited over a year to seek medical attention.[23] The combination of clinical common sense, the apparent efficacy of surgery, the correlation between early stage and survival, and the observation of delay (construed as room for improvement) represented a powerful argument for a public health campaign focused on reducing delay.

While Lane-Claypon's work was sometimes cited in the (small) cancer epidemiology literature in the 1920–1950 period, the frequent quantitative claims in both the medical and public education literature about the magnitude of the benefit when cancer was "taken in time" were mostly unsubstantiated and exaggerated. For example, as late as 1945 an article in a women's magazine could proclaim that "medical authorities tell us that *without discovery of a single new fact*, 30 to 50 percent of potential cancer victims can be saved. That means 4,000,000 to 6,500,000 living Americans."[24] A 1950s movie intended to change the attitudes and practices of physicians – specifically to increase their index of suspicion when interpreting seemingly benign symptoms and to conduct more periodic health exams – visually depicted breast and other cancers as individuals casting two shadows. Small solid ones represented site-specific cancer mortality "when diagnosis and treatment were early" and large nebulous shadows represented the gruesome contemporary situation. The specific claim for the early detection of breast cancer was a reduction in 5-year mortality from 75 to 25 percent.[25]

Since the start of the twentieth century, the purveyors of the "delay" message also claimed interim population-level success and used such claims to argue for the efficacy of surgery. "The impressive increase in the number of cures reported in 1941 as compared with 1920," began a typical popular report, "is owing to the improvement of diagnostic technique, the growing number of cancer clinics approved by the American College of Surgeons – from 13 in 1928 to 368 in 1943 – and, what is vitally important, the fact that people are more and more heeding the symptoms of cancer when they first appear."[26] Looking forward in time, cancer education materials frequently claimed that more compliance with the "delay" message would lead to an even greater number of cures. According to a 1956 cancer publication, "authorities confidently believe that this rate of cure (one in four) could be doubled if more persons could be induced to seek medical help when the first signs or symptoms of cancer arose or would submit themselves to regular cancer detection examinations."[27]

Assumptions about the natural history of breast and other cancers, such as that cancer is uniformly and rapidly fatal, permitted observers to claim – in the absence of adequate controls – that surgery was responsible for apparent cures and prolonged survivals afterward. "It is obvious

that the mortality from untreated cancer is 100 per cent," wrote one surgeon in the 1930s.[28] James Ewing, the preeminent cancer pathologist of
the first half of the twentieth century, reportedly taught that "if a woman
neglects a cancerous lump in her breast, involvement of the axilla, or
armpit, will occur in approximately six months time."[29] Statements such
as Ewing's reflected the widely held assumption that breast cancer always
spread in an orderly, incremental, and local manner.

"Delay" and the Existential, Moral, and Medical Uncertainties of Doctors and Patients

The success of the campaign was not only a matter of promoting surgical efficacy. It is also important to see how the entire "delay" cluster of
assumptions – about time, cancer's orderly and local growth, its uniformity – "worked" at the clinical level. These ideas and language provided
a framework with which doctors among themselves or in their dealings
with patients could more easily negotiate responsibility for cancer. The
inability to cure cancer could be blamed on another physician's temporizing or on a patient coming to medical attention too late. Time played a
complementary role to extensive surgery. Progression of cancer and death
could be and was blamed on failure to hew the proper line, either by
delaying or by incomplete surgery.

"Delay" also served a similar purpose for patients and the lay public,
who, as we saw earlier, not only feared cancer but understood it to strike
or progress at random, without any effective way to avoid it. Lay persons'
fears of cancer could be mitigated by knowledge that there was something
to do to prevent it – seek early medical attention for suspicious cancer
signs. "Delay" linked individual responsibility for disease with good outcomes. Individuals were told that heightened awareness and early medical attention represented an insurance policy against cancer.

While the "delay" message thus made women more responsible for
their disease, it minimized for clinicians some of the existential, moral,
and medical uncertainties of taking care of patients with cancer. Few clinicians, even surgeons, saw enough patients with cancer, breast or otherwise, to have more than a fragmentary personal angle on the kind of
aggregate picture of the disease built up by years of accumulated clinical
experience and recorded in textbooks or by the kinds of statistical models
that were being constructed by epidemiologists. Nevertheless, clinicians

had to reconcile the needs and demands of, and anxieties raised by, individual patients with this aggregate reality.

In 1907, surgeon E. B. Hayworth wrote to Halsted about a disturbing case. A Yonkers doctor had criticized Hayworth for the way he cared for Mrs. Connoly. Ten years before consulting Hayworth, Connoly had an incomplete breast amputation (the axilla was not opened) for suspected cancer. At the time of her first visit to Hayworth a year earlier, he discovered that all her glands were enlarged, "two being size of hen eggs and adherent to adjacent tissues etc." Hayworth operated on Connolly and found extensive disease in the axilla, neck, and around the heart and removed what he could (he was unable to remove all of the extensive disease). "To let the patient down easily, I told her the examination showed them to be semi-malignant and that x-ray treatment should be followed to prevent a return." She returned 2 months later with disease along the edge of the chest wall muscles that Hayworth had removed. He continued:

> The patient has never yet presented herself for a course of x-ray treatment. The case is interesting from the long period existing between the removal of the breast and the involvement of the axillary glands. If you think my handling of the case was proper I would be glad to have you so express yourself to Mrs. Connoly – as I believe from the criticisms of her Yonkers physician she is under the impression that the surgical treatment she received at my hand was improperly performed.[30]

In this short letter, Dr. Hayworth managed to criticize the surgeon who first operated on Mrs. Connoly for not removing her axillary glands, express amazement at the long interval between her initial presentation of breast cancer and her later recurrence, convey worry and frustration at his own inability to completely excise all cancerous tissue in the operation he performed, and implicitly blame the patient for waiting until her lymph nodes were the size of hen eggs before seeking medical care and later for not getting x-ray treatments.

Along with Halstedian beliefs about completeness, the "delay" cluster of ideas provided a framework to order and rationalize the moral complexities inherent in the routine care of women with breast cancer. Apportioning blame and responsibility played so large a role in part because of the gaps between the particular circumstances of Mrs. Connoly's case and different aspects of the breast cancer ideal-type: between the first surgeon's decision "not to open the axilla" and the Halstedian surgical ideal of removing all cancerous tissue and then some en bloc, itself justified by a localistic, orderly model of the natural history of breast cancer; between Dr. Hayworth's inability to remove all cancerous tissue during surgery and that same ideal; and between the patient's implied delay and her failure to present for x-ray treatments, on the one hand, and medical expectations of the compliant patient, assumptions about the natural history of cancer, and a positivism about existing treatments, on the other.

The "delay" narrative did not close these gaps but provided a way to simplify the very precarious moral implications of choices made in situations that did not always conform to idealized pictures of disease, doctors, or patients. "Delay" provided a way for doctors not only to shift blame toward each other and onto patients, but also to make a simple connection between the idiosyncrasies of a specific individual's case and a model of the disease's typical course (as in Dr. Hayworth's surprise over the long interval between Mrs. Connoly's initial surgery and her first recurrence) – and therefore bring order to a morally perilous situation ("the case is interesting . . .",). The "delay" message allowed physicians to blame time or the patient rather than their surgery or disease concepts if bad outcomes ensued. Dr. Hayworth and other doctors could reassure themselves that some unanticipated and feared events were exceptions to the rule and thus not their fault.

The apportioning of blame that is evidenced in Dr. Hayworth's letter was common but not always offered in such a transparently condescending style. Another of Halsted's correspondents introduced a patient to him in 1914, writing "I know, Dr. Halsted, that you will do everything possible for her. I am only sorry that she did not come to me sooner, but this is the best we could do."[31] Regret and sadness for the patient as well as some gesture of joint responsibility soften but do not fundamentally alter the assumption that delay had led to worse consequences for the patient.

There was a halting progression to a less overt style of victim blaming (although not necessarily changed in substance) in cancer education materials as the twentieth century progressed. In 1920, the ASCC arranged a diorama exhibit on cancer built on a simplistic and overtly moralistic choice faced by a woman with a breast lump – the right way and the wrong way. In the diorama depicting the right way, one woman says to the other, "All persistent lumps or other unusual conditions in

women are suspicious....It might be cancer....Please see a good doctor." The second woman goes to the doctor and gets a correct diagnosis
and treatment. After 2 weeks in the hospital, she tells her friends, "Yes
the doctor says I am cured. Now I shall help spread the message of early
treatment." In the diorama depicting the wrong way, a woman delays and
ends up not only with cancer but broke. "Two years have exhausted all
our savings," she pleads to a bank officer. "I must get a position to support
my children."[32]

As late as 1944, C. C. Little, an ASCC executive and the principal
initiator of its Women's Field Army (WFA) volunteers, depicted delay
and popular fears of cancer as a "profound psychosis" in WFA training
material. WFA training was built on the "creation and maintenance of
personal responsibility. This is the most important matter of all. The Field
Army worker must appreciate that she has undertaken more than an ordinary share of individual responsibility in the fight against cancer."[33] As
pioneers in personal responsibility, WFA volunteers were supposed to get
at least biyearly cancer examinations.

By the 1940s, however, the blame-giving message was usually presented in a more sophisticated, although no less moralistic, manner. "If
she does not watch for those signs, or if, after discovering them, she does
not seek competent medical care until cancer has passed its early most
curable stage," an author of an article in a women's magazine in 1945
asserted, "she has no one to blame for the consequences but herself."[34]
"There were the usual problems that arise in all families, the sons' mar-
riages and the widowhood of one," another typical popular article related,
"whose wife, tragically enough, suspected that she was a victim of cancer but told nobody, and paid the ultimate price for her secret."[35] In a
1948 popular article, typical of a gentler variant of the "delay" narrative,
a woman wrote about the guilt and indecision that surrounded her delay
in seeking care for a lump in her right shoulder blade. When it turned
out to be benign, she regretted the 2 years of self-inflicted agony.[36]

By the 1950s, the American Cancer Society (ACS), the successor
organization to the ASCC, had begun its "little red door" campaign, an
attempt to make walking into an ACS office less threatening, as part of
its attempt to modulate the fear-inspiring effects of the "delay" message.
In some "delay" educational materials, the ACS changed the label of the
delaying group from "certain to die" to "dependent on new discoveries."
The ACS also encouraged more nuanced delay narratives by offering a

$500 prize for the best breast cancer story, defined as one about "noticing" the first symptom, which could then be popularized.[37]

Both to hammer home the issue of personal responsibility and to stress the mechanistic and orderly vision of cancer that was the basis for the "delay" message, popular writers frequently used analogies to familiar technologies. This enabled them to point out the seemingly absurd situation that people often take better care of their machines, possessions, and surroundings than their bodies. A 1923 ASCC poster showed a picture of a forest fire accompanied by the following text: "As With a Fire So With Cancer. Prompt and efficient action is necessary to prevent spreading and final Destruction!"[38] "If a water pipe breaks in your house," similarly analogized *Journal of the American Association* editor Morris Fishbein about cancer delay in 1947, "you call a plumber just as soon as the first few drops of water seep through the ceiling."[39] A 1952 cartoon film, *Man Alive*, was built on an analogy between cars and bodies, mechanical trouble and cancer. The movie lampooned men who would take preventative precautions with their car but not their own bodies.[40] Other "delay" public health literature made analogies between proper lawn care and care of one's own body.[41]

Other stylistic qualities of the early detection message as it appeared in voluntary and public health campaigns also help explain the centrality and durability of the "delay" message. As others have frequently pointed out, this message was consistently and intentionally enveloped in images and narratives that emphasized the dangers of delay, that is, the message was built on fears of cancer.[42] These images and narratives were gripping, direct, and easily understood. In 1948, the American Cancer Society launched a "1 every 3 minutes" (someone dies of cancer) poster campaign.[43] In later decades, they employed a similar and progressing "one in N" campaign about cancer incidence. In 1949, ACS publicity director James Hauck wrote philanthropist and cancer activist Mary Lasker about his worries over the ACS's statistically oriented fear campaign after a satirical article on ACS campaigns titled "one out of one will die" appeared in the popular press.[44] Cancer activists dealt with these objections in print as well. "There have been some comments to the effect that these cancer-detection clinics, all the talk of cancer, the cancer campaigns, are breeding a race of 'cancerophobes,'" a popular piece recounted. "It is true that some people overdo the cancer hunt and can worry themselves into an illness trying to avoid one. But most observers agree that the lives saved by intelligent preventive measures more than make up for the few additions to the ranks of hypochondriacs."[45]

A more Freudian version of the "delay" narrative appeared in the 1950s and 1960s. In a 1964 report of psychiatric evaluations of women with breast cancer who delayed (which was defined as either admitting delay or – with great circularity – having presented to medical attention in the late stages of cancer), the long history of the "delay" campaign was itself cited as evidence of these women's failure to take adequate responsibility. "Although there have been intensive efforts to inform the public through periodicals, radio, television, and other media," the psychiatrist-author recounts, "many women with obvious signs of disease of the breast present themselves for treatment when the disease is so far advanced that only palliation is possible." According to the author, the main reasons for delay are to be found in women's retarded psychosocial development, specifically a failure to develop pleasurable breast sensations and associations. And in what reads like a cruel parody, centuries-old fears of breast cancer surgery were now reconfigured as individual pathology. When one woman asserts, "I was worried about being disfigured," this was understood as "evidence both of her narcissism and her low self-esteem."[46]

The Self-Reinforcing Cycle of Perceived Efficacy and Behavior Change

The mass campaign was effective in changing the attitudes of many women and some general practitioners about cancer. Increased fear of cancer and less skepticism about surgery did lead to an increased number of women reporting to their doctors with suspicious cancer signs. More women got biopsies (which had supplanted Halstedian surgical diagnosis). Breast lumps were much more commonly benign or had a more favorable prognosis than in previous eras. There are many lines of evidence to support this contention.

As early as the 1920s, physicians had observed a dramatic decline in women's self-report of delay in seeking medical attention for cancer symptoms. A mid-1930s discussion of cancer education compared women's delay in 1911, when the average duration between onset of symptoms and medical visits was 16.7 months, to 1933, when the duration was 8.1 months.[47] In the late 1940s, the ACS reported that surveys had found a more modest decline in the relative numbers of women who delayed seeking cancer care between 1923–1938 (79.3 percent) and 1946–1947 (70.6 percent).[48]

Not only did women appear to be delaying less as the century wore on, they were presenting with fewer symptoms, smaller lumps, and with more benign disease. Deaver, writing in the 1920s, was astounded by the changing composition of women who presented with breast lumps, observing that women now, "due to propaganda," often present with "imaginary" breast lumps.[49] As noted earlier, Bloodgood remarked with astonishment in 1922 that he was advising no surgery in over half the patients with breast complaints.[50] Bloodgood also observed that the negative breast biopsy rate on the Hopkins surgical service, about 1 percent in the 1890s, had risen to 75 percent by 1923.[51] Robert Greenough, writing in 1935 about breast cancer patients presenting to Massachusetts General Hospital, noted that while 74 percent of cases showed axillary involvement (a bad prognostic factor) in 1914 that figure had dropped to 40 percent. "This, I believe," Greenough concluded, "is a clear indication of the value of public education."[52]

Women's decision not to delay interacted with pathological practice in other ways as well. The increasing use of new methods of intraoperative diagnosis such as frozen sections lessened lay and medical fears of unnecessary "complete operations." Observers also noted that pathologists in the first few decades of this century had lowered their threshold as to what constituted cancer.[53] Pathologists also developed new concepts of early and "precancerous" entities, such as Foote and Stewart's description of lobular carcinoma in situ in 1941, which raised the number of pathological diagnoses for women who had better prognoses, thereby increasing the apparent efficacy of treatment (see Chapter 7 for fuller discussion).[54]

Women's decisions to present to their doctors in greater numbers and with less delay made the management of breast lumps more difficult in some ways. In 1935, Bloodgood noted that it had become harder in recent years to distinguish benign from malignant disease on clinical grounds and there was more unnecessary surgery than in earlier decades.[55]

The larger and healthier subset of women presenting to doctors with cancer-related complaints strengthened the belief that both modern treatments and the public health campaign built on the "delay" message worked. Some public health activists even argued that it was a woman's duty to report immediately to a doctor with a suspicious lump because such actions on a large scale would lead to better statistics, less fear of cancer, and even more early detection. "If you have a lump in your breast," wrote the author of a 1935 "delay" piece for lay persons, "you have a duty to other women. Every time a woman comes early and joins the numbers of the intelligent woman whose examination revealed that there was no need of operation or whose lives were saved by early operation, the lifesaving gospel of early attention gains further prestige with the public and spreads to save more lives."[56]

Because of the larger and healthier denominator (due to more women complying with the "delay" message and changed diagnostic practices) the ratio of breast cancer deaths (which was either stable or increasing at a much lower rate than new diagnoses) over women with breast cancer (sometimes called the case fatality ratio) dramatically decreased in those early decades. Put another way, an individual's chances of surviving breast cancer had increased. This decreased case fatality rate or its corollary increased survival rate created the impression that cancer education, via decreased delay along with effective surgery, had led to a genuine improvement in the health of ordinary women. This in turn led more women to seek "early" medical attention, resulting in more diagnoses, and to a further increase in the impression of effectiveness.

Thus, there existed by mid-century a self-sustaining feedback loop in which attitudes and beliefs about the natural history and treatment of breast cancer and the efficacy of early detection led to behavioral changes that changed popular and medical perception of aggregate data about cancer, which in turn sustained attitudinal and behavioral changes. This powerful set of reinforcing perceptions and behaviors managed to keep the "delay" message at center stage through most of the twentieth century even as skeptical voices questioned the efficacy (especially using the unchanged mortality from cancer), style, and implications of the campaign.[57]

SEVEN

"Prophets of Doom"

Skeptics of the Cancer Establishment at Mid-Century

Mrs. Bronson's Fears of Breast Cancer

In the mid-1950s, Mrs. Bronson had a horrible dream. A male voice repeatedly uttered "cancer," telling her that cancer was a "gangster in the body" that "grows and grows ... a horror that never stops." The voice continued: "Is it contagious? Is it inherited? Will my kids have it too? What will happen to me? Will I die?" Waking up from this nightmare as her own voice pounded out the words "cancer, cancer," Mrs. Bronson experienced no relief. Her waking life had itself become a nightmare ever since she had perceived a lump in her breast a few weeks earlier.

Mrs. Bronson's family knew nothing about her breast lump or her fears. After getting her husband off to work and her children to school, she set out on some errands in the tidy, middle-sized American town in which she had lived all of her life. In her local pharmacy, she bought some milk. Distracted and impatient, she dropped it on the pharmacy floor. Frozen with embarrassment and fear, Mrs. Bronson was transfixed on the growing puddle until she abruptly ran out of the door, leaving the drug-gist, her long-time neighbor, shrugging his shoulders in disbelief. Walking quickly down the street, not knowing where to go or what to do, Mrs. Bronson found herself in front of the local branch of the Women's Field Army (WFA) of the American Cancer Society (ACS, the newly renamed ASCC). She stared at the posters that contained messages like "Only you can prevent cancer" and "With a check-up and a check," sum-moned up her courage, and opened the door.

Inside the office, an unassuming WFA volunteer of about Mrs. Bronson's age and social background greeted her, invited her into a well-lit office, and listened to Mrs. Bronson's story. The volunteer told

Mrs. Bronson that she had come to the right place and that her fears would soon be allayed. She also told Mrs. Bronson about the mission of the ACS and gave her an overview of the many ACS research and educational programs. The ACS message was that no one is immune to cancer. One American in eight will die of cancer, more than 175,000 per year, more Americans than were killed in the entire World War II. But with early detection and modern treatment, more and more Americans were being saved from this curse. Mrs. Bronson's visit was to be more than educational. Before she left, the ACS volunteer picked up the phone and made an appointment for Mrs. Bronson with a family doctor in private practice.

The doctor found time to see Mrs. Bronson almost immediately. His brightly lit office was reassuring. Drawing a simple diagram of the breast and surrounding tissues, the doctor explained that cancer is a disease of errant cells that grow in size within the breast for a long period before spreading to the lymph glands in the armpit, from where it sadly can spread throughout the entire body if not caught in time. He explained that the only way to know if Mrs. Bronson had cancer was to do a biopsy, which he characterized as a minor procedure. He hinted but did not exactly say that if the biopsy showed cancer the surgeon would proceed at once to a complete cancer operation, the details of which were not spelled out. Mrs. Brown agreed to the biopsy. There was no formal consent process and no discussion of the risks and benefits of the biopsy or subsequent surgery.

In what seemed like another instant, Mrs. Bronson was anesthetized and undergoing surgery in a large, brightly lit amphitheater with many doctors and nurses in attendance. The surgeon removed a small piece of Mrs. Bronson's breast lump, which an assistant carried to the nearby pathology laboratory. With their gloved hands extended in the air, the entire operating staff waited in suspense for the verdict from the pathologist. The pathologist quickly froze the specimen and took razor thin slices using a specialized machine. The tissue slices were then quickly fixed and mounted on slides. The clock in the operating room ticked loudly. "Which will it be?" the pathologist and the whole operating team wondered. The pathologist reviewed the slide and sent a message to the operating room – the lump was benign, no need for a complete operation. After the anesthesia had worn off, the surgeon and the family doctor told Mrs. Bronson the good news. Not only was she greatly relieved but she was also thankful for the help of the American Cancer Society and the private family doctor and surgeon to whom they had referred her. In appreciation, Mrs. Bronson became a member of the Women's Field Army and was soon making bandages, fund raising, typing blood, visiting children with terminal disease, bringing neighbors to ACS educational programs, and counseling other scared women with the message that "time is life."

MRS. BRONSON, OF COURSE, IS OR WAS A CELLULOID CHARACTER. HER story formed the central plot in an educational film, "Time is life," jointly produced by the American Cancer Society and the U.S. Government sometime in the 1950s.[1] It was shown to women's groups and other lay audiences until it was retired in 1969. It was remarkably similar in plot structure to an ASCC film "Choose to Live" that was produced 20 years earlier.[2] The newer film had the same core "do not delay" message but presented it with scarier and technically more polished Hitchcockian effects, such as the way the camera in the opening scene panned over the shadowy town into Mrs. Bronson's bedroom (separate marital beds of course) and Freudian plot devices such as the use of the growing puddle of spilled milk to signal unconscious distress.

The one and revealing major plot shift was that the woman in the earlier film did have cancer, necessitating one-stop surgery, while Mrs. Bronson's biopsy was normal.[3] In addition to falling back from the excesses of the campaign of fear, the normal biopsy in the newer film reflected the fact that as more women sought medical attention for breast lumps, a far greater number of them would have negative biopsies. Mrs. Bronson's narrative of fear and release was becoming increasingly prevalent. Many lay people lived with the terror that they had cancer as a direct result of public health messages and screening programs only to learn later, through other medical interventions, that their fears were baseless. This experience often gave men and women a sense of meaning and purpose, leaving them with few regrets about all that they had experienced.

While "Mrs. Bronson" represented the climax of the "do not delay" effort, each and every aspect of her composite reality was by 1950 inspiring a good deal of dissent, much of it passionate. A small number of surgeons, pathologists, epidemiologists, public health workers, and lay persons were voicing their doubts about the different cancer beliefs and practices that constituted Mrs. Bronson: the manipulation of public fear in service of attitudinal and behavior change; the moralism surrounding the one correct clinical approach; the burden of responsibility for surveillance and early detection of cancer placed on individuals; the epidemiological perception that cancer was a growing threat to the nation's health; the orderly, localistic, ontologic model of cancer's natural history and the radical surgery it rationalized; and the optimism and sense of progress about present and future treatments and public health interventions. The very alliance between the ACS and the National Cancer Institute that made possible the filming of "Time is life" itself became the object of a mid-century counterreaction. These skeptical voices were in the minority, diverse, and ill-organized, especially in comparison to the centralized, nationwide efforts of the ACS and the National Cancer Institute. Skeptics came from different quarters, had different agendas, and often drew upon questions, ideas, and practices that preceded the Halstedian surgical revolution and the early detection public health efforts. What is typically recalled about this dissent is the opposition to radical cancer surgery. This is understandable because the extent of surgery became the explicit focus and rallying cry for many medical and lay critics in the 1960s and afterward. But not only has the story of opposition to the radical mastectomy been told repeatedly and well, we also reduce and distort a larger set of developments and their implications for the present if we understand the skepticism in the pre-1960 period as one exclusively over the best type of surgery for women with diagnosed breast cancer. So in the sections below I trace a series of parallel and interacting countercurrents of beliefs and practices, deliberately playing down the more frequently told story of the opposition to the radical mastectomy.[4]

Progress Against Cancer?

A half-century of publically promoted optimism, behavioral and attitudinal change, and the diffusion of early, radical surgery had not delivered on the turn-of-the century promise that progress against cancer would soon be made. The falling twentieth century "case-fatality" ratio was the good news about cancer's aggregate impact. A woman diagnosed with breast cancer had much better odds of surviving at the middle of the twentieth century than one at its beginning. "Thirty years ago, a woman having cancer of the breast was almost certain to die of it," one observer emphasized in 1948. "Today, due to early diagnosis and greater refinement in surgery and treatment, cures have jumped and cancer doesn't mean a death sentence."[5]

But the falling case-fatality ratio was only one way of perceiving progress. Cancer mortality rates were generally increasing or at best stable during this period. This stable or increased mortality rate eventually deflated the cascade of changed behavior and perception of success that had long driven the "do not delay" campaign.[6] The absence of a perceptible decline in age-adjusted cancer mortality could be and was interpreted by some observers as a sign of clinical, public health, and societal failure. "The persistence of uniform level trends in rates derived from such diverse and changing circumstances," vocal critic N. E. Mckinnon wrote in 1955, "thus leaves no doubt that control programs providing earlier and more treatment have not achieved any decisive reduction in mortality."[7]

Some clinicians, having witnessed the improved chances that their breast cancer patients would survive compared to those in previous eras, were affronted by skeptical inferences from cancer statistics such as those drawn by Mckinnon and others. "There are those who on a purely *statistical basis*," surgeon Robert Janes disdainfully noted in 1944 (italics mine), "tell us that we have not in anyway influenced the mortality rate from carcinoma of the breast in all these years."[8] For Janes and other defenders of the "delay" campaign, it was the aggregate statistical impression, rather than the clinical gaze, that was illusory.

There was a widespread perception that cancer statistics were misleading.[9] The numbers that the statistician or epidemiologist counted were of course only as good as what had been recorded as cause of death and how accurately cancer had been diagnosed in the first place. Some observers pointed to the way that older inaccuracies in registering cancer deaths (such as registering affected organs rather than the organ in which cancer originated as the cause of cancer death) and the greater life-span of current cohorts relative to the past could explain the apparent increased rates of certain cancers and cancer in general.

"When the death return comes from anyone but a physician, the cause of death is seldom reported as cancer," Willcox observed in 1917.[10] One physician, writing in 1921, made an analogy between the "apparent increase" in cancer mortality "where no real one exists" and the recorded 40 percent increase in mortality from appendicitis between 1900 and 1915. The "real rate," suggested this physician, was undoubtedly "decreasing in this period because of surgical advance and readiness to resort to surgery."[11]

Better population-level statistics and analysis were needed. One source of innovation was the burgeoning life insurance industry. Life insurance companies needed to accurately predict the likely mortality experience of policyholders and had an economic interest in reducing cancer mortality. Two of the most prolific American researchers studying population trends in cancer were Louis Dublin, who worked for Metropolitan Life Insurance, and Frederick Hoffman, who worked for Prudential. Hoffman was involved with the ASCC from its beginnings and Dublin was an active member in the organization later on. In its early years, a significant portion of the ASCC budget came from the Metropolitan Life Insurance Company.[12]

In 1925, Dublin had noted the rising cancer mortality among Metropolitan policyholders, observing that cancer had risen to one eleventh of Metropolitan payouts, and argued for a national response.[13] Hoffman conducted intensive studies of cancer mortality throughout the world and made many causal inferences. His studies of breast cancer supported a general correlation between "civilization" and breast cancer mortality. In one study, for example, he noted the unusually low proportion of breast cancer deaths/total cancer deaths ratio in Chile, compared to the much higher rate in New Zealand. Hoffman similarly noted that breast cancer was virtually unknown in Japan "except among the higher types of the race who live practically European lives."[14]

Another innovation was the establishment of cancer registries. State laws increasingly mandated that uniform and complete reporting of clinical and pathological data about all new cancer diagnoses be sent to centralized state offices. The first such registry in the United States was in Connecticut in 1936. Cancer registries provided a more reliable way of evaluating cancer's distribution in a population, secular trends, and miscellaneous correlations that might offer clues to cancer's causes, as well as cementing the centrality of hospitals and hospital-based pathologists in cancer clinical care and research.

At mid-century, most Americans did not need to wait on more accurate cancer statistics and better analyses to perceive that there was something very worrying about cancer trends. Viewed in terms of what was likely to cause individual death, cancer was palpably perceived to be a much greater threat not only in the early twentieth century relative to the nineteenth century but at the middle of the twentieth century compared to its beginning. Without knowing the exact numbers, Americans could readily perceive the dramatic relative mortality shift between 1900 (which already represented a greatly increased mortality from 50 years earlier) and 1950. In 1900, cancer was the ninth leading cause of mortality in the United States (as recorded by death certificates). The annual cancer mortality rate was 64 deaths per 100,000 people while the overall American mortality rate was 1,719 deaths per 100,000 people. By 1950, the annual cancer mortality rate was now 140 per 100,000 people at a time when the overall mortality rate had fallen to 964 deaths per 100,000 people.

The combination of the more than doubling of cancer mortality and the near halving of overall mortality resulted in a quadrupling of cancer's relative proportion of deaths, from approximately 4 percent to over 15 percent of the total mortality burden over the course of the first half of the twentieth century.[15] Americans understood that their individual odds of dying from cancer as opposed to some other cause had radically increased in the first half of the twentieth century.

The increasing odds of dying from cancer were all the more disturbing when perceived against the declining population impact of acute infectious disease. In contrast to acute, infectious diseases, there was no apparent decline in American breast cancer rates either with the progression of time or by escape from the material and social conditions of poverty (in fact, the opposite trend in social class seemed operative). As both medical and social problems, breast and other cancers seemed not only intractable but ran counter to the prevailing trends that generally associated modernization and entry into middle class life with progress against disease. "During the same period of years that witnessed remarkable progress in the control of tuberculosis, typhoid fever, malaria, and other important diseases, where rationally conceived preventive measures have been effective," Dublin argued, "the cancer control movement has apparently made no impress."[16] In 1942, Haagensen observed a similar lack of progress in breast cancer mortality and used this observation to argue for more radical surgery rather than as evidence that current treatments and public health campaigns were ineffective.[17]

From the late 1920s onward, other critics of the ASCC campaign demonstrated the ineffectiveness of the ASCC's "delay" campaign on its own terms. Philadelphia physicians Stanley Reimann and Frederick

Safford in 1928 showed that the onset of the ASCC campaign in 1914 was not associated with any change in the steady decline since 1900 in the period of time women "delayed" seeking medical attention after noticing a breast lump. Since the campaign might not even have positively influenced women's behavior, they decried the "campaign of fear" waged against the public:

> Should the propaganda be increased, until every newspaper every day carries some warning, until every radio set in every home every day enunciates at least once, "be careful of cancer," until every week is cancer week? This is obviously a reductio ad absurdum. Popular cancer propaganda in the United States, and we suspect in other countries also, has some undesirable aspects. It has unduly disturbed the peace of mind of many normal individuals and made veritable 'cancerophobes' of many.[18]

Clinicians traded stories with each other about how the campaign made healthy patients fear they had cancer, so much so that excessive fear was a useful diagnostic sign that the patient did not have cancer (and vice versa). "A prominent surgeon says that when a patient comes to him and tells him that she is worried to death about a lump which appeared in her breast a short time ago and is causing severe pain, he is fairly sure that she does not have cancer," a medical journalist in 1945 reported. "But when a patient comes in apologizing for taking up his time and saying that she is coming only because her daughter or some friend insists on her doing so . . . he immediately gets another grey hair, for he is fairly sure the patient has cancer."[19]

Pessimism about cancer detection was also part of the criticism of the overselling of cancer fear and the effectiveness of treatment. Writing about centralized cancer detection and treatment efforts, Cleveland surgeon George Crile Jr. wrote

> Great clinics will be built for the detection of cancer. Billions will be spent, and for what purpose? Have we proved that more facilities will cure more cancers? Out efforts in the last twenty years have failed to reduce the rate of death from cancer. Is cancer when detected early more curable than when treated a little late? These are questions that must be answered. We must not live on in a dream of wishful thought. If we do, we are like our primitive ancestors, building temples to our ignorance and making sacrifices to the gods of fear.[20]

"We finally had to conclude," Dr. Raymond Kaiser, long time United States Public Health Service (USPHS) cancer control director recalled, "that from the standpoint of finding cancer in any form, that the amount of effort and expenditure didn't support our findings. We didn't find enough cancer by this means." And, as Kaiser put it in another context, "actually there was very little we could apply to control because we didn't have cancer detection procedures and methods that really worked."[21]

In the early decades of the "delay" campaign, cancer activists frequently acknowledged that prevention campaigns and practices necessarily increased fear of cancer, but accepted that to make an omelette one had to crack some eggs. In 1927, Halsted's protégée Joseph Bloodgood, for example, acknowledged, even celebrated, this trade-off, writing that "they [his cancer patients] come because of that little element of fear, so we can safely make the statement that fear in the beginning of disease will help you. The fact that an individual consults his physician because of fear of disease marks one of the greatest triumphs of the art of medicine."[22]

But by mid-century, many ACS affiliated cancer activists were increasingly critical of the use of fear, in part because fear-inspiring messages had increased and reached potentially inappropriate audiences such as children. In 1948, an ACS official announced a decision to withdraw a child-oriented pamphlet, the "Changing of the Guard," because it targeted the under-twelve set with frightening messages such as that "some women die of cancer when they are about as old as your mother is," "Cancer kills more fathers and mothers than any other sickness," or "If a mother or father dies (of cancer), a home is broken up."[23]

The Rediscovery of Idiosyncrasy

In contrast to received ideas about cancer's local origins and the power of surgery to effectively cure "early" cancer, mid-twentieth-century skeptics stressed breast cancer's idiosyncratic nature and the poor correlation between pathological diagnosis and subsequent clinical course. They often repeated the nineteenth-century observation that many women who had small tumors that were detected "early" and who underwent complete operations nevertheless died of metastatic disease, while other women who had "delayed" for years nevertheless survived their disease, often with no intervention or having had less-than-complete operations.

The authors of a 1932 clinical series from Johns Hopkins expressed their "great uncertainty as to whether or not the biological characteristics of a malignant growth can be prognosticated from an objective histological examination." These authors contrasted two patients, one of whom had a small tumor that "existed for forty years before operation, after which the patient lived for many years" and another whose tumor was "very large," of 3 months duration, and who "died from generalized metastases within 6 months. However, both tumors were infiltrating scirrhus carcinomata indistinguishable in their microscopical pattern."[24]

This rediscovery of cancer's idiosyncrasy was not confined to a small number of peripheral critics. Many elite surgeons and pathologists recognized the great variability in breast cancer's natural history and the imperfect connection between clinical and pathological staging (systems for gauging degree of cancer spread) and subsequent events. Leading pathologist and cancer theorist James Ewing (1866–1943) summed up idiosyncrasy in breast cancer and its disturbing implications in 1928: "I have drawn the impression that in dealing with mammary cancer, surgery meets with more peculiar difficulties and uncertainties than with almost any other form of the disease. The anatomical types are so numerous, the variations in clinical course so wide, the paths of dissemination so free and diverse, the difficulties of determining the actual conditions so complex, and the sacrifice of tissue so great, as to render impossible in a majority of cases a reasonably accurate adjustment of means to an end."[25]

The medical literature in the first half of the twentieth century was replete with similar observations about breast cancer's idiosyncrasy. Like Ewing, most observers did not take their frustration to the point of rejecting the received, "localist" natural history dogma. They hoped that more research and clinical and technological improvements could rationalize and improve upon the disturbing inability to predict the clinical course of cancer from pathological findings. One physician in 1948 noted that cancer often looked identical to embryonic tissue and observed, as Paget did in the nineteenth century, that cancer was ultimately a biological, not a morphological, entity. But instead of rejecting pathological cancer staging, he hoped for new biological tests for cancer, such as one that would test tissues' ability to survive transplantation, that would replace existing, that is, static and morphological, diagnostic practices.[26]

Throughout the twentieth century, many clinicians were frustrated by the inability to find predisposing or exciting factors. "When we come to cancer of the breast, the most prevalent type of the disease in the female, we cannot find so evident a cause," Philadelphia surgeon J. B. Deaver wrote sometime in the early part of the century. "Most cases of breast cancer, strange to say, attack healthy, robust women. Here we must incline to the theory of susceptibility, although we cannot as yet account for the susceptibility nor can we combat it."[27]

Predeterminism – Questioning the Received Model of Cancer's Natural History

Some mid-twentieth-century American surgeons, pathologists, and others offered a more programmatic and radical critique of the cancer status quo. Most notable was Los Angeles surgeon Ian MacDonald who became associated with a set of critical ideas that he and others labeled "predeterminism." According to MacDonald, the biological characteristics of breast and other tumors, mostly genetic but also related to as yet poorly-understood host-tumor interactions, rather than the apparent stage of disease, determined the tumor's subsequent clinical course. MacDonald linked this predeterminist view to idiosyncrasy, saying that "each patient is an individual problem; the attack on a specific neoplasm [tumor or growth] should be conditioned upon a knowledge of its usual biologic pattern and the best evaluation possible of its behavior in the individual."[28] He also called for "a radical change in the clinician's philosophy of cancer therapy. Rigid ideas of prognosis in terms of duration and dimension should be abandoned in favor of an attempt to evaluate the biological potential of a neoplasm in an individual host."[29]

The problem that MacDonald and other "predeterminists" faced was that there was little knowledge about and few tools with which to divine – and effectively intervene in – the unique biological features of tumors or the host–tumor interaction. So despite some rhetorical efforts to deny it, predeterminism, in line with the term's everyday meaning, had a decidedly nihilistic meaning and oppositional character. Black and Speer's 1953 formulation of the predeterminist counterdogma captured these qualities. "It is implied in data prepared for lay consumption as well as in medical writings that early diagnosis of breast carcinoma and radical mastectomy would result in almost universal control of the disease," they wrote. "This latter utopian state is presumed to be attainable by greater public education and physician awareness in order to bring the patient to surgery as soon as possible after the appearance of the breast mass." Delivering their coup de grace to received ideas and practices, Black and Speer concluded that "the tacitly assumed uniformity of biologic behavior and autonomy which is the basis and 'raison d'être' of current teachings and practices in regard to breast carcinoma is untenable."[30]

Most skeptics did not go so far as Black and Spear in rejecting the orderly natural history of cancer, but they acknowledged, as one observer put it, the "lamentable fact that the very early stage of the most active cancers are probably present without the patient's knowledge, and with all our present diagnostic equipments are undetectable and represent an absolute subclinical picture which we have at present no known method of recognizing."[31] MacDonald brought his clinical experience to bear on claims made about the effectiveness of the "delay" campaign, pointing out to his fellow clinicians that there was no objective way to measure when patients first began to suffer symptoms from cancer. He observed that "it is readily apparent that no method is available by which the duration of human cancer can be determined with accuracy. Even in the visible palpable lesions the clinical history is clouded by tricks of memory and retrospective association with other events, and occasionally by deliberate falsification. This historical uncertainty becomes deepened for the inaccessible sites where vague departures from the normal state of physiological unawareness of visceral function are the only 'early' symptoms of cancer."[32]

MacDonald and other predeterminists pointed out the biases and systematic problems that sustained the conventional view of breast and other cancers' natural history and curability. They pointed out that what we would today call negative publication bias contributed to the misapprehension that breast and other cancers had an orderly natural history. Studies that showed no effect of "early" surgery or no association between stage and survival were less likely to be published. Responding to MacDonald's observation of this problem, one clinician at a medical conference said that he "had a similar experience. Our material showed no relationship and therefore it was never published."[33]

More generally, MacDonald was critical of the poor quality of statistical data and inference in most surgical publications, as well as the weak scientific basis of most surgical practice. MacDonald reviewed 236 articles that purported to study the effectiveness of early treatment. He believed that only 16 of these studies contained data that could possibly be considered reliable. Almost all of these studies "failed to establish any significant value for early treatment, and a few of them expressed some disbelief of their inability to do so. Other than these few authors, the literature offered many stereotyped allusions to the desirability of early treatment and a general inclination to explain bad results in terms of delayed treatment."[34]

MacDonald and others disparaged their colleagues' overestimation of the efficacy of existing cancer treatments. One pair of predeterminists expressed their disbelief in surgeons' mystical faith in the orderly, localist model of cancer and the value of early, radical treatment by quoting in full the following passage from a published clinical trial:

> Statistics are peculiar things. It is also found that the average time between the discovery of the "lump" and the operation of those that died of recurrence is practically the same as of those that have remained free of the disease. These apparently contradictory figures should not lessen our determination to operate as early as possible in every case.[35]

For predeterminist critics, these authors' active dismissal of their own "contradictory figures" by asserting the peculiarity of statistics reflected a disturbing flight from scientific reality. Predeterminists self-consciously grabbed the scientific high ground by frequently using the language of statistical inference to lay out their argument. "In order to investigate the absolute curability of the breast," Park and Lees wrote, "it is necessary to start with the null hypothesis that cancer is incurable until it is proved to be curable; and the difficulties of this proof are great."[36]

An important strand of predeterminism was skepticism about radical surgery. Throughout the early twentieth century, there were some surgeons who never adopted the complete operation, experimented with ancillary radiation therapy, and/or carried out more limited surgery. For many surgeons in the first half of the century, the discomfort with the Halstedian paradigm was not so much a complete rejection of early, radical surgery but a belief that it was too uniformly applied. In 1953, Williams et al. captured this sentiment by noting, "Ewing pointed out many years ago that the radical operation was, on the one hand, performed too often on comparatively innocent growths, such as encapsulated adenocarcinoma, and localized duct cancers which may be ablated by simple mastectomy; and, on the other hand, on highly malignant forms of the disease which are invariably fatal. The good result in the first type of case is ascribed falsely to sacrifice of tissue, whilst in the other type of case the extreme limits of tissue removal will not save the patient."[37]

At mid-century, many clinicians were rediscovering the limited or absent power of radical breast cancer surgery to make an impact on the course of metastatic disease and cancer mortality, observations that had been acknowledged by Halsted. An increasing number of reviews were noting that radical surgery had limited impact on mortality. One review concluded that "the radical mastectomy operation leaves much to be desired from the standpoint of long term survivals. It appears that mortality in cancer is a constant process, little affected by treatment. Between 24 and 38 percent of patients with cancer behave as if cured with respect to mortality, regardless of method and treatment."[38] Reflecting this rediscovery of the limited impact of surgery on mortality and metastatic disease, MacDonald in 1951 argued that when talking about surgical end results in cancer we should speak of "controlled" rather than "cured" cancer.[39] Park and Lees similarly trumpeted that the "radical mastectomy has no influence in diminishing the incidence of distant metastases nor in preventing or postponing death from the growth of such distant metastases."[40]

MacDonald and colleagues also took direct aim at other surgeons' efforts to be sure that every last bit of cancer was extirpated. MacDonald caricatured such surgical practices as a neurotic anxiety that tried but could not extinguish itself by being ever more extensive. "It is not irrelevant to complain," MacDonald argued, "even to this audience, that the principal cause of this failure is the clinicians frenetic state of therapeutic over anxiety; not content to observe the effects of oophorectomy alone, he uses additive hormonal therapy, or corticosteroids, or ex-radiation, or even combinations of these as the ugliest manifestation of this 'belt and suspenders' complex in therapeutics."[41]

Mckinnon in 1949 explained the way surgical moralism led to pressures on pathologists and surgeons to diagnose cancer whenever there was any doubt.

> Not only is the diagnosis one of opinion; when treatment is made dependent on the pathological report, it is sometimes one of forced opinion. The pressure of circumstances is then, as everyone knows, for "Cancer" or "Not Cancer." Possibly surrounded by the conviction, though not always convinced himself, that early and complete treatment is of supreme malignancy, the pathologist can hardly fail to give

the patient the full benefit of any doubt even in his own mind...It could be that the dominance of the concept of the supreme importance of early treatment has created a circle of events from which it is difficult to become disentangled.[42]

MacDonald and colleagues' dissent also drew on the received wisdom of the previous generation, which had explicitly recognized that pathological diagnosis of cancer was not a cut-and-dried, objective process. They also recognized that the threshold for diagnosing cancer had been significantly lowered as the twentieth century progressed. Park and Lees concluded in 1951 that the gradual increase of calling borderline conditions cancer explained the paradox of improved surgical cure rates for breast cancer while the mortality rate remained constant. Park and Lees restated and made explicit the older pathological wisdom that there was a continuum from the noncancerous to the cancerous. They observed that a good pathologist can generally be certain that a specimen is benign. "In cancer of the breast, however," they wrote, "one has to worry so often whether to call a tumor malignant or not; there is so much difference between opinions on borderline cases; and so much of the "probably not cancer but safer away" type of diagnosis, that there can be doubt that many tumors treated as if they were malignant were, in fact, not malignant at all."[43]

In the medical literature of the 1950s and early 1960s, there was a fierce counterattack to predeterminism and its implications by mainstream surgeons and pathologists. Surgeon Louis Notkin in 1959 derided predeterminism as defeatist, fatalist, and mystical. He ridiculed the logical leap from observing that some women who present with apparent late disease survive for a long time to predeterminism as an Alice-in-Wonderland-like logic, whose slogan might well as be "the later, the earlier." Notkin and others appealed to the clinical experience of surgeons, to their distrust of statistics, and to common sense. Notkin objected to the psychic harm predeterminism might cause to the cancer patient as "it does convey a sense of frustration, hopelessness and mysticism, and unless clarified to the point of lucidity and usefulness should be dropped."[44]

Other critics similarly noted the nihilistic implications of predeterminism and felt that abandoning current prevention and treatment practices was equivalent to abandoning patients and women in general. As late as 1969, one observer tried to separate the extreme implications of predeterminism (abandoning screening and surgery), arguing that (quoting

William Blackstone): "Mankind will not be reasoned out of feelings of humanity."[45]

McDonald was stung by the criticism that predeterminism was akin to admitting defeat in the fight against cancer, since he believed that the problem was finding new treatments or modifying existing ones, not completely abandoning breast and other cancer surgery. Less convincingly, he argued that predeterminism should not make patients feel hopeless, arguing that predeterminism did not mean predestination. He argued that he was not a "prophet of doom" (as he was called by those he characterized as believing in "the triumph of hope over experience") and that "the limited usefulness of conventional methods is as distressing to converts to predeterminism as to the skeptics, but the educational sedation provided by the failure to recognize such limitations prevents a wider understanding of the total problem."[46] He also acknowledged that a few cancers besides breast cancer, such as those of the uterine cervix, do have "a natural history which generally conforms to the traditional doctrine that curability is directly related to the 'earliness' of diagnosis and the 'immediacy' and effectiveness of treatment."[47]

Precancers?

At mid-century, the war against time led to the discovery, definition, and increased diagnosis of precancerous conditions – as well as a counterreaction. Until the early decades of the twentieth century, pathologists and clinicians believed that almost any benign lump or injury could transform itself into true invasive breast cancer under the "right" conditions. In 1941, a long simmering controversy over the meaning and significance of early cancer diagnoses erupted in the wake of Foote and Stewart's article in a pathology journal entitled "Lobular carcinoma in situ [cancer in position]: a rare form of mammary cancer."[48] These authors' innovation was to identify and legitimate a specific precursor to invasive cancer, parallel to precancers named at other sites, and to link this new diagnosis in a precise if probabilistic way to frankly invasive cancer. Lobular carcinoma in situ (LCIS) was quickly embraced by some surgeons as an important advance because it might be an opportunity to surgically intervene prior to the point of biological predeterminism. Some surgeons advocated and performed mastectomies, sometimes bilateral, on women with LCIS, because there was a growing consensus that LCIS was often a diffuse process in both breasts.[49] The aggressive approach to these in situ cancers was rationalized by the observation that invasive cancers, so many of which were unsuccessfully treated by even the most radical surgery, had to come from somewhere. The underlying momentum behind this quest was captured by Fred Stewart's reported quip that "the female breast is a precancerous organ."[50]

While "precancerous" diagnoses were made in the era prior to the discovery and promotion of "in situ" cancers, they had largely served as a rationale for operating on benign, if suspicious, growths. For those who upheld a clear-cut boundary between cancer and noncancer, these labels were useful in dealing with patients but were not objective categories. In the early twentieth century, Philadelphia surgeon J. B. Deaver for example wrote that "the word 'precancerous' is a useful word to use in advising the patient to have the benign growth removed, but in a scientific sense the word is a misnomer, as the particular growth, to my mind, is either cancerous, or it is not cancerous."[51]

Ideas about and responses to LCIS had parallels in cervical cancer, a disease whose anatomy and natural history had permitted more research into putative "precancerous" stages (e.g., by repeat sampling of cervical tissue using colposcopy or PAP smears, discussed in the next chapter). Nevertheless, there was considerable controversy over the meaning of precancer in cervical cancer. Skeptics of an aggressive approach to screening and treatment noted the much higher prevalence of precancerous lesions than clinically diagnosed cervical cancer or cervical cancer mortality, arguing that the natural history of many or most of these precancers did not lead to frank cancer or cancer death. There was great pathological controversy over the criterion for labeling and categorizing in situ cervical cancers and dysplasia and the relation between these categories and the risk of developing cervical cancer.[52]

Controversy also extended to the naming of these cervical lesions, a development that would have its parallel in breast cancer. Dr. Lewis Robbins recalled that the public health officials in charge of jump starting Pap smears around the country understood that the word "carcinoma" inside the "cervical carcinoma in situ" term was inherently controversial because "the Pap smear isn't diagnosing cancer, it's diagnosing a precursor. Why do they call it cancer than? Because nobody would pay any attention if they called it dysplasia. If you call it carcinoma in situ, then they will examine it, do something with it."[53] At one level, the existence of these precancerous states seemed self-evident. Cancer must derive from cells that were once normal and normal cells did not become cancerous instantaneously. As Fred Stewart reportedly put it, "cervical cancer comes from carcinoma in situ because where else could it come from?"[54]

From the beginning of its promotion, there was skepticism about the diagnosis and surgical approach to LCIS from doctors who came from the predeterminist camp. N. E. McKinnon in 1955, for example, voiced skepticism about the surgical approach to carcinoma in situ, placing it in the older history of surgical approaches to all kinds of other lumps and conditions "considered possibly "pre-cancerous"," which have failed because "curing non-lethal lesions does not reduce mortality."[55]

Other observers questioned the wisdom of removing the breasts of women with LCIS because most of these lesions presumably did not develop into frank cancer and those that did had an "unusually favorable" prognosis. Writing in 1972, long after the predeterminist heyday had passed, the authors of an epidemiological report observed that the "expanded recognition of precancerous breast lesions poses the question of the most appropriate therapy."[56]

Other criticisms of the status, meaning, and implications of LCIS came from surgeon Cushman Haagensen, who remained a champion of the radical mastectomy long after data from randomized clinical trials had severely damaged its status as conventional treatment. Writing in 1981, Haagensen pointed out that Foote and Stewart's initial report of patients diagnosed with LCIS did not demonstrate evidence of coexisting cancer or metastases. Haagensen believed that simply taking the lesion out seemed curative. He noted that LCIS typically occurred among premenopausal women, frequently regressed after menopause, and had a very favorable prognosis. As a consequence, Haagensen argued that these lesions be called lobular neoplasia rather than carcinoma in situ. "The correct choice of a name for a disease is very important," Haagensen concluded, "not only because it identifies it, but also because it prejudices the choice of treatment. Lobular carcinoma in situ is a misleading and unfortunate name for this benign, noninfiltrating, special microscopical form of lobular proliferation of the mammary epithelium. The name *carcinoma* denotes an epithelial lesion that, once established, grows progressively locally and often metastasizes. Most surgeons amputate breasts when the lesion is classified as carcinoma, even though the name used includes the qualifying phrase in situ."[57]

"Failing to Correspond Closely With Hopes or Expectations"

For skeptical physicians at mid-century, public cancer education campaigns, radical surgery, and modern medicine had failed to deliver on the promise that had been promoted since the beginning of the century. In many ways, the ideas that constituted this skepticism were not that different from assumptions about cancer that were widely held prior to the promotion of localist views of breast and other cancers, radical surgery, and the "delay" campaign.

First, there was a historically familiar recognition that despite advances in understanding cancer, there was still no unambiguous definition of, or way to diagnose, breast cancer that reliably distinguished between tumors that would ultimately kill patients from those that were more benign. As in the nineteenth century, mid-twentieth century skeptic James Lees observed that the medical world still had "difficulty" agreeing on "what we mean by cancer. Do we mean by a cancer a disease which kills within five years? Do we mean by cancer a disease which kills eventually, which metastasizes, which infiltrates? Do we mean a histological appearance, or do we mean the histological appearances which we have learned to associate with a future malignant behavior?"[58]

Second, the greater claims for efficacy of breast cancer surgery in the twentieth century than in the nineteenth had arguably unleashed a more nihilistic and bitter counterreaction. Although controversies had been continuing "for decades even generations" because treatments were "equally effective," Lees argued that "the commonest cause of continued controversy is, in fact, equal ineffectiveness."[59]

This pessimism extended not only to surgical treatment but also to the optimism that was at the heart of the "delay" campaign and organized cancer control efforts. Mckinnon noted that in light of the "tremendous" efforts in publicity and propaganda for early diagnosis and treatment, including subsidized cancer clinics, "some decline in the rates might have been anticipated. However, ... no one should be greatly surprised to find them failing to correspond closely with hopes or expectations."[60] Furthermore, medical science seemed no closer to finding a biological explanation for who got cancer and when. Despite the discovery of chromosomes and insights into human immunology, medical science had not made much progress over earlier constitutional explanations of cancer predisposition and idiosyncrasy. As a 1945 *Saturday Evening Post* article commented on cancer predisposition:

> What, then, according to the geneticist, is inherited? A "susceptibility," a "tendency," a defect in the "constitution," is his answer. What he means by these mystic terms he cannot tell you. Is paper "susceptible" to tearing because it is thin? Is iron "susceptible" to rusting just because it is iron? Engineers and chemist scrapped such explanations long ago and use more precise language. Such loose words as "susceptibility," "tendency," and "constitution" carry us back to the seventeenth century, when physicians reported that John Doe "died of a humor" and thereby explained nothing. Such vagueness reflects a backward state of medicine. Yet we shall have to make the most of "susceptibility," "tendency," and "constitution" in cancer. There is nothing more precise to offer.[61]

While mid-century predeterminists remained in the minority, many people in the cancer mainstream increasingly acknowledged that there was something seriously wrong with contemporary efforts to control breast and other cancers, especially the overselling of cancer fears and the failure to significantly reduce cancer mortality. As a result, a great deal of experimentation with new types of cancer prevention began in the 1950s and 1960s. But before considering the rise of *cancer surveillance*, let us consider how mid-twentieth-century skepticism, along with other continuities and changes in American medicine and society, was shaping the experience of women with breast cancer, especially their decision-making and relations with doctors.

EIGHT

Balancing Hope, Trust, and Truth

Rachel Carson

In 1987, Dr. George "Barney" Crile, Jr. (1907–1992) was asked to review "for accuracy in emotional level and content" a screenplay for a proposed television docudrama about environmentalist Rachel Carson (1907–1964).[1] Crile had been one of Carson's physicians during her struggle with breast cancer. After reading those parts of the screenplay that concerned his relationship with Carson, Crile wrote the producer that "I completely disapprove of it. I would not allow it to be shown as is."[2] Crile's first and major objection was to the following scene:

> Dr. Crile: Apparently the tumor metastasized. They missed it last April.
> Rachel: So it was malignant.
> Angle: Dr. George Crile Jr., nodding confirmation.[3]

Crile wrote the producer he "would never have said 'They missed it last April,' they didn't miss it at all. They just didn't tell Miss Carson that it was a definite malignancy. This of course, was a mistake. But I hardly see how a person of Miss Carson's intelligence could have undergone a radical mastectomy and not been certain that the tumor that she had been treated for was malignant."[4]

Crile was objecting to a simplistic and perhaps anachronistic rendering of more complicated and nuanced events. He believed that Carson's surgeon was guilty neither of misdiagnosis or outright lying, but a softening of the cancer diagnosis's impact by introducing some uncertainty. This may have been a moral or tactical mistake from Crile's perspective, but patients of "Miss Carson's intelligence" could easily infer from the context – devastating, radical surgery – whatever level of detail and truth they could handle and at their own pace. As we shall see as we look at Carson's personal history of cancer and her relations with physicians and others, the normative evasion of the cancer diagnosis was shifting and contested by the early 1960s, buffeted by changes in society and medicine. But there has also existed a less widely appreciated continuity in the efforts of patients, physicians, and others to find some balance among sustaining hope, retaining trust, and honesty.

It is not hard to understand why a television producer in the late 1980s might cast Crile as a physician more forthright than his peers and Carson as a patient championing her right to make autonomous clinical decisions based on accurate medical facts. Crile had been a prominent skeptic of received clinical practices and beliefs about cancer in the 1950s and 1960s, including physician paternalism. Rachel Carson had almost single-handedly brought Americans and others into a new consciousness about the dangers of industrial pollution and had inspired a new lay activism about cancer. But despite her prominent role as an environmental activist and social critic, and her exposure to the way human efforts to control nature had contributed to the "one in four" lifetime cancer risk in the United States, Carson was publicly silent about her own cancer. Moreover, Crile's and Carson's delicate negotiations surrounding Carson's diagnosis, treatment, and prognosis had their own evasions, denials, and ambiguities. Their relationship, especially as it concerned Carson's prognosis and decisions about treating "incurable" cancer, often resembled a delicate pas de deux in which Carson and Crile together balanced hope against increasingly discouraging realities and unsatisfying clinical options.

"A New Ailment"

According to Linda Lear, in her comprehensive and insightful biography *Rachel Carson: Witness for Nature*, Carson had a small breast cyst removed in 1946 and in 1950 a medical examination revealed a tumor in her left breast. After what Lear described as a "casual" search for a surgeon, she underwent surgery in September 1950. She was told that the tumor was benign and received no further treatment.[5]

In January 1960, Carson was diagnosed as having a duodenal ulcer. Her most trusted friend Dorothy Freeman wrote her that upon learning Carson had "developed a new ailment," she was "so afraid – and I might as well name the fear – that you were going to say cancer that the words duodenal ulcer came almost as a relief."[6] Revealing the depths of the general fear of cancer and their continuities with Halsted's patients, Freeman and Carson only rarely used the word *cancer* during their many discussions of different aspects of Carson's cancer in subsequent years. Also in the same letter, Freeman presented the pros and cons of telling her husband about Carson's ulcer diagnosis, evidence of the wide zone of privacy generally accorded any serious illness in this and other periods.[7]

In March 1960, while drafting material for what would become the cancer chapter of *Silent Spring*, Carson discovered several cysts in her left breast. Her internist, Dr. Healy, immediately made arrangements for Carson to see a surgeon, Dr. Sanderson, who operated on Carson in early April.[8] "It was discovered that I had two more [cysts] in the same breast," Carson later recounted about the decision-making and information flow around the time of surgery. "An operation was advised. The preliminary sections in the operating room aroused enough suspicion that a radical mastectomy was performed. However, the permanent sections did not reveal definite malignancy, although something was said about 'changes.' No follow-up with radiation was considered necessary."[9] It was possible that there was some diagnostic uncertainty by the pathologists, but Sanderson was offering a conventional "middle ground" evasion of cancer realities (more later).

It is not clear if Healy agreed with Sanderson's evasions, but he later bemoaned its consequences for Carson's treatment. "Because of her being informed that there was no malignancy," Healy wrote Crile eight months after Carson's surgery, "her present management is quite difficult."[10]

In the immediate aftermath of her radical mastectomy, Carson believed that "the only possible attitude seems to be to feel thankful this discovery was made so early. I think there need be no apprehension for the future." Beginning a pattern of active efforts to hide her cancer diagnosis, sickness, and medical care, she asked friends to keep news of her operation private. Her stated motivations subsumed a desire to maintain her privacy and a concern about damaging her public role as an environmental activist, perhaps because her struggle with cancer might suggest vulnerability or less-than-scientific motivations for her work. "I have no wish to read of my ailments in literary gossip columns," Carson explained. "Too much comfort to the chemical companies."[11]

Some of Carson's friends were concerned with her doctors' decision to give no further treatment besides her radical mastectomy. Their concerns were understandable given the considerable visibility of new (chemotherapy) and old (radiation) cancer treatments and the American Cancer Society (ACS) campaigns that emphasized the effectiveness of multiple modalities of cancer treatment. However, Carson's surgeon's behavior was entirely consistent with Halstedian fatalism about the possibility of metastatic disease and skepticism about the efficacy of any initial treatment besides radical surgery.

Unfortunately, complications soon developed. In November 1960, Carson noted a "curious, hard swelling on the third or fourth rib on the operated side, at or near the junction with the sternum." She had a crisis of confidence brought to a head by her doctors' apparent evasions about the nature of this new swollen area. Although her doctors had "professed to be puzzled" about the nature of the new problem, they were giving her radiation treatments.[12] Carson concluded that she had not "been told the truth last spring" and decided to get in touch with Barney Crile.[13]

Barney Crile and Mid-Century Skepticism About Cancer

Carson had some acquaintance with Crile before this December 1960 crisis in confidence. She had met Jane Crile, Barney's wife, at a reception for an earlier (Carson) book in Jane's family's Cleveland department store in 1952. Crile later attributed his writing career – both his 1955 controversial anti-(medical) establishment book on cancer, *Cancer and Common Sense*, and the nature adventure books he wrote with Jane – to this meeting because Carson had introduced the Criles to her literary agent and friend Marie Rodell, who would become the Criles' literary agent as well.[14]

Crile was the son of the Cleveland Clinic's founder, surgeon George Crile, Sr. Crile Sr. had been Halsted's contemporary but was neither enthralled with him nor his surgical approach to cancer. Crile Sr. had never performed a radical mastectomy. "Halsted is an obsessional fuddy-duddy," Crile Jr. recalled his father saying, "who takes all day to do an operation that should never be done at all."[15]

Crile Jr. was born into wealth and privilege. After an undergraduate degree at Yale and medical school at Harvard, Crile took up surgical training at Barnes Hospital and the Cleveland Clinic, where he stayed throughout his long and distinguished surgical career. Crile's skepticism of prevailing surgical practices in cancer stemmed from astute clinical and sociological observations as a trainee. Crile had observed that less extensive surgery was often done on the sly, while radical operations were frequently done on hopelessly ill poor people. He was horrified by the operating room deaths of many patients with advanced cases of cancer (good "teaching material"). He learned that prevailing cancer statistics were unreliable, observing that his fellow clinicians frequently did not distinguish between primary and secondary tumors on death certificates.

Later, from the perch of his salaried position at the Cleveland Clinic, Crile criticized his fellow "fee for service" surgeons for performing more radical operations because they earned more from them.[16] In less confrontational moments, Crile pointed out that his fellow surgeons, like other craftsmen, were more comfortable with, and had more confidence in, their own rather than others' tools. "Neither is a surgeon dishonest because he thinks that his way of treating this is good," Crile observed. "But you're not going to have a surgeon, if you come in with a little lump in your breast, you're not going to have him say, 'All you need is a lumpectomy and radiation. We have this wonderful radiation therapist down there. The results will be just as good as if I did a modified radical mastectomy.' They don't say that because they don't believe it."[17]

Through his work at the Cleveland Clinic, contacts in professional circles, publications, and publicity such as a 1955 Life Magazine article, Crile's skeptical message about cancer beliefs and practices had reached a wide medical and popular audience.[18] Crile was part of the larger current of medical and surgical discontent with reigning cancer ideas at mid-century explored in the previous chapter. Crile advocated less radical surgery as well as the use of radiation therapy, as did his friends and distant colleagues Oliver Cope, Reginald Murley, and Geoffrey Keynes. But Crile's criticisms had a more general focus on excessive fear of cancer and medical hubris, a message that he delivered to both medical and lay audiences.

Crile's main message in *Cancer and Common Sense* was that twentieth-century clinical and public health efforts had created unnatural and destructive fears of cancer. Medical and public health leaders "have portrayed cancer as insidious, dreadful, relentless invader. With religious fervor they have fashioned a devil out of cancer. They have bred in a sensitive public a fear that is approaching hysteria. They have created a new disease, cancerphobia, a contagious disease that spreads from the mouth to ear. It is possible that today cancerphobia causes more suffering than cancer itself."[19] In addition to being an iatrogenic, psychological and bodily insult, cancerphobia was costly in strict economic terms. "When patients indoctrinated with this propaganda demand unnecessary and expensive tests, physicians are afraid not to give them. The demand for these tests stems from the philosophy of fear. As long as public education is made up of threats and false promises, fear and irrational demands for superfluous and expensive tests will result."[20]

Crile argued that fear had filled the void created by our ignorance of cancer's natural history and causes. He was critical of the tendency to label all kinds of noncancerous pathological entities as "precancerous" and then to fear them and treat these conditions aggressively. Cancer was frequently depicted as an alien process taking over the individual's body from without, rather than as a biological process from within. "Since we know so little about the factors that cause cancer," Crile wrote, "we can do little to avoid getting it. We must accept the possibility of cancer as we do the possibility of being struck by lightning. It is something that we should not court by taking foolish risks, but neither should we devote our lives to avoiding it."[21]

Cancer definition was a major problem. Crile believed that many physicians were falsely confident that they could predict something uniform and accurate about the future from the particular stage and grade of a tumor. "Even pathologists may not agree as to whether a tissue is or is not a cancer," Crile wrote. "Their science is a biologic science and, as such, is inexact." Echoing the predeterminist critique, Crile believed that "every cancer is a separate problem which should be dealt with in an individual way and no generalization as to treatment should be made."[22] More generally, Crile questioned whether "every cancer, even a harmless microscopic cancer with which a patient might live for a lifetime, be included in the statistics? Or should we count only those cancers which have progressed to the stage of invading tissue, of causing symptoms, of threatening life? The problem is with the concept of the word 'cancer' and with the lack of a precise definition. This is the major problem with which the physician is faced in the analysis of statistics. This is the reason why professional perfectionists have been fooled into foolishness, fooled by statistics which bear no resemblance to the clinical facts."[23]

Crile's skepticism was deep, although his publications had a less nihilistic tone than Ian McDonald's and other predeterminists' writings. In a letter to a physician reader, Crile let down his more balanced public face, writing that he was not only skeptical that radical surgery offered no additional benefit than less extensive surgery but that there was little evidence that surgery of any sort made a difference. "I can assure you that we have done our level best to play down the real basis of controversy," Crile concluded "which is whether our attempts to cure cancer are doing more harm than good."[24]

Crile's skepticism toward received societal, medical, and public health ideas and practices vis-à-vis cancer derived mostly from his clinical experiences and personal observations rather than his own or others' research. His style of argumentation combined personal anecdote, casual review of his own and others' clinical experiences, and "common sense," in sum, a formula not all that different from Rachel Carson's style. Others – notably the clinical researcher Bernard Fisher – would in subsequent decades provide an empirical basis for widespread change in surgical approaches to breast and other cancers. Although Crile's critical stance toward existing medical practices resonated with the new ways of evaluating and testing medical practices, he did not himself use or even understand the tools of the new evaluative sciences.[25]

Crile called for psychological approaches, not medical or surgical ones, to problems – like fear of cancer – that were essentially psychological. "Perhaps, in our attempts to be scientific, we have neglected the psychology of patients who are emotionally disturbed. Is it quackery, the dispensing of sugar pills?"[26] In the doctor–patient relationship in cancer, Crile championed the need to preserve hope and relieve suffering, especially when cure was not possible given current understandings and interventions. "It is not death itself that the patient fears," Crile wrote quoting J. E. Dunphy, "it is not suffering of which he is afraid. The thing that the patient with incurable cancer dreads the most is that he will be abandoned by his physician."[27]

The goal of treatment was to keep the patient in a state of equanimity. "Surely the medical profession can teach the people who have incurable cancer to live with their cancers in equanimity. When faith is strong there comes a time of peace."[28] While he counseled the importance of always being able to do or offer something to cancer patients, it was clear that Crile did not believe mutilating surgery and other extreme treatment modalities should be offered to cancer patients for their symbolic value only. Less extreme measures would certainly do in situations in which there was no efficacious treatment.

Crile was also concerned with the way that the overselling of cancer fears turned both physician and patient away from the essentially spiritual character of suffering and the care of the sick. "No physician, sleepless and worried about a patient, can return to the hospital in the midnight hours without feeling the importance of this faith," Crile wrote about the spirit of healing. "The dim corridor is silent. The doors are closed. At the end of the corridor, in the glow of the desk lamp, the nurse watches over those who sleep or lie lonely and awake behind the closed white doors. No physician entering the hospital in these quiet hours can help feeling that the medical institution of which he is a part is in essence religious, that it is built on trust. No physician can fail to be proud that he is a part of his patients' faith."[29]

"Now Which of You Is in Charge of Not Giving Up?"

Carson initially contacted Crile for general advice and a recommendation for new Washington, D.C. doctors. She wanted "a new evaluation of the whole thing by someone else." She was afraid of finding herself in the hands of an "overzealous" surgeon and understood that "radiation and chemotherapy" were "two-edged swords." Friends had urged her to go for treatment at a cancer clinic in which NIH sponsored clinical trials were occurring. But Carson worried – echoing her concerns about industry, chemicals, and environmental damage – that the NIH was "eager to have more and more chemicals tested, and all this makes me feel like a guinea pig." She was also desperate to get on with her research and writing and not "spend the rest of my life in hospitals."[30]

Carson ended up going to Cleveland to be evaluated by Crile. After her visit, she wrote him that in retrospect it was "strange that in the very beginning I did not think in large enough terms to think of going to Cleveland and to you." Carson was relieved that "the direction of her treatment [is] in your hands." Carson particularly valued Crile's "scientific" awareness, by which she meant Crile's "unwillingness to rush in with procedures that may disrupt that unknown but all-important ecology of body cells." This was one of the few times that Carson connected her criticism of the way social and economic behavior were disrupting ecological relations throughout nature to to her cancer. Carson also valued Crile's "frank" discussion of "the facts, even though I might wish they were different."[31] In his reply, Crile endorsed the ideal of truth telling, but added that he "always believed that *intelligent people in responsible positions* [my italics] not only wish to know as much as possible about any ailment they have, but also that such people are entitled to know everything that is known about such ailments."[32]

Crile began his role as director (Carson's view) or advisor (Crile's characterization) by suggesting to Healy that Carson be sterilized, either by surgery or with radiation. If sterilization induced regression of Carson's disease, then one could assume that Carson's breast cancer was endocrine dependent, opening the door to endocrine ablation therapy (stopping the body's production of estrogen by destroying the organs involved in producing the hormone: ovaries, adrenal glands, and the pituitary gland) at some point in the future. Crile was an advocate of endocrine manipulation in breast cancer not only because he believed it worked, but because it was a more systemic and biologically specific intervention than either radiation or chemotherapy. While Crile also recommended focused radiation to the involved internal mammary nodes, he urged no radiation to the axilla where Carson already had a "very complete operation." Crile was concerned that axillary radiation might lead to lymphedema. In the years since Halsted, Crile and other surgeons had no problem with the idea that axillary surgery and radiation could cause lymphedema.

Crile believed that treatment should be directed at Carson's cancer recurrences and symptoms as they arose, rather than giving prophylactic (or what we today would call *adjuvant*) chemotherapy or wide-field radiation. He believed that such anticipatory treatment could cause serious side effects while lowering "systemic resistance" to disease.[33] In his books and papers, Crile lambasted his fellow surgeons for their use of radical surgery and other extreme and ultimately futile treatments in situations in which they were not going to cure the patient of cancer.

We are not privy to exactly what Crile told Carson about her prognosis at this first visit, but the larger pattern of communication suggests that he told her that the treatment plan was aimed at controlling rather than curing cancer. In his autobiography, Crile recalled that Carson came to see him for "an incurable recurrence of her cancer" for which he gave "not lifesaving but comfort-sustaining advice."[34] In an approach similar to Halsted's, Crile never explicitly told Carson that her disease was fatal or that she had a certain number of months or years to live. Neither did Crile state that any treatment or maneuver would cure her cancer. For Crile, sustaining comfort meant not extinguishing Carson's hope for survival or at least a long period of survival. As advisor, Crile not only made recommendations to Carson's D.C.-area physicians, but also managed her expectations, hopes, and fears.

Understandably, Carson and her friends did articulate this hope for cure. Dorothy Freeman wrote Carson that she "truthfully" had found it easier to "think happier thoughts" after Carson had found Crile, "even to the point of real faith that this shadow will be conquered."[35]

At the time of her local recurrence, Carson clearly understood and feared that treatment might not work and that she might die from her cancer. In January 1961, for example, she explained to Freeman that she wanted to take her nephew Roger, who had lost his parents and was in Carson's charge, with her on a trip to California because "If it must be that his world has to be shattered again before he reaches manhood, at least I want while there is time to share as many 'wonders' as possible with him."[36]

Carson eventually was referred to a new radiation therapist, Dr. Caulk, who radiated her ovaries and began a prolonged course of treatments directed at the clinically apparent disease in her left chest. During this same period, Carson was also afflicted with severe, disabling arthritis of unclear etiology.[37] The pain and physical limitations of her arthritis, the energy devoted to doctor visits, radiation treatments, and hospitalizations, left her wheelchair bound, unable to write, and isolated. In the midst of this nightmarish situation, Carson, like Emlen monitoring her compression therapy, examined her body for signs of a response to the radiation, initially seeing no change, tentatively recognizing some improvement later, and finally seeing a clear response.[38]

Carson's disease experience had certainly been transformed by treatment – not only by the bodily mutilation from surgery and the nausea and other side effects of radiation, but by the maze of difficult responses to her concomitant illnesses, such as the way her arthritis led to the removal of fluid from her joints, antibiotics, and injected steroids.[39] "What a strange, bleak world I'm living in right now," Carson wrote Freeman.[40]

In her negotiations around arthritis treatments, Carson appeared to reinvent herself as a less passive patient and consumer of medical information than earlier in her illness when she left it to her internist to choose her surgeon. She chose to make her rheumatologist's recommendation of gold treatment for arthritis the line in the sand over which she would not cross. Carson did her own research on gold treatment and found that one of its potential side effects was bone marrow suppression. She wrote to Freeman about her growing skepticism toward doctors in general and her desire to no longer be "submitting" to treatment.[41] "As you know," Carson wrote Crile of her skeptical thoughts, "I'm not an especially tractable patient, and don't just go along with such things without doing some inquiring and thinking on my own."[42] In another letter to Crile, she wrote that a leading – and witty and skeptical – pharmacology text had characterized treating rheumatoid arthritis with gold as "treating a disease of unknown etiology with a drug of unknown action."[43]

Crile contacted Carson's D.C. doctors and consulted local authorities in Cleveland. He told Carson that he did not "take such a long range pessimistic view about this because a great deal can be done for rheumatoid problems today." He concluded that gold treatment was defensible but so were other options. Crile trusted the judgment of a rheumatologist in Cleveland who had advised him that short-term treatment with gold was reasonable in Carson's case. This specialist had also raised the possibility of nitrogen mustard and cortisone injections into Carson's joints.[44] But even Crile's support did not dissuade Carson from refusing to take gold. In a carefully scripted encounter, Carson confronted her rheumatologist with the evidence against gold and gave him a face-saving excuse to rescind his suggestion – she was getting better. In many ways, this encounter over gold connected Carson's environmental activist persona with her life as cancer patient and foreshadowed an awakening of a larger consumer and patient's rights orientation in American society.

Carson's health appeared to improve over the spring and summer of 1961 as she was finishing *Silent Spring*, although she developed a new problem, iritis (an eye inflammation), that made it difficult for her to see and edit her drafts.[45] Looking back at the preceding 2 years in early 1962, she wrote Freeman, "Yes, there is quite a story behind *Silent Spring*, isn't there? Such a catalogue of illnesses! If one were superstitious, it would be easy to believe in some malevolent influence at work, determined by some means to keep the book from being finished."[46]

In February 1962, Carson discovered new swellings in her right armpit. She decided to fly to Cleveland to consult again with Crile. He excised a lymph node that was quickly determined to be cancerous. Crile believed it "foolish" to do radical surgery on the newly involved right side of her chest and suggested to Caulk that radiating the right armpit and collarbone would effectively control the disease. Revealing that there were limits to what clinical information he would disclose even to the right type of patient, as well as being respectful of Caulk's expertise with radiation treatment, he wrote Caulk that "This [the areas to be irradiated] I am leaving entirely to your judgment, and have not discussed it in any detail with Miss Carson."[47]

Carson would later write Freeman that in the aftermath of the need for more radiation treatment that her "courage had deserted me for a time." Carson found some encouragement from Morton Biskind, a physician whose research on chemicals and cancer she had previously used in her research. Biskind gave Carson practical advice for managing nausea and other side effects of radiation treatment.[48] Carson at the time had a deepening ambivalence about the meaning and experience of the "2-million volt monster.... For even while it is killing the cancer I know what it is doing to me.... But under the circumstances I have no choice but to accept the hazards of radiation."[49]

In other conversations with Biskind, Carson began to consider remedies and treatments that were outside the medical mainstream. Biskind had recommended liver compounds and B-complex vitamins. Carson wrote Freeman that Biskind's recommendations were "borne out by research I'm familiar with –animal studies, I mean. Dr. B has had patients on such a program who have simply had no recurrences, even though the cancer had metastasized at surgery. Of course one should also make a strong effort to eliminate the chlorinated hydrocarbons from one's food, because they cause loss of the B vitamins and also damage the liver. But civilization has made it so very difficult to do that."

On the one hand, Carson's reaching out to therapies outside of the mainstream was similar to the efforts of Emlen and women after her to do something more than whatever was then considered mainstream therapeutics, especially with their disease progressing despite the best therapy. On the other hand, Carson's actions very much reflected her professional stance. The reliance on out of the mainstream but credible scientists, the casual extrapolation from animal studies to humans, the stringing together of suggestive and eclectic bits of data were common elements to both Carson's life as cancer patient and the substance and style of *Silent Spring*.

Carson described her moods as "mercurial" during this period, noting that it was hard to be "philosophic or courageous when one's feeling sick at one's stomach."[50] Her struggle with advancing disease led to fears for the future as well as more mundane concerns, such as finding a wig after radiation treatment left her bald. In April 1962, Carson discovered "something" in her right armpit that Caulk felt was cancer and treatable. At the same time, Caulk did not think her new neck and back pains were the result of cancer although cancer would later be implicated. "The trouble with this business," Carson wrote Freeman, echoing the sentiments of Emlen and Smith but under more intense and invasive medical and self-surveillance and treatment, "is that every perfectly ordinary little ailment looks like a hobgoblin, and one lives in a private little hell until the thing is examined and found to be nothing much."[51]

Carson continued to make sure that knowledge of her cancer did not extend beyond her small circle of intimates. She instructed Freeman to tell people who asked about her "you never saw me look better." Carson could not bear small talk about her illness and incapacity. "As to those few people you have felt it necessary to tell, will you please try to impress on them how I feel about it?"[52]

Silent Spring appeared in September 1962. Carson was immediately caught up in a world of speaking engagements, interviews, and world-wide attention. She made a visit to Cleveland in October, but saw Crile and his wife Jane (who was suffering and would soon die from breast cancer) only at a social engagement. The juxtaposition of her literary success and her hidden cancer life seemed strange to Carson herself, who wrote Freeman, "All this is written as though the menacing shadow did not exist, yet the day before I left (for Cleveland) it seemed as though time was standing still and there might even be no tomorrow."[53]

By the start of the new year (1963), Caulk had concluded that Carson needed radiation treatment for her continued back pain. Carson's recollection to friends of the exact reasons for this treatment were reminiscent of the evasions and ambiguities that surrounded her original cancer diagnosis, about which she had been angry and regretful in retrospect. Carson wrote Freeman that Caulk had done x-rays and "although nothing shows, he felt it advisable to use some radiation. The point is that early stages of trouble in a vertebra may cause some pain but changes visible on x-ray may not appear for several months, by which time it is more difficult to handle."[54] Carson offered a delicate balance of truth, fear, and hope to Freeman about these new findings, saying it was safest to assume the worst, but drew some hope that they caught these new metastases early. She later recounted to Crile that she had concluded herself that her back pain was due to metastatic disease, noting that "Dr. C. says not necessarily, but I think he's just trying to reassure me."[55]

In early 1963, Carson also had a fainting episode, which was soon understood as the first installment of a new medical problem, angina pectoris and underlying heart disease. These new heart problems might (Dr. Healy's theory) or might not have been caused by her radiation to the chest.[56] Because of the angina, Carson was "virtually under house arrest."[57]

More cancer problems soon developed. New swellings appeared above "the collar bone, midway to the shoulder, on the left side" in February 1963. Carson summoned up the courage of Jane Crile, who had just died in January. During Jane Crile's last hospitalization, she reportedly had looked at the assembled doctors and asked, "Now which of you is in charge of not giving up?"[58] Carson wrote Crile about the new collarbone swellings and the need for further radiation treatments, as well as the additional finding of cancerous destruction of her scapula. Crile was ready again to be in charge of "not giving up" for Carson. Crile had telephoned Carson and told her (as she related to Freeman) that "radiation has taken care of it before and it will again. So that is what we must believe. He also sounded optimistic about the heart."[59] Crile telephoned Caulk and discussed the overall direction of the latest radiation treatment and also laid out a plan of androgen treatments (male sex hormone).[60]

The constant, if stuttering, treatment of newly discovered disease with additional radiation treatment had become a typical feature of mid-twentieth-century breast cancer therapeutics, but it had a direct parallel in the repeated localized breast cancer surgeries that were often performed on patients in the pre-radiation era, especially before radical cancer surgery became the norm. One of the great appeals of radical cancer surgery was to put an end to this unsatisfying situation. The original meaning and context for the name given to radical cancer surgery – *the complete operation* – was that there would be no need for future surgery. For Crile and other mid-century skeptics, however, common sense in cancer meant accepting the incompleteness of cancer therapeutics.

With advancing disease, Carson drew hope from where and from whom she could, and coped with nausea and other side effects of treatments. She also more frequently articulated her apprehension of the future. In February 1963, she asked Crile directly,

> Doesn't this all mean the disease has moved into a new phase and will now move more rapidly to its conclusion? ... If this is the correct

interpretation I feel I need to know. I seem to have so many matters I need to arrange and tidy up, and it is easy to feel that in such matters there is plenty of time. I still believe in the old Churchillian determination to fight each battle as it comes ("We will fight on the beaches –" etc. And I think a determination to win may well postpone the final battle.) But still a certain amount of realism is indicated, too. So I need your honest appraisal of where I stand.[61]

"We both know that my time is limited," she wrote Freeman in early March 1963, "and why shouldn't we face it together, freely and openly? I know that you must have dark thoughts and 'hard nights' – how could it be otherwise?"[62]

In early April 1963, Carson wrote Crile, discouraged by the progression of her disease and the renewed radiation to her spine, first to discuss her objections to hormonal manipulations – androgen therapy, followed by either removal of her adrenal glands or destruction of her pituitary gland – that Crile had apparently suggested as possible next steps. She was "unable to feel any enthusiasm for the hormonal approach" not only because of the problems associated with adrenalectomy or pituitary ablation in themselves, but also because "neither promises a great deal, really, in terms of prolongation of life," according to articles she had recently read in the *Journal of the American Medical Association.*

Carson had her own new idea, one recommended to her by her trusted colleague Dr. Biskind and one which she was "99% sure" Crile would disapprove: Krebiozen. As she explained:

> I want to give it a trial. I'm not expecting miracles. I'm well aware there is no claim it is a cure, and also aware it is a 50–50 chance as to whether I'd be helped at all. But if I'm in the lucky 50% bracket, I feel I might live more comfortably and perhaps somewhat longer than otherwise and avoid the side effects of hormones. . . . I am well aware of the controversy over Krebiozen and of the A.M.A.'s long-standing war against the Foundation and Dr. Ivy – but then I have seldom if ever found myself in agreement with the A.M.A. Their attacks on Krebiozen resemble so closely some of the methods used against those critical of pesticides that the parallel is quite suggestive.

Carson hoped to convince Healy to inject her. She wanted to get Crile's approval, noting that Caulk had already voiced his disapproval "simply for the reason that he doubts it will do any good. My answer was that as far as I've been able to learn it will do no harm, so what do I have to lose?"[63]

About the same time, Carson explained to Freeman that Krebiozen was not really a drug and did not attack local manifestations of disease like radiation. Instead, "it really helps the whole body resist."[64] In a later letter, Carson made clear to Freeman that the urgency around starting Krebiozen followed from her desire to "recover some of the optimism I've lost."[65]

In 1963 everything about Krebiozen was surrounded by controversy. In the 1940s, Krebiozen had been initially described as a bull blood derivative with effectiveness in lowering blood pressure. In the 1950s, it was described as a horse serum derivative that had been immunologically stimulated to be an effective anticancer substance. By late 1963, Federal officials believed that in powder form it was made up of the amino acid creatine and in liquid form a combination of mineral oil mixed with small amounts of other common chemicals.

However, what Krebiozen was or might have been as a substance does not reveal very much about its meaning to Carson or others. Most important for Carson, as she implied in her letter to Crile, was that Andrew Ivy's crusade for using Krebiozen to treat cancer patients contained many parallels to her own work. Since 1951, the story of Krebiozen had been linked to Ivy's fate. Ivy was a physician research scientist who was then vice-president of the University of Illinois, Chicago. Ivy had championed Krebiozen after being convinced by data on its effectiveness in inducing regression of cancer in animals. He became entangled in a decades-long public and scientific debate that involved the University of Illinois (whose chancellor was forced to resign at one point because of his opposition to Ivy), the Illinois State Legislature, the U.S. Congress, the judicial system, the American Medical Society (AMA), the Federal Drug Administration (FDA), the media, and countless patients and clinicians. At the time Carson was considering the use of Krebiozen, March 1963, the FDA was investigating Krebiozen in the shadow of the thalidomide tragedy and the Kefauver–Harris regulatory legislation that ensued.[66]

Carson saw Ivy, like herself, as a credible David fighting a scientific and policy Goliath. Carson also shared with Ivy a boundary problem. Ivy had crossed from laboratory science, the field from which his scientific credibility derived, to clinical medicine, the latter being the field that typically evaluated claims of therapeutic efficacy. Carson had crossed from her role as a government field scientist engaged in research, publications, and policy making, a woman whose training had fallen short of obtaining the Ph.D. credential, to being a scientific authority on, and public advocate for, the environment. While Ivy had avoided standard clinical trials, publications, and government review in his promotion of Krebiozen, Carson's method and style of interpreting evidence was also a challenge to normal ways of making inference about scientific data. *Silent Spring*'s cancer chapter, for example, juxtaposed summaries of laboratory experiments, testaments of prominent occupational cancer researchers like William Hueper, and selective retellings of particular etiological cancer theories such as those of Otto Warburg, that had never been well received by American cancer specialists.

Carson and Ivy each challenged typical ways that normative science reached consensus, evaluated evidence, and communicated with the larger society. Carson's and Ivy's crusades represented parts of a larger critique of normative science, although Ivy's battles over Krebiozen were more contested and heated. In March 1963, Carson was beginning to feel the chemical industry's counterattack on *Silent Spring*, and felt a deep sympathy for Ivy's situation, especially the "bickerings, struggle for power, bigotry" of Ivy's detractors.[67] More specifically, Carson felt a deep sympathy for Ivy on the basis of his being an enemy of her enemy – the American Medical Association (AMA). Carson had drawn attention to the AMA's practice of referring doctors to a pesticide trade association for information on the health effects of pesticides.[68]

Carson's interest in Krebiozen also reflected many aspects of her particular situation vis-à-vis cancer. She had earlier decided to avoid chemotherapy because of its anticipated ill effects on the "ecology of cells." She continued to worry about the implications and side effects of radiation. Looming in the background were Crile's suggestions to further manipulate her internal hormonal environment with adrenal or pituitary ablation. Carson was understandably looking for a treatment that was not only less toxic but one that might have a better fit with her view of the body and the environment. Carson understood Krebiozen as a "living tissue" substance, rather than a drug, as a means to have "the whole body resist" rather than as a systemic poison. It was analogous to organic methods of pest control, like crop rotation, rather than pesticides. Carson's situation, like that of many patients who failed first line treatments, was desperate.

Crile responded to Carson that he did not blame her for wanting to "employ some agent which has the possibility of effecting systemic control." He offered her the standard reasons for mainstream medical skepticism of Krebiozen: no one knew what it was or how it worked, there were no clinical trials, it was expensive, and there were no standard preparations. Crile personally had experience with fifteen cancer patients who had used Krebiozen, none of whom had apparently benefitted. Crile nevertheless concluded, "the main thing in the treatment of this disease is to keep busy doing something, and certainly Krebiozen would be as good as anything else except hormones."[69]

Crile made it clear that he preferred hormonal treatments as the next step. While Krebiozen had no track record, there were many "well documented" remissions due to hormonal manipulation in cases of advanced breast cancer.[70] Crile noted that twenty patients had tried the new pituitary ablation procedure in Cleveland, and there had been no associated morbidity and mortality. Moreover, this procedure (the radioactive implant that would destroy the pituitary gland was placed via an incision in the upper palate) was done by a respected neurosurgeon. "What I would do if I were you would be to go right ahead with Krebiozen for the present, and I hope that you will be fortunate enough to obtain a remission from its use," Crile wrote Carson. "If not, however, I would certainly go directly to Yttrium implantation which involves none of the side effects of the use of male hormones and gives the maximum chance for prolonged remission."

Crile concluded the letter by suggesting that his own stance on cancer was closer to Carson's perspective on the environment than Ivy's. After praising a recent television appearance by Carson as a "beautiful program," Crile urged Carson to "remember that the scientific approach to the problem of breast cancer employs alterations in the specific chemicals that control growth of specific tumors. This is the type of biological specificity that you are looking for in your ecological problems and that to date have shown the greatest promise in the control of malignant tumors."[71] In other words, the hormonal manipulation that Crile was proposing was not only more scientific (data existed, credible clinical reports, no secrecy) but also more consistent with an ecological mindset.[72]

Crile was not concerned with fighting the Ivys of the world. He may have had, like Carson, some sympathy for Ivy on the basis of the attacks on him by organized medicine. Caulk, on the other hand, was concerned about the larger battle between mainstream therapeutics and the fringe.

He wrote Crile that he hoped "that we can avoid having her receive the Krebiozen, because if any coincidental improvement should accrue, such benefit by a well known person, as she, would give the sponsors of this product unwarranted support."[73]

Carson had Healy talk directly to Dr. Durovic, who "developed the method [of Krebiozen treatment]," and who was able to send a supply of Krebiozen and dosage instructions.[74] She took Krebiozen during the spring of 1963 without apparent improvement. Even early on in the treatment she voiced some doubts about using it and delaying the hormonal manipulations that Crile had been suggesting. "Krebiozen is still a hope, but only that," Carson wrote Freeman in early May. "I wonder if I should submit to Barney's operation. I guess I must talk to him soon."[75]

It is instructive to compare Carson's use of Krebiozen and the situation in which Halsted's breast cancer patient Mrs. W. E. Burgess found herself in 1914 (see Chapter 5). Burgess had been told by one of Halsted's trainees that her situation was "hopeless." Halsted himself had first raised the possibility of trying Coley's serum – which like Krebiozen had an immunological rationale and a promoter, Coley, who had some credibility but whose foray into therapeutics was considered marginal by the cancer establishment of the day. Halsted later communicated to Burgess, as Crile did to Carson, that this treatment was not likely to be efficacious but stopped short of actively discouraging it. Like Carson, Burgess and her husband sought out Coley and Coley's toxins themselves.

However, unlike Ivy 50 years later, Coley actively tried to establish his credentials with Halsted and others and took a conciliatory, almost apologetic, tone about the most contentious aspects of the treatment, such as its aggressive marketing by pharmaceutical companies, the potential for personal profit, and the often false hopes read into it by patients. Halsted treated Coley with courtesy and respect. Between Coley's time and Ivy's, however, the public controversy around "quack" treatments in cancer as well as the negotiations among different physicians over such fringe treatment had become more contested and less civil.[76] In part, this was due to the fact that by 1963 there were more norms for establishing therapeutic efficacy than there had been in 1914. On the other hand, the essence of the negotiations between surgeons and terminal cancer patients around this "alternative" treatment was remarkably similar, if only because the meanings attached to different aspects of terminal care had not changed that significantly. There remained a need for patients to recover optimism, to sustain hope, and ultimately, as Crile put it, "to keep busy doing something."

For Carson, like Emlen and other women before her, the advance of cancer and the apparent failure of treatment created space for reflection on spiritual matters and mortality. In March 1963, Carson had mused to Freeman about three different types of immortality – *material immortality*, related to the survival of the living world in constantly changing form (in her first 1937 publication, Carson had written that "against this cosmic background the life span of a particular plant or animal appears not as a drama complete in itself, but only as a brief interlude in a panorama of endless change"[77]); the *immortality of memory*, instantiated by the idea that Carson herself would live on in the memory of others "largely through the association with things that are beautiful and lovely"; and finally, a *personal immortality*, the kind of traditional life-after-death, provided for by religion and seemingly so much at odds with the secular and scientific world that Carson inhabited. Carson was comforted that personal immortality was a possibility, that "we do not really 'know' and I am content that it should be so."[78] Carson could not expect the deathbed epiphany that Emlen's friends and family recorded. She could nevertheless take some comfort from knowing that the limit of life was something "we all share." She was also comforted by her physician and friend's wisdom. "Barney's comparison of the life–death relationship to rivers flowing into the sea," she concluded her thoughts about her own mortality to Freeman, "is to me not only beautiful but somehow a source of great comfort and strength."[79]

Carson was able to return to her beloved cottage in Maine in 1963. At the end of the summer, she alluded to the need to accept that this was her last stay there. Writing Freeman about their joint witnessing of the migration of Monarch butterflies, she noted, "it had been a happy spectacle, that we had felt no sadness when we spoke of the fact that there would be no return. And rightly – for when any living thing has come to the end of its life cycle we accept that end as natural."[80]

Back in Washington, x-rays had confirmed what Carson had suspected. Cancer had spread to her pelvic bones, leading to more radiation, a trial of testosterone injections, and more serious consideration of Crile's plan to implant radioactive seeds in her pituitary gland. "This *has* to work," Carson wrote Freeman about the testosterone injections in early October.[81] After a good day in late October, Carson wrote Freeman that "it [the slight improvement in walking] seemed like just a tiny bit of thaw during a long winter's night – but whether it really means anything I'm not sure."[82] Soon afterward, when it was clearer that the disease in the bones was progressing despite the testosterone, she was started on a trial of prednisone, which gave her some temporary relief from pain and improvement in function. Following Crile's advice, she also consulted a neurologist for her hand and arm pain. Like Caulk and her rheumatologist at their initial visits, he suggested that there might be noncancerous causes of her new problems. Carson derived some temporary hope from this consultation as well as the temporary reprieve from more radiation or pituitary ablation.[83] Less than 2 weeks later, however, Carson came to believe that her hand and arm problems were due to cancer in the neck and prepared herself to submit to more x-ray treatments.[84]

In early 1964, with her disease advancing, Carson remained concerned about shielding friends and others from the depressing reality. Writing to Freeman about a friend who last heard more optimistic reports of Carson's health, Carson urged her not to give "any new details about my health problem. The last she knew the curve was up, and I'd rather keep her thinking that as long as possible. This is now for *my* protection more than hers."[85] Carson developed more neurological problems, such as loss of taste and smell, leading to more tests and more explicit communication with her doctors about her prognosis, but still with conclusions left for Carson to draw herself. She wrote Freeman that Caulk had said to her, "'I do hate to be the purveyor of so much bad news to you.' Then he added,' But you know, it is three years since you first came to me, and you had very serious problems then.' I felt that he left unsaid, 'Don't expect too much more time.'"[86] It's reasonable to believe that this was exactly what Caulk, in the interest of honesty yet preserving hope, was trying to suggest.

More problems soon ensued. At the end of January 1964, Carson was hospitalized for a lung infection and developed meningitis and shingles. She also became anemic requiring transfusions. By March, Carson finally consented to having her pituitary gland ablated by means of a radioactive implant. After considering having the procedure done in Washington, D.C., she decided to have it done in Cleveland under Crile's watchful eye, despite the apparent disapproval of Freeman and other friends. On March 18, she had the Yttrium-90 implanted. At the time, Carson was near death, jaundiced from liver metastases, and with heart irregularities.

She returned to her home on April 6 and died in the late afternoon of April 14, apparently of a heart attack.[87]

THE WAY RACHEL CARSON LIVED AND DIED WITH BREAST CANCER reflected many aspects of late-twentieth-century medical and social realities as well as some unique aspects of Carson's situation. The very existence of the rich set of correspondence around Carson's cancer derives from her literary gifts and prominence, as well as from her decision to seek guidance from Crile in Cleveland. Unlike Halsted's distant correspondents, Carson sought out Crile because of his public role as a skeptic of received cancer ideas and practices as much or more than his clinical expertise.

Early in the course of her cancer treatment, Carson had been a typically compliant patient, accepting her internist's choice of surgeon, and the surgeon's choice of surgery. But by late 1960, she was regretting ever having played this role. Carson had lost confidence in some of her treating physicians because her disease was advancing, the available options were disturbing, and the euphemisms surrounding her diagnosis and prognosis had worn thin.

It is not possible to fully reconstruct Carson's knowledge of, and desires for, the truth about her cancer diagnosis and prognosis at different points. But it is probably fair to say that some purposeful and adaptive ambiguity existed in her doctors' representation of truth, in her own understanding, and in her relations with her doctors.

Carson's experience shared many elements with Halsted's patients and other women living in earlier periods. Physicians had been explicitly concerned with not telling the truth to sick and especially terminally ill patients since antiquity. The ethics of avoiding truthful diagnoses, if done for patients' overall benefit, was enshrined in the AMA's 1847 *Code of Ethics*.[88] By the 1950s in the United States, however, whether to tell cancer patients their diagnosis was the subject of considerable research and debate.[89] Studies reported that patients wanted to know their diagnosis, while surveys of physicians showed that evasion of the diagnosis remained the norm.[90]

When Dr. Sanderson told Carson in the wake of her mastectomy that both the frozen and permanent section pathology revealed *borderline* cancer, accompanied by hints that the cancer was caught early, he was employing a strategy that was common at the time, an era in which cancer was defined by pathology rather the clinician's judgment. In 1955, Samuel Standard articulated the traditional ethical position that evasion of truthful diagnoses was justified if it would improve the patient's prospects for recovery and that such evasions allowed patients to draw inferences in their own way and at their own pace. But he also offered a generation-specific "middle ground" way of carrying out the evasion that constituted the script, scene directions, and rationale for Sanderson's actions. Standard urged that patients be told that their cancerous tumors were benign but on the verge of malignancy and that their "early" surgery was therefore a prophylactic measure. Although he surmised that a patient knew she had cancer when she "awakes without the breast," this "middle ground" formulation helped her live "without the sword of Damocles over her head."[91]

While Crile believed that Sanderson's use of this strategy had been a "mistake," he also believed that Carson must have understood she had cancer in the wake of her mastectomy. Carson, on the other hand, wrote to friends and colleagues that she felt deceived by Sanderson after later learning more accurate medical details from Crile and others. Despite these explicit statements however, it is still possible that Crile's assessment was in part or wholly accurate. Probably Carson understood that her pathology was very likely to have been cancer yet inferred something hopeful from her surgeon's statement that there was some pathological uncertainty over its exact nature. There are a number of hints from Carson's subsequent behavior that she believed deception was sometimes justified and that she was capable of self-deception in order to maintain hope. Carson remained with her general internist, Dr. Healy, for example, despite his collusion in the original evasions. Carson herself actively evaded the truth of her diagnosis with almost everyone outside of her inner circle of intimates. While Carson was appreciative of Crile's "frank" communication about her diagnosis, there was still a pattern of collusion with Crile in the evasion of the exact nature of her prognosis.

The inference that Carson understood that she had cancer at the time of her initial surgery also has some empirical support in what has been observed about others in similar situations. A 1995 study of nurses' observations about physician–patient truth telling in terminal diagnosis reported that nurses estimated that in those cases when physicians refused to tell their patients that they are dying, a majority of patients knew of, or referred to, their impending death. Thirty-four percent of nurses estimated that up to 70 percent patients knew about their impending death, and 23 percent estimated even up to 90 percent patients did. Ethnographic studies of truth telling in terminal illness from the 1960s have similarly revealed a complex reality in which different versions of the truth and patterns of patient and physician communication coexisted.[92]

With the rise of legal precedents, patient rights, consumerism, and many other societal and medical developments the norms and expectations about truthful cancer diagnoses would change greatly in the years after Carson's death.[93] But the extent of the perceived shift in truth telling in terminal diagnosis may be overstated while obscuring continuities in physician, patient, and family efforts to balance hope, trust, and truth. In a 1988 study, for example, Canadian physicians reported that they routinely informed their patients about the results of breast biopsies. But an observational study showed that "despite their perceptions of their behavior, very few of the physicians actually communicated positive biopsy results to patients in a clear and direct manner."[94]

In addition to negotiations over diagnosis and prognosis, Carson and Crile needed to navigate among complex and unsatisfactory treatment options. Carson's convictions about society and the environment contributed to her discomfort with extant treatment options. Carson was concerned about the crudity of, and unseen damage caused by, the "2-million volt monster" that delivered focused radiation to worrisome growths and the potential damage to the "ecology of cells" by the recent introduction of cancer-destroying chemicals. Carson's argument was in part a response to the shadow of the cold war and the threat of nuclear annihilation. Fear of this potential holocaust had also infused Carson's message about the hidden, insidious, and boundary-less dangers of pesticides.[95]

Crile's dissent had different origins. He was part of an antiauthoritarian countercurrent within a much smaller microcosm of American society – the world of surgeons, surgical practice, and hospitals (described in the previous chapter). Crile recoiled against the style and substance of Halstedian certainties and moral imperatives. He had inherited from his father – a contemporary and competitor of Halsted – a cynical view of the pretensions to scientific truth of surgical practices such as the complete operation for breast cancer. Crile's dissent was not based on the high-culture critique of existing therapeutics that was just stirring in the 1950s and 1960s – the need for evidence in the form of randomized clinical trials and the like (taken up in the next two chapters) – but on a near visceral reaction to the received "false consciousness" about cancer that he observed and experienced as a surgeon and medical trainee. His critique was formed around observations of the incongruous behavior of his fellow surgeons and medical colleagues, the cancer establishment, and the fears and actions of ordinary people.

Crile argued that society had placed too much stock in speculative, localist models of the definition, meaning, and natural history of cancer. And because of our fears of cancer (which like Carson's environmentalism resonated with cold war fears of communism and personal/communal annihilation), we had made a fetish of extreme but ineffective radical treatments, oversold existing means of prevention, made cancer an *unnatural* enemy from without, and had lost track of the reasonable goals of the doctor–patient relationship and the spiritual nature of suffering and dying.

While Carson would later become a symbol for breast cancer activism, she was publicly silent about her cancer and never even imagined that her position as a breast cancer patient or victim would be a source of credibility or authority. Carson worried about just the opposite situation, that is, the widespread knowledge of her breast cancer would damage her credibility because it would give her message a narrow, personal motive. Both the style and substance of environmental and disease advocacy would soon change radically.[96]

In retrospect and to some of Carson's friends at the time, the decision to bring Carson to Cleveland for radioactive ablation of her pituitary gland did not seem in tune with either Crile's "common sense" approach to cancer nor Carson's desire to see her cancer, suffering, and dying as part of a natural process. Crile's caricature of the older and current clinical practices, which he felt were responsible for exaggerated societal fears of cancer, was perilously close to the clinical experiences of Rachel Carson, many of which he directed:

> When the breast panel were all through, they were still back to the days of Halsted and Willy Meyers' father and could offer nothing better than a radical mastectomy followed by x-ray therapy. When this failed they resorted to castration, estrogens, androgens and then with further failure, to adrenalectomy and hypophysectomy. This transition

of a living being to an animal has done more to cause fear of cancer than anything I have experienced in the past 35 years of practice.[97]

One way to understand and reconcile Carson's and Crile's actual decisions with their stated views and values is to recognize that the negotiations between Carson and Crile were more informed, open, and egalitarian than those which occurred in many older and contemporary clinical situations, even if the outcome was similar. Also, Crile valued the radioactive pituitary implant ablation as less invasive than some existing practices, such as a surgical removal of the pituitary gland, itself illustrative of a more general way that adjectives like "radical" and "conservative" are applied and used in relative not absolute terms. Crile also privileged almost any hormonal manipulation over other existing modes of therapy because hormones possessed more biological specificity in breast cancer.

Nevertheless, the fact that Carson's last weeks of life involved this aggressive treatment far from home and her loved ones at the hands of the leading advocate for common sense and cancer also needs to be understood as reflecting powerful cultural forces both within medicine and the general society: the therapeutic imperative to do something to preserve life or mitigate suffering from disease, the tendency to express hope through medical "action," and the fact that in real time both patients and doctors have often reached for treatments that have some theoretical chance of helping sustain life or relieve suffering even though the living will often regret these treatments after patients or loved ones die.[98]

In some profound sense, the meaning of the cancer diagnosis per se was shifting radically throughout the twentieth century. The cancer diagnosis was increasingly attached to all kinds of cancers picked up by screening, often at "earlier," "precancerous" putative stages of disease. As a result of these changes, the shift to greater honesty in the diagnosis and naming of the disease perhaps represents not so much ethical progress as a changed clinical reality. The initial diagnosis of cancer, by the time of Carson's diagnosis, was much less of an absolute death sentence than was generally the case in earlier eras. In effect, the locus of evasion shifted from initial diagnosis to negotiations over the prognosis of disease that all parties agreed and recognized as cancer. These continuities deserve emphasis because they are still with us, they underscore complex inertial forces that still need to be better understood, and they present dilemmas that are not likely to yield to simplistic solutions.[99]

Not surprisingly, Carson's name and experience as cancer patient have been appropriated by environmental cancer activists. A prominent breast cancer advocacy group focused on the environmental etiology of breast cancer on Cape Cod is called the *Silent Spring Institute*. An HBO documentary on a group of women with breast cancer and their work as advocates, especially in the domain of agitating for greater environmental research and interventions, was called *Rachel's daughters*.

These groups sometimes suggest that if Carson were alive today and suffering from breast cancer, she would not have been silent about her own cancer and would have taken a more activist stance about cancer advocacy. Yet there are clues in Carson's experiences that she might look askance at some of the ways her life and work has been appropriated. She might have objected to the kitsch sentimentality of pink ribbons in a disease she understood as her "private little hell."[100] Carson also never questioned the authority and credibility of standard science, only that its findings had been distorted and silenced by narrow interests. Carson knew that as an unmarried female and as someone challenging powerful interests, she was vulnerable to personal attacks that might trivialize her message by concentrating on her personal life rather than her writings. She eschewed victimhood and fiercely protected her privacy.

Carson took greater control of her own treatment when it was not going well and when she worried that her physicians' evasions might be leading to untoward clinical consequences. The trust Carson placed in Crile and retained for some of her other physicians was largely based on their implied promise to not give up on her. Hope for survival and relief from suffering, trust that doctors and friends will not abandon you, and truth telling – a difficult matter given medical uncertainty and cancer progression – have been and continue to be competing goods to be balanced by cancer patients and the people who care for and support them.

NINE

The Rise of Surveillance

By the 1960s, it was clear to more than Barney Crile and other medical skeptics that little progress had been made against breast cancer, despite half a century of the "do not delay" campaign and the increased investments in medical research and health care since World War II. American women were still dying of breast cancer at about the same high rate as earlier in the century. Although the greater numbers of women diagnosed with breast cancer meant the diagnosis was less of a death sentence, women with metastatic breast cancer, such as Rachel Carson, continued to suffer greatly from both the disease and ever-more-intensive medical interventions.

The major public health response to this disturbing stalemate was to extend the war against time from "do not delay" style exhortation to the mass surveillance of otherwise symptom-less and sign-less women.[1] Cancer activists would ultimately use the term *screening* to refer to disease testing on individuals without symptoms or at no special risk. In most cases, cancer-screening practices emerged from diagnostic tests. How and why doctors and cancer activists imagined new uses for older technologies and changed their context of use is the central story in this chapter.

Cancer surveillance shared many assumptions with the earlier educational campaign. It extended the quest for the definition, identification, and intervention in cancer to a putatively "earlier" point in breast cancer's natural history as well as earlier in women's personal history of breast cancer. The rapid succession of different programs and technologies discussed in this chapter – cancer detection clinics, cancer blood tests, cytological screening in other cancer sites, self-breast examination, and mammography – did similar work and were shaped by similar assumptions and expectations. Cancer activists searched for some effective means of prevention that was more technological, was less dependent on women themselves, answered the skepticism and fatalism of predeterminists and other critics, paid back the public in the "here and now" for their investment in cancer research, and fit the organizational needs of the cancer establishment and the realities of American private, fee-for-service medical practice.

The Making and Unmaking of Cancer Clinics

A way station from the "delay" campaign to screening was the creation and promotion of cancer clinics subsidized and run by public health services and voluntary organizations such as the ASCC/ACS. The main business of these clinics was to detect cancer using existing clinical practices and technology among both healthy women and women with suspicious cancer symptoms and, secondarily, to provide treatment. Cancer activists had multiple, compelling reasons for promoting such clinics. Few private doctors possessed the expertise or technology to provide high-quality cancer diagnostics and treatment. While this was most obvious in the provision of radium, where use was dangerous and the available supply was dramatically limited, x-ray detection of gastrointestinal cancers or detecting cervical cancer with colposcopy (microscopic examination of the cervix, first developed in the 1920s) posed similar challenges.

Cancer activists also believed that detection clinics were necessary so that the soon-to-be-discovered cures for cancer could be given to everyone who needed them. "Suppose that right now – today – a scientist somewhere developed a drug that would arrest cancer," the author of a 1950 popular cancer article imagined. "Could your state quickly reach every one of its cancer victims? Or suppose some laboratory developed a drug that would control cancer pain in one part of the body. Could your state hurry the drug to those it might help?"[2] Most physicians and researchers understood, however, that cancer cures were a long way off. The provision of cancer detection services was understood as a way to return something tangible to the public for their financial (through taxes and contributions) investment in cancer research. This "payback" rationale was especially compelling after attempts to create a national health insurance program during the New Deal failed.

Subsidized cancer clinics were also felt to fill an obvious gap in the "delay" campaign. What use was there haranguing the public to not delay when some women could not afford medical care? In addition, agencies such as the ASCC/ACS wanted to create opportunities for service among their many volunteers, which would also create a reservoir of emotional and human capital for the future.[3] Hoping for a cascade effect, the ACS placed articles in magazines and newspapers in which women were implored to agitate for cancer detection centers, even encouraging their own doctors to form one.[4]

ASCC/ASC activists believed that the biggest obstacles to the success of cancer detection clinics was the doctor in private practice, who was not generally doing nor enthusiastic about cancer detection. "The reason for this," the head of the ACS's Women's Field Army (WFA) in the 1940s said, "is that ordinarily, general practitioners do not see many cases of actual cancer per year and in the past have chiefly seen only those cases which were advanced and incurable. As a result, the doctor, especially if he is isolated from a modern, up-to-date cancer clinic, is inclined to be pessimistic."[5]

Despite some protestations to the contrary, it is clear that the cancer detection clinic movement was an end run around usual fee-for-service, private care. In an ACS report summarizing the state of cancer detection clinics in 1947, the author wrote, "while every effort should be made to encourage physicians to send their patients to these clinics, to refuse applicants unless referred by their physicians would not be desirable." Dr. Schram stated in the report on 2,552 persons examined in the clinics in Philadelphia that only "one man and seven women were referred to the clinic by physicians."[6]

Cancer activists hoped that physicians in practice would tolerate such clinics because cancer detection services were neither popular among, nor fee generating for most physicians. WFA leaders urged their minions to agitate for specialized cancer hospitals and detection clinics. In WFA training materials, James Ewing argued for a major role of specialized cancer clinics and hospitals and advised WFA volunteers to raise money for them and to encourage patients to use them. Leaders were aware that such efforts would be greeted with suspicion by some general practitioners who feared economic competition and viewed the provision of any medical services outside of fee-for-service private practice as the first step toward socialized medicine. Volunteers were taught to respectfully overcome these potential concerns. "In many states," the WFA training material warned, "you will find that the mere mention of aiding indigent patients by transportation and other means will arouse suspicion and antagonism." Volunteers were told that by carefully balancing the needs of general practitioners with those of the larger society the "WFA is one of the greatest guarantees that has yet been devised for maintaining the influence of the general practitioner and for protecting his interests."[7]

Cancer detection clinics, such as the Cancer Prevention Clinic for Women in New York City, which was started in 1937 with considerable ASCC support, responded to local needs and the gaps in the contemporary medical system. Elise L'Esperance, a physician and cancer activist who directed the Cancer Prevention Clinic, explained that the clinic was started because the New York Infirmary's tumor clinic, which provided cancer treatment and diagnostic services to people with cancer symptoms, was overwhelmed by women "eager to know if they had cancer." This prevention clinic was to be run by women doctors and volunteers in order to encourage more women with breast lumps and other symptoms to seek care.[8]

Before it was tested by experience, public health officials placed a great deal of hope in the periodic cancer detection examination, assuming not only that it would be effective but also might pay for itself by evading costly late-stage cancer treatment. In 1936, for example, prominent cancer researcher and ASCC official C. C. Little discussed with U.S. Surgeon General Thomas Parran an insurance scheme in which the ASCC would guarantee a $1,000 payment for the cost of cancer treatment if women paid a tiny premium ($1 per year) but underwent yearly cancer detection examinations.[9]

While the ASCC/ACS promoted cancer detection clinics in films and other propaganda, few such clinics actually materialized and those that did served only small numbers of women even in their heyday. L'Esperance's Cancer Prevention Clinic, for example, served less than a thousand new patients in 1945. The many more women who wanted examinations were put on long waiting lists.[10] A survey conducted in 1945 by the American Cancer Society reported that only 14 percent of the population had had a cancer examination while 45 percent had had a special tuberculosis examination.[11]

By mid-century, the ACS's enthusiasm for cancer detection clinics had cooled. Along with jettisoning its small budget, physician dominance, and "ladies home garden" mentality, the mid-century transition from the

ASCC into the ACS solidified a commitment to private fee-for-service practice.[12] ACS leaders had also grown increasingly skeptical of the effectiveness and expense of cancer clinics.

Not everyone within the cancer establishment in this period was equally pessimistic. Epidemiologist and Metropolitan Life actuary Louis Dublin was among those ACS leaders who were wary of the shift in the 1940s and early 1950s from traditional cancer activism – including cancer detection clinics – to research. In an address to the ACS board of directors in 1949, Dublin argued that the ACS was in danger of making a fetish out of research and losing touch with its audience and fund raising base – the man and woman in the street, who "want to see evidence of service. They want to know that there is a place where they can go to get the kind of examination that we have been ballyhooing about all these years and until we have built up that kind of service here, there, and everywhere, the people don't know that the cancer movement means anything."[13]

ACS official John Kilpatrick responded that Dublin had a "complete lack of understanding of this problem. Here in New York where we have more detection centers than any in the world. The meager results do not justify the amount of money that these clinics receive, and in small population centers where "mass production" is impossible the cost would be fantastic, with no assurance that the results would be any more satisfactory." Kilpatrick went on to quantify these inefficiencies. In 1948, "the 14 detection centers partially supported by the New York City Cancer Committee made 10,895 examinations and discovered only 20 cancers, at a cost of approximately $5000 each. Many of the same people keep coming back to those centers after periods of six months to one year, so that in effect many perfectly well people keep having the examinations over and over again at the partial expense of the society."[14] Even the staunchest ACS advocates of the success of existing clinics reported detecting cancers in only 0.5–2 percent of asymptomatic women attending such clinics.[15]

Some of the low yield from cancer detection clinics and programs was the direct result of concerns about infringing upon private, fee-for-service medicine. For example, Philadelphia physician Catherine MacFarlane (1902–1971) organized a campaign in the 1930s to detect cervical cancer among asymptomatic women using pelvic examinations. She ran into opposition, however, from local obstetrician-gynecologists who were skeptical of both the rationale for screening and the socialistic tendencies of her activism. As a result, the Women's Medical College, where Mac-Farlane worked, insisted that study participants had to have the approval of their private physicians. MacFarlane further avoided the appearance of socialized medicine by drawing volunteers from women's clubs and limiting enrollment to white women. These restrictions led to a systematic mistargeting of the detection campaign, as cervical cancer was and is much more prevalent among poorer women, who were unlikely to have a private physician or to be members of all-white women's clubs. Not surprisingly, the yield of MacFarlane's experiment was low (four cervical cancers per 1,000 women in the initial screen, none in subsequent screens).[16]

In addition to problems of efficacy and competition with private practice, cancer detection as practiced in the 1940s and 1950s was very intensive and demanding for both health providers and patients. A 1944 article in *Reader's Digest* favorably depicted the authors' experiences at a cancer detection clinic, a process that necessitated three visits: one for an interview with a social worker and a gynecological examination, a second for fluoroscopy of heart and lungs and tests of her eyes and ears, and a third for a visit with a private physician. The physician told the author that she was cancer-free, leading her to celebrate as "there is no other sensation equal it."[17] While many patients may have shared this exuberance, cancer detection services at mid-century were widely perceived by cancer activists and physicians as not worth the intensive medical effort.[18] A prominent cancer researcher recalled being "completely turned off" by the cancer detection clinic "because it just didn't have any possibility as I could see it. We didn't have anything that specific that we could offer. Physicians were having to do all the examinations. It's just one of these things. You can't use physician time for screening, it's just too expensive and too boring for the physician eventually."[19]

The cancer establishment's declining support for subsidized cancer clinics resulted in the post–World War II promotion of "every physician's office a cancer detection center." The ACS promoted in films and pamphlets the notion that the periodic physical examination presented many opportunities for cancer detection for the vigilant physician in private practice, because, as a popular ACS message emphasized, "half of all cancer involves sites [are] accessible to direct examination."[20] The ACS also tried to convince private practitioners that cancer detection could be

economically viable. The publicity material for a 1950s cancer prevention film aimed at general practitioners, for example, noted the added
economic value for doctors in encouraging apparently healthy people to
submit to cancer examinations: while only 1 percent of patients submitting to cancer examinations might turn out to have cancer, half were
likely have other medical problems.[21]

At mid-century, however, the promise of detecting cancer in truly
asymptomatic, apparently healthy individuals was unrealized and not
supported by experience. Whether in the public clinic feared by private practitioners or in the private doctor's office, cancer detection had
failed to impress contemporaries as effective. "I must admit that cancer
detection centers have not proven overwhelmingly successful," Charles
C. Cameron, medical and scientific director of the ACS between 1946
and 1956 later recalled, "but neither has the old cliché about 'every doctor's office is a cancer detection center.'"[22]

The Cancer Detection Blood Test – the Simple Solution on the Horizon

One response to the apparent technological limitations of cancer detection services was a quest to create a simple, preferably blood-based, cancer
detection test. Many promoters self-consciously drew an analogy to the
Wasserman reaction, an early-twentieth-century immunological blood
test for syphilis that has served and still serves (in revised form) important research, public health, and clinical purposes.[23] Immunologist and
historian of science Ludwik Fleck in the 1930s argued that the discovery of the Wasserman reaction had been influenced by centuries of social
thought about syphilis that stressed it was a disease of the blood (as well
as other overlapping conceptions, such as its being a carnal scourge).[24]
In a comparable way, the many putative cancer detection blood tests that
appeared in the 1940s and 1950s in the United States can be understood
as a response to long held popular and medical beliefs in cancer's constitutional and blood-borne character (beliefs that were nevertheless tem-
pered by more localist conceptions of cancer).

Specific twentieth-century insights into the nature of cancer were,
however, perhaps more important in shaping the quest for cancer detection blood tests. The hormonal research of Charles Huggins (for which
Huggins shared the Nobel prize in medicine in 1966) suggested that it

might be possible to detect circulating hormones or other biologically active substances in the blood that were clues to cancer. Other biological insights that supported this quest included increased acceptance of blood-borne metastases (which directly or indirectly might leave traces in the blood) and the stirring of interest in cancer chemotherapy, heralded by Alfred Gilman's and Louis S. Goodman's partially successful test of nitrogen mustard on a lymphoma patient in 1942.[25] If cancer could be cured through injection into the blood, there was reason to believe that cancer could be detected in the blood.

While there were attempts to find serological markers "in the blood" for breast and other cancers early in the twentieth century, such as Ernst Freund and Gisa Kaminer's 1911 putative cancer blood test, efforts did not really pick up in the United States until after World War II.[26] In 1948, the National Cancer Institute formally introduced a research initiative aimed at discovering simple cancer detection tests.[27] As they did with cancer detection clinics, promoters rationalized this initiative with the argument that the federal and voluntary effort to discover new cancer treatments would be wasted if there was no reliable way to find people with cancer who would benefit when discoveries were made. "Even if the cause and cure (of cancer) were unexpectedly found tomorrow," NCI official Jacob Heller declared, "there would still be need for effective diagnostic tests."[28]

Over the next decade, science magazines and the popular press reported on a range of cancer diagnostic tests, including tests that measured electrical currents across the stomach,[29] clotting times and factors,[30] radioactive tracers injected into the body,[31] dyes injected into the blood system and sensed by ultraviolet light,[32] electrical contacts that had been swallowed,[33] and the reaction of animals injected with human blood.[34] Other studies used supervoltage x-rays (to detect lung cancer)[35] and polaroid photography.[36] These tests were often reported as more than promising but less than a reality. "If this test is found to be what these early results indicate," a typical report in Reader's Digest began, "it will mark the greatest single blow against cancer since the discovery of radium and x rays. It would become a routine procedure in every physical examination, which, if done at frequent intervals, would detect the presence of any hidden cancer at an early and still curable stage."[37]

By 1960, however, the scientific community had judged the quest to find a simple cancer detection test a failure and one with negative implications for cancer prevention. A 1955 internal NCI memo concluded that blood diagnosis of cancer had been "plagued by many problems among which have been overly enthusiastic persons reporting false results before adequate clinical trials, too high a percentage of 'false negatives' and 'false positives,' poor public relations in handling the publicity, exploitation of tests by certain laboratories and physicians, and many other problems."[38]

Looking back at many of the scientific and popular accounts of these tests, the boundary with quackery was blurry, especially in the incessant reports of just-on-the-horizon quick fixes in the here and now for the cancer problem. At the same time, there continued to be unsatisfied expectations for a reliable means of mass detection of cancer that used novel technology and could be easily assimilated into medical practice.

The Pap Smear

One cancer detection test did appear in the 1940s that would eventually be widely perceived as effective, and useable in private practice – the Pap test for cervical cancer. While at the Cornell Medical Center in New York City in the 1910s, George Papanicolaou (1883–1962), after whom the test was named, collected vaginal specimens with a nasal speculum from guinea pigs and examined the resulting loose cells microscopically (the whole process was called a vaginal smear) for evidence of where his animal subjects were in their estrous cycle. In 1928, he made a presentation of his research using human vaginal smears to a conference on "Race Betterment." Papanicolaou's work was of interest to eugenics researchers because improved means for determining ovulatory status was important for contraception and population control.

But Papanicolaou took his cytological work in another direction, toward cancer diagnostics. Working with Cornell colleagues, Papanicolaou tested and refined the vaginal smear as a cancer detection test for women admitted to New York Hospital. If the cells on the smear looked malignant, biopsies could be taken using colposcopy. If cancer was found, then women were potentially cured by hysterectomy. Many problems had to be overcome, however, from the lack of criteria for diagnosing cancer on the basis of loose cells and pathologists' unwillingness, even if competent in examining cells, to look at so many normal tissue samples in order to find the occasional abnormal ones. The practicality and feasibility of testing healthy women for a rare cancer also had to be actively constructed. In the 1940s, for example, Massachusetts cancer control officials evaluated Papanicolaou's technique "from an administrative point of view." Because the positive diagnosis rate among asymptomatic women was only 1 percent, as opposed to the much higher rates among bleeding women and women with other gynecological symptoms, it was not deemed "feasible."[39]

The resources necessary to overcome such clinical and public health "common sense" about applying so much effort and resources to detect so few cancers came in 1945, when the ACS began championing the use of Pap smears on a mass scale to detect cervical cancer. The ACS funded training programs, clinical trials, patient education, and routine screening in clinics and hospitals. This infusion of activism and resources changed physician and lay behavior, which in turn helped reverse conventional wisdom about the unfeasibility of cervical cancer screening. Some observers of ACS involvement have suggested that not only was the ACS crucial in the success of the Pap test, but the Pap test represented a lifeline for the ACS by providing it with a raison dêtre, consistent with their constituencies and outlook.[40] This powerful synergy echoed the momentum of the still continuing "do not delay" campaign and later ACS and NCI mammography efforts.

Neither Papanicolaou's nor the ACS efforts were themselves without precedent in cervical cancer. Before 1940, there had been concerted efforts to reduce cervical cancer mortality through "do not delay" type exhortations, community-based screening programs with pelvic examinations like the one in Philadelphia led by Catherine MacFarlane, and work at the boundary of diagnosis and screening, such as films aimed at increasing physician's level of alertness and competence in diagnosing cervical cancer.[41]

In addition to ACS support in jump-starting its use, other modifications to the Pap technology had to be taken before the Pap smear could be widely diffused in American medical practice. As Monica Casper and Adele Clarke have demonstrated, many small innovations – "tinkering" as they characterized them – had to occur to make the basic technology do the massive screening job expected of it.[42] For example, pathologists did not want to look at loose cells and lots of normal slides or even the normal areas of slides that might contain an abnormality. Pathologists did not think their job was to apply their diagnostic acumen in a highly probabilistic manner, essentially scanning and sampling from the great numbers of normal cells in most Pap specimens.

In order to overcome these obstacles, a whole new class of worker and work was created – the (largely low-paid female) cytotechnician who worked in a shop-floor-like environment, scanning and sampling massive numbers of slides for cancer. "I guess the pathologists didn't want to be looking at a thousand or ten thousand slides to find one positive and all the rest negative," recalled Dr. Arthur Holleb, who directed ACS efforts to promote the Pap smear starting in 1947, about the early obstacles. "The suggestion was made that we could train technicians to read slides, that the pathologist would look only at questionable cells. This was a disturbing concept: technicians can't know pathology, only pathologists know pathology."[43] As disturbing as it was, the new cytotechnician-based industry of Pap smear evaluation was created and was a crucial step in the widespread diffusion of the Pap smear.

Besides such professional innovations, ACS activists had learned that the manipulation of lay demand for PAP tests was the best way to change medical practice and physician beliefs. "You've gone to the wrong people," physician Dudley Jackson recalled about efforts to sell the Pap smear directly to physicians. "You were going to the leaders of organized medicine. They will block everything you should do in cancer...you should talk to cancer patients...you've got to go to the public first."[44] "Mainly the doctors were skeptical: the test was not going to work," Holleb recalled. "It was entirely too simple. After all, those cells had been lying around for years. Why hadn't somebody found this before? The physicians thought this way, and they were fearful that we would educate the public to create a demand for which we could not supply the professional competence. But the lay members on the American Cancer Society board were all for it."[45]

In hindsight and to some contemporary observers, there were two crucial differences between the Pap smear and its relation to cervical cancer and screening and diagnosis of breast and most other cancers. First, the cervix is anatomically atypical. The examiner with only simple tools can reach cancerous and precancerous cells. Excisional biopsies of the cervix and even hysterectomies, the next steps after positive Pap smears, are also less mutilating to women than comparable breast surgery. Second, the natural history of cervical cancer is unusual. There appears to be a long duration of time (often many years) in which clues (such as those picked up in the Pap smear) of more destructive malignancy are present and during which wide surgical excision of cancerous or precancerous tissue often leads to "cure," that is, no future local, regional, or distant spread.

Papanicolaou himself, among others, would later carry out experiments to see whether breast cancer could be detected through cytological examination of fluid obtained from mammary ducts and ran into the predictable problem that such cells were extremely difficult to find and sample.[46] Other screening technologies would have to be developed to do for breast cancer what the Pap smear had done for cervical cancer.[47]

Unlike the situation in breast cancer, cervical cancer mortality in the United State has been declining throughout much of the twentieth century. For most doctors and laymen, the declining death rates from cervical cancer in the decades after the introduction of the Pap smear constituted proof that detecting cancer at a precancerous or other "early" stage was effective in a more conclusive way than the many exaggerated and unsubstantiated statistical claims that were part of the "do not delay" campaign. The success in preventing what had once been the most prevalent female cancer also created great hope and expectation for a similar screening technology that could be used to prevent the new leading cause of female cancer death.[48]

The successful push to incorporate the Pap smear into the routines of medical care and women's lives also played a crucial role in the history of breast cancer screening by creating a precedent for a practical and effective test that could be used in the course of routine medical practice. The Pap smear campaign also helped create a new nexus of beliefs and behaviors: the compliant, healthy American woman who was willing to submit to regular examinations of her most intimate anatomy for the purpose of preventing cancer.

It is important to point out that although it was very successful, neither the ultimate shape of Pap smear technology nor its context of use was inevitable. One intriguing direction that has been tried in the past but never widely adopted is programs for women to do their own Pap smears. Whether or not such technology would work to reduce cervical cancer mortality, one can speculate that self-administered Pap tests would not have done all the other kinds of work eventually accomplished by the Pap smear – from its role in sustaining the ACS and fee-for-service medicine to the creation of the compliant female screening object.[49]

Self Breast Examination

Cancer activists began in the 1930s to promote the idea that healthy women should regularly examine their own breasts for suspicious lumps and other signs of breast cancer, what came to be called self breast examination (SBE). In the years following World War II, the ACS produced SBE movies, planted articles in the press, sent speakers around the country, and developed teaching material to be used by physicians, ACS volunteers, and the lay population.[50] While individual women had surveyed their breasts for signs of cancer in earlier eras, there had been no organized movement for them to do so.[51] The ACS promotion of SBE was nevertheless an incremental innovation from the "delay" campaign, as it was only a small step from promoting heightened awareness of suspicious cancer signs to urging self-surveillance.

SBE was a logical outgrowth of physician directed cancer detection clinics and programs. For example, Catherine MacFarlane added physician directed breast examinations to her cancer detection clinic in 1942. She soon promoted SBE as a means of detection in the interval between cancer detection clinic appointments. One reason for this effort was that very few breast cancers were detected in routine visits to the clinic – in only 11 among the 11,203 cancer detection visits at MacFarlane's clinic up until 1955 were new breast cancer diagnosis made on the basis of physical examination alone.[52]

Although SBE was unlike the Pap smear in that it was self-administered and did not involve any novel technology, it was often promoted – awkwardly at times – as a specific and technical detection procedure. Given this lack of technological innovation, it hardly requires pointing out that the mid-century promotion of SBE reflected social more than biomedical or technical developments.

As exhorting women to simply "not delay" had not produced a decline in cancer mortality, cancer activists were looking for different ways of having an impact. SBE rested on similar assumptions as the "do not delay" campaign: an orderly ontological model of breast cancer's natural history and belief that individuals should bear responsibility for detecting cancer. SBE was plausible and compelling because clinicians had long known that almost all breast masses that were proven to be cancerous were first detected by women themselves and only afterward confirmed by their physicians. SBE also seemed attractive because it preserved a woman's privacy by not involving others, especially male physicians.[53]

Promotion of SBE was directed by the ACS, not by grassroots movements, and it ultimately served to displace responsibility for detecting cancer from physicians onto ordinary women. At the same time, however, one can also see in the exhortations over SBE the stirring of the patient autonomy and consumer movements in medicine in which women would take more responsibility for their health and health care.

There was almost no discussion of the efficacy of SBE until the 1970s. Later observers would decry that SBE had been promoted in an evidence-free environment. "The breast self examination is being promoted with films. Of course, this is another example of the thing that so often happens," cancer control official John Dunn recalled in 1975. "It sounds like a good idea and lets promote it and show woman these films and tell them that they ought to be doing this, but nobody ever evaluated this thing."[54]

In 1977, Philip Strax, one of the earliest proponents of screening mammography, noted that, despite SBE's compelling rationale and its promotion in films and pamphlets, "the net result of all this effort has been insignificant. Gallup polls have indicated that only a small percentage of women exposed to these pamphlets or movies have responded with regular self-examination. Most women admit to not understanding this routine, being averse to the thought of examining themselves, being too anxious even to begin the study, or simply not having the inclination to be bothered."[55] Prominent New York surgeon Cushman Haagensen and his colleagues similarly believed that "recent exploitation of breast carcinoma by the media has so badly frightened many women that they can no longer examine their breast objectively." In addition, after years of teaching patients to perform SBE (including writing papers and making a movie), Haagensen concluded that "very few of them have continued to practice it for very long."[56]

Breast X-Rays Done Since the Early Twentieth Century, But Not for Screening

Screening for cancer using breast x-rays emerged in the 1950s and 1960s in large measure because two previously separate trends caught up with each other. One was the growing demand for an effective screening test for breast cancer. The other was a half-century of tinkering with radiological techniques to aid in breast cancer diagnosis. Then and now, a limiting influence on any radiological aid to breast cancer diagnosis is that once cancer is suspected, given the dangers of missing the cancer diagnosis or subjecting a patient to radical surgery for no reason, it needs to be confirmed by pathological examination. So innovators largely limited themselves to trying diagnostic x-rays in situations where there was not enough clinical suspicion to warrant a surgical biopsy or where some diagnostic uncertainty remained after pathological examination.

While most accounts of the history of mammography, which have generally been done by radiologists, have woven a tale of gradual technological improvements that finally led to a test that was reliable enough to use for diagnosis and later screening, a more accurate assessment might be that the growing demand for effective means of prevention encouraged new uses for – and extended the run of – technological innovation in breast x-rays. This demand was so compelling by the late 1950s and early 1960s because of the cumulative failure of the "delay" campaign, cancer detection clinics, cancer blood tests, and SBE and the relative success of the Pap smear. In other words, what is most striking about the history of breast x-rays is the imagined new uses of – and constituency for – the breast x-ray as a mass screening tool.[57]

The first reported use of radiographs of the human breast (done on pathological specimens) date from 1910, only 15 years after the first x-rays of human tissue by Wilhelm Conrad Roentgen (1845–1923).[58] In the 1930s, some physicians attempted transillumination of the breast (shining nonionizing light of different wavelengths through the breast) as an aid to cancer diagnosis.[59] Around this time, American radiologist Stafford Warren started using breast x-rays, perhaps the first American to use them in clinical diagnosis, touting them as a superior to transillumination for distinguishing cancer from chronic mastitis because they visualized the breast capsule, the structure of breast masses, and calcifications (not seen on transillumination) as well as leaving a three-dimensional, permanent record. Warren also noted that breast x-rays could make a definite clinical contribution among women who had fatty breasts. While fat impeded palpation, it improved the diagnostic resolution of breast x-rays. Warren also presented mammography as a way of following women who had been examined by surgeons and felt not to have cancer. He reported finding cancers among such women using breast x-rays.[60]

Warren's work, however, was apparently greeted with skepticism and apathy.[61] Years later, mammography pioneer Robert Egan would explain that after Warren "there followed 30 years of disinterest and actual disrepute."[62] But another view came from the author of an official history of the American Cancer Society who believed that Warren's success was not seized upon by others because he had not created a viable niche for breast x-rays within surgical practice. Surgeons still believed that palpation was "all that was needed."[63]

Radiologists in subsequent decades combined breast x-rays with other techniques in attempt to find a niche for them in breast cancer diagnosis. In 1945, Raul Leborgne injected contrast into breast ducts and took x-rays of breast anatomy, a practice thought unsafe in earlier periods (some believed that tumors might follow).[64] Leborgne thought that this innovation would give x-rays a niche in the diagnostic work-up of breast cancer because it "will often enable the surgeon to operate sooner in cancer of the breast and to perform small, conservative, prophylactic operations in simple intraductal papillomas which have been well localized."[65]

Dr. Jacob Gershon-Cohen: "It's There, Don't You See It?"

Most accounts of the history of mammography have depicted Dr. Jacob Gershon-Cohen (1899–1971) of Philadelphia as a tireless advocate for breast x-rays in both cancer diagnosis and screening, but imply that his published results were not replicated or for other reasons not believed. As a result, Gershon-Cohen's efforts were not directly responsible for the rapid uptake of screening mammography in the early 1960s. Typically, such histories give credit to Robert Egan's later technological innovations. But Gershon-Cohen arguably did more than any other single individual to promote the visibility of and rationale for using breast x-rays as a screening tool. Gershon-Cohen's efforts also provide a window into the practical obstacles that needed to be overcome before mammography could be widely deployed and some of the ways the technology might fit clinical practice besides being an effective diagnostic and screening tool.

In many ways, Gershon-Cohen was on the academic periphery. He was a practicing radiologist at a community (albeit large and university-affiliated) hospital, Albert Einstein in Philadelphia. His eclectic and wide-ranging interests – spanning the viral etiology of cancer to, at the end of his career, tele- and video diagnosis – were increasingly out of tune with the growing specialization of academic medical careers.[66] While the model of a busy clinician publishing results from the clinical outcomes of his private patients was an accepted and prestigious model in the era before rapid expansion of the U.S. research efforts after World War II (for example, the distinguished career of cardiologist Paul Dudley White at Harvard), by the 1960s this type of research and resulting knowledge was much less important than clinical trials generated from a wider and less selected pool of potential research subjects.

Gershon-Cohen had been experimenting with breast x-rays for cancer diagnosis since 1937. He would eventually write over 125 articles on breast x-rays. His analysis of why breast x-rays had not been assimilated into medical practice despite his own and others' efforts did not emphasize purely technical obstacles. Instead, he pointed to the need to overcome the inertia created by the mindset, routines, and economic context of the practices of other radiologists and surgeons. The biggest obstacle was surgeons, who generally were skeptical about radiologists' ability to detect cancers.[67] In a handwritten note on an offprint of a 1965 paper that Gershon-Cohen gave to prominent Philadelphia surgeon I.S. Ravdin, he wrote that "the contents of this report require an awareness of its implications which you have already attained in contrast to most of your colleagues." Gershon-Cohen believed that most surgeons, unlike Ravdin, could not see outside the narrow clinical parameters of the individual patient–surgeon relationship and give credit to contributions from other types of doctors. In the article itself, Gershon-Cohen gave a case history in which there had been "a delay of 24 months that need not have occurred if the roentgenologist's report had been taken seriously."[68]

Steeped in the "do not delay" rhetoric but also knowledgeable about clinical realities, Gershon-Cohen began a 1955 paper by observing that after noticing a breast lump on SBE, many women simply wait and do nothing. He argued that the supervised aspect of breast x-ray, by removing the responsibility from women and placing it onto the medical system, might prevent this delay.[69]

Gershon-Cohen understood the potential value of breast x-rays in their clinical context rather than in the more idealized way NIH bureaucrats and others further removed from the doctor–patient encounter often viewed technology. Gershon-Cohen argued, for example, that for doctors and women confronted with the possibility of breast cancer, breast x-rays provided a "brief respite from the final decision to act"; that the allure of technology would be a powerful positive motivator to encourage women to be screened; and that negative breast x-rays, much more than benign physical examinations, would prove reassuring to many patients, especially those with "cancerphobia."[70]

Gershon-Cohen also promoted new clinical niches for diagnostic breast x-rays. They might, for example, be routinely used to detect cancer in the unaffected breast of women already diagnosed and treated for breast cancer. If a serum-based cancer detection test was ever found to work, then x-rays of the breast would further localize the cancer.[71]

Most importantly, Gershon Cohen may (in a 1956 paper) have been one of the first American physicians to clearly articulate the goal of using breast x-rays to screen adult women for cancer. He and colleagues quickly followed up with a trial of screening breast x-rays. This trial did not have a control group and was dependent on patient volunteers from Gershon-Cohen's clinical practice. In addition, it did not use vigorous inclusion and exclusion criteria and employed enthusiastic radiologists who admittedly "over-read the films."[72] Gershon-Cohen later reported an incidence rate of detected cancer in this trial that was much higher than one would expect from the distribution of breast cancer in the general population. Out of 1,055 screened women, 115 women had an abnormality that required a biopsy; 23 of these proved to be malignant.[73]

Since many of these women must have been previously diagnosed, had lumps or worrisome symptoms, or were at higher risk than the average women, Gershon-Cohen's study did not in itself constitute compelling evidence for mass screening. Gershon-Cohen himself was more concerned with finding solutions to more practical obstacles to the mass diffusion of breast x-rays. He noted that radiologists commonly misdiagnosed films and that breast x-rays were so unpleasant for some women (pain and forced reckoning with one's mortality) that women would often not repeat the experience. In the report of his "screening" study, Gershon-Cohen noted that while most patients with cysts were reassured after being told they had a normal x-ray, "at least 11 volunteers have refused to return for reexamination because they were emotionally disturbed by the procedure. Unquestionably a number of women are unable to withstand the strain of a periodic check-up of this type, especially since it involves a certain time lag (usually a week) between examination and report."[74]

Gershon-Cohen believed that breast x-rays might illuminate the natural history of cancer. In a 1958 paper, he suggested correlating some precancerous states with mammography in order to better understand the relationship between physiologic changes such as dysplasia and cancer.[75] He believed that deploying breast x-rays on a mass scale might not just detect early, small cancers, but also find precancerous tissue before it had become cancer. He was well aware of, and motivated by, the dismal record of existing practices to have an impact on breast cancer mortality.[76]

Gershon-Cohen had a very difficult time finding money to support his research and tinkering. Lewis Robbins, the chief of the cancer control program for the Public Health service, later recalled the many objections to Gershon-Cohen's 1960s application for a $15,000 grant to continue his screening program: Gershon-Cohen was "almost alone in his interest in mammography"; reviewers were critical (for reasons discussed above) that the study was diagnostic rather than screening as Gershon-Cohen had claimed; and negative x-rays would give women a "false sense of security." One reviewer presciently "urged that we check for unnecessary exposure in this study." The only thing that saved this application was when I. S. Ravdin offered the information that Gershon-Cohen had discovered two occult cancers that he had been unable to palpate.[77]

According to the recollections of a prominent mammographer, Gershon-Cohen "more than anyone else ... foresaw the great potential value of periodic repetitive screening in the control of breast cancer."[78] This enthusiasm for screening was evidently part of his problem, coming before its time from a radiologist with marginal academic credentials and a private practice orientation. Ravdin repeatedly advised Gershon-Cohen to tone down his enthusiasm.[79] Ravdin also urged Gershon-Cohen not to infringe on surgeons' turf by publishing in radiological not surgical journals.[80]

Years later, Robbins would recall Ravdin's description of Gershon-Cohen that captured the surprising power of Gershon-Cohen's breast x-rays to see cancer where Ravdin, the surgeon, could not, as well as the skepticism that surrounded this divination by a marginal academic player in the late 1950s and early 1960s. "But his point was that Gershon-Cohen could see something, nobody else could. Gershon-Cohen would hold it under a bright light and take a glass and look and others couldn't find anything, but Gershon-Cohen said, it's there, don't you see it? Nobody saw it. Radiologists couldn't see it. Nobody believed him. They thought it was – I don't know what they thought it was."[81]

Gershon-Cohen's efforts to find an effective screening tool for breast cancer did not stop with mammography. He was a leading innovator or tinkerer in other techniques, such as thermography, as well.[82] He claimed that increased mammometric heat was present in 70 percent of thirty-six proven breast cancers.[83] At the end of his life, Gershon Cohen was investigating putting a series of half-ounce thermographic dials on the surface of women's breasts, which he dubbed mammometry, looking for surface signs (heat) of deeper trouble. In this and other tinkering, it is difficult to distinguish between the bold and innovative and the merely foolish and idiosyncratic.

Fitting Breast X-Rays Into Clinical Practice

It would take direct Federal involvement in the 1960s to overcome the many obstacles and make visible the many benefits that Gershon-Cohen had observed about mammography. As a technology not previously the focus of much NIH research support, diagnostic and screening uses of breast x-rays were initially the turf of the United States Public Health Service (USPHS) cancer control program. As in earlier periods, the scope of cancer control was the leftover clinical and preventive activities that were not the focus of NIH and NCI research.

In addition to the small grant it gave to Gershon-Cohen, the USPHS cancer control program funded radiologist Robert Egan, who worked at the MD Anderson Cancer Center in Houston. Egan, who had a background in metallurgy, and had been experimenting with breast x-rays since 1956. Unlike Gershon-Cohen, Egan worked at a major cancer research institution and focused his research efforts in a more single-minded way on technological innovations, such as using higher amounts of radiation and hot lighting of images (special lights providing more illumination of images), that would improve breast x-ray's diagnostic accuracy.[84]

Robbins recalled that his enthusiasm for breast x-rays was piqued during a site visit to Egan's project in Houston where he met a radiologist who had spent a week with Egan and who now claimed he would have no trouble finding cancer in his own cases. "Suddenly, I could see radiologists all over the country learning this within a short period of time and doing it," Robbins recalled. Prominent radiologists were impressed with Egan's films.[85] Robbins became convinced that the federal government had an important opportunity to jump-start a powerful new tool for both breast cancer diagnosis and screening (the latter being most important). Robbins understood that a prerequisite for widespread radiologic diagnosis and mass screening was a workforce of radiologists who were both capable of performing and interpreting breast x-rays and who were enthusiastic about this kind of work and could overcome surgeons' skepticism. Starting in 1960, Federal Cancer Control money supported a quest to create such a capable and enthusiastic workforce.[86]

In his initial research, Egan took advantage of a radiological interlude that was part of usual preoperative practice. Prior to breast cancer biopsy, women routinely had chest x-rays in order to determine their preoperative risk and the need for any adjustments to surgery. While patients were down in the x-ray department, Egan took additional films of the breast, and later, the axilla. Egan's 1960 report of highly accurate mammograms was important in convincing fellow radiologists that mammography was an efficacious diagnostic technology (it would eventually result in requests for 15,000 reprints).[87]

The technological improvements associated with Robert Egan's work were only the prerequisite for breast x-rays' gaining widespread credibility as a diagnostic and screening tool; they were not sufficient in themselves. Egan claimed he had renamed the procedure *mammography* in order to emphasize that the technological improvements in sum resembled a new procedure that was much more efficacious than prior radiological techniques. The term, however, as noted earlier, had been used previously.[88]

Federal support of mammography in the 1960s proceeded along a fault line that would influence future developments in important ways. Robbins's cancer control office understood its role as that of promoting immediate change in clinical practices for diagnosing and treating cancer. They did not feel that the promotion of mammography could wait until there was a scientific consensus about its efficacy. Robbins was aware of the difficult challenge of changing attitudes, spreading knowledge, and building the infrastructure that would be necessary for screening mammography to diffuse in medical practice. He also knew that research into efficacy was problematic and time consuming, and in any case, it was the responsibility of the larger research community. Robbins efforts were practical and activist. He aimed to change the minds and practices of radiologists by funding training and demonstration projects. Most prominently, cancer control monies subsidized a large number of radiologists to get 1 week of training in reading mammograms, including travel and living expenses.[89]

Finding out whether mammography really "worked" was the responsibility of NCI, which had begun at almost the same time to plan for a large, high-profile, and unprecedented prospective clinical trial of mammography (discussed in the next section). These distinct, parallel, and minimally interacting federal efforts set a precedent that would persist throughout the next decades. The fact that cancer control and cancer research occupied distinct and often oppositional bureaucratic and ideological niches within federal efforts in part explains why research into whether mammography really worked followed rather than preceded centralized efforts to jump-start mammography use in the United States. Other factors also help explain why the cart was put before the horse here, including the general bottom up, decentralized character of technological innovation and diffusion in American medicine and the considerable societal pressure to do something immediately about the cancer problem.

In creating an active and capable radiologist workforce devoted to cancer diagnosis, cancer control officials had to overcome the conventional wisdom among radiologists in the early 1960s that screening was impractical and unrealistic. Egan himself had not imagined in his first papers that screening would become usual practice. It is not clear that he even understood the full dimensions and meaning of screening as opposed to diagnosis. For example, Egan used a woman with a suspected cancer to illustrate the uses of mammography for screening.[90]

In the early- to mid-1960s, many radiologists reported their clinical experiences with breast x-rays and concluded that given the costs, burdens, and risks of x-raying women without symptoms, the low yield of cancer cases meant that screening was not practical.[91] "If anything, the experience of this study might be interpreted as placing mammography for screening some years away," the authors of an Egan replication study reported in 1965. "The conventional x-ray unit permits convenient study of only fifteen to twenty patients a day by mammography. Furthermore, the six views of the breast require far more study for reliable interpretation than did the old screening for tuberculosis. There is real danger that tumors will be missed if there is an attempt to give a 'one-minute review' to mammograms. The decision regarding the use of mammography for screening should be left to those studies designed to evaluate the application of the procedure for this purpose."[92]

Radiologists' skepticism about screening breast x-rays paralleled pathologists' attitudes toward Pap smears a decade earlier. For both groups, the idea of screening meant learning new skills and paying detailed attention to many normal specimens. Before mammography might be accepted by large numbers of radiologists, they had to accept and assimilate a much more probabilistic style of image interpretation. Even with the technical improvements of the last few decades, cancer is still not definitively diagnosed or ruled out by mammography alone. Instead, radiologists find *suspicious lesions*, which are then explored further, or *no definite evidence of malignancy*.

Cancer control officials and mammography supporters like Egan hoped to overcome surgeons' skepticism of any diagnostic procedures besides physical examination and biopsy as well as pathologists' skepticism by funding radiologists to use the new technology and therefore creating many opportunities for surgeons and pathologists to see its utility. "There was considerable skepticism among clinicians and surgeons as to the value of mammography – in many cases open antagonism," Egan explained. "As further mammograms were taken, the pathologists at first were amused, then interested, when positive diagnoses began to appear prior to breast biopsy on lesions difficult to locate in the biopsy specimen. Clinicians began to take more interest in the procedure when some non-palpable carcinomas began to be diagnosed on mammography."[93]

HIP: Proving the Efficacy and Limitations of Screening Mammography

As cancer control officials were changing the attitudes and routines of radiologists about mammography, the NCI, in 1963, under the direction of Dr. Michael Shimkin, Chief of the Biometry and Epidemiology Branch and Associate Director for Field Studies, began to plan a randomized clinical trial of the effectiveness of screening mammography. The very idea of such a trial was unprecedented in its methods, scope, logistics, and implications. Shimkin was well versed in predeterminist skepticism about cancer treatment and public health practices. "It is even very hard to demonstrate the effect of any therapy in breast cancer," Shimkin argued in response to a question at a 1961 conference. "We need randomized, designed studies of breast cancer more than in any other neoplastic disease."[94]

The ensuing study was perhaps the first large-scale, randomized clinical trial for any disease comparing screening to no screening over a long period using disease-specific mortality as the primary endpoint. Because the technology's penetration into clinical practice was still minimal, it was ethically and practically possible to conduct a trial using a nonscreened control group. The situation would be very different just a few years later. "Within 5 years, mammography has moved from the realm of a discarded procedure to the threshold of widespread application," the authors of a mammography study would assert in 1966.[95]

The study took advantage of the methodological innovations that were developed in other large clinical trials and epidemiological studies of the 1950s and early 1960s.[96] But a clinical experiment of screening had its own special problems. Whether screening "works" or not ultimately depends on the effectiveness (or ineffectiveness) of treatment. Diagnostic technology is not in itself beneficial to patients although it may directly confer risks such as radiation exposure.

In 1963, Shimkin discussed with Sam Shapiro, a statistician who served as the research director of the New York Health Insurance Plan of Greater New York (HIP), a staff model health maintenance organization in New York City, and Phillip Strax, a HIP radiologist, the idea of conducting a randomized trial of mammography using HIP patients and doctors. Planning was in part inspired by Gershon Cohen's 1961 pseudo-screening experiment and the first Egan papers.[97] Shapiro later recalled that the special features of HIP – its large size, membership stability, clinical databases, and newly developed computer programs – made it possible to accomplish the task.[98] Health maintenance organizations like HIP were relatively new and were trying to create a market and ideological niche as progressive, cost-efficient, and population-oriented purveyors of health care. Using HIP as a site for preventive research therefore had considerable appeal to such an organization.

After an exploratory visit from Shimkin, Shapiro, Strax (whose wife had died of breast cancer 16 years earlier), and surgeon Louis Venet decided to test mammography and physical examination (the study group) against no screening (the control group).[99] A total of 62,000 volunteers (a sample size of adequate statistical power to detect a 20 percent reduction in mortality due to screening) were randomized. The study enrolled women between the ages of 40 and 64 from December 1963 until June 1966. Surgeons generally performed the physical examinations. The 65 percent of the study group who showed up for the initial examination were offered three additional examinations (all but 12 percent had at least one additional examination).[100]

The investigators wanted to know if mammography and physical examination could detect cancer not already known to patients and their doctors. So entry was limited to women who did not report existing symptoms or prior diagnoses of breast cancer. HIP investigators were aware that uncontrolled and less sophisticated trials such as those done by Gershon-Cohen had reported high detection rates that could only be explained by the fact that many women already had and knew they had suspicious signs or actual diagnoses of cancer and entered trials in disproportionate numbers. The desire to measure only new cases also led investigators to throw out cancer cases uncovered during the study period that were determined to have had been diagnosed before the study began. This procedure, however, would later prove problematic because there would be many more such exclusions in the study group due to more frequent contact with investigators and thus more scrutiny. This procedure raised the possibility that any putative mortality benefit in the study group could be due to greater exclusion of already existing breast cancer cases.[101]

Because of the long preclinical and clinical phases of breast cancer it was not until 1971 that the HIP investigators were able to reliably report mortality results. As of October 1969, there were 31 breast cancer deaths in the study group and 52 in the control group, a 40 percent mortality reduction. There was no statistically significant mortality difference between study and control groups among women who were under 50 at the time of initial screening.[102] It was difficult to assign the relative contributions of mammography and physical examination to the observed difference.[103]

HIP investigators believed that their study was the death sentence for biological predeterminism. "The principle of 'biologic predeterminism' in breast cancer that led to pessimistic attitudes toward detection has been abrogated with the data from the Health Insurance Plan," HIP investigator Phillip Strax concluded.[104] Although Strax believed that the HIP study was the death knell of predeterminist critics and pessimistic attitudes, the transformation of "breast cancer" into a mass disease, in part catalyzed by HIP, would inspire a whole new generation of cancer skeptics.

TEN

Crisis in Prevention

(1) Such confusion at this late stage of the project underscores the folly of waging an all-out "war on cancer" before it is even known whether the weapon may be as deadly as the disease.

Unsigned editorial, New York Times.

(2) Ode to a Millirad:
We're taught we must find breast Ca
Before it starts to grow,
for that's our only hope today
To overcome the foe.
We often need mammography
To spot the one we seek:
When it's too small to feel or see,
When it's quite lean and weak.
But now a clamor rings alarm:
Will bad exceed the good?
Will x-ray hazard produce harm
And hurt more than it should?
We could push numbers to and fro
And hope the fright will fade,
But why not cut the dose so low
That fears are all allayed?

Phillip Strax, prominent mammographer

(3) In our preoccupation with statistical and epidemiological data, with lead times and length biases, we must often stop and remind ourselves that we are dealing with anxious, frightened, and often terrified human beings.

Morton Goldman, NCI official

(4) Now if a butcher who short-weighs a pound of bologna is performing an unlawful act, why is there no such legal protection preventing excessive irradiation to women's breasts?

Rose Kushner, breast cancer activist

(5) I am convinced that if we among the profession here can't even understand what we are saying to each other, that we are going to have troubles.

Samuel Thier, prominent academic internist [1]

Launching the Breast Cancer Detection and Demonstration Projects

In 1972, Arthur Holleb, a senior vice-president at ACS, and Phillip Strax, the HIP study coinvestigator, discussed the possibility of a wide-scale, national breast cancer screening demonstration program that would be supported by both the ACS and the NCI.[2] Holleb and the ACS were eager to repeat their success with Pap smear promotion. Cancer control, which had languished as a central United States Public Health Service (USPHS) activity (Robbins' promotion of radiologist training in mammography was one of its last acts), had recently become a central mission of NCI as a result of wording added at the end of the legislative process that resulted in Nixon's 1971 Cancer Act.[3] NCI officials visited Strax's Guttman Institute, a NYC cancer screening center that had mammography as its centerpiece, and decided that promoting mammography on a wide scale was feasible. Earlier USPHS efforts to build a capable and enthusiastic radiologist workforce had laid the groundwork. The recent publication of HIP results showing a 40 percent lower death rate in the screened group provided a scientific rationale.[4] There was also considerable excitement about the mutual benefits to both the NCI and the ACS for cosponsoring and cofunding a project that would jump-start mammography. As one observer at the time noted, "both the ACS and NCI will gain a great deal of favorable publicity because they are bringing 'research findings to the public' and 'applying them.' This will assist in obtaining more research funds for basic and clinical research which is sorely needed."[5] The ACS and the NCI struck a deal in March 1973 about funding the project in which the ACS would pay one-third and the NCI two-thirds of the total cost.[6]

Despite being under the aegis of the NCI, the resulting Breast Cancer Detection and Demonstration Projects (BCDDP) had a lot more in common with – and in some sense inherited – the activist agenda of earlier UPHS cancer control programs rather than the research tradition of the NCI, which had shepherded the HIP study. BCDDP was part of a much older tradition of public health demonstration projects that had been carried out by federal and state governments as well as private foundations earlier in the century. These projects marketed new public health practices to community groups, medical specialists, and local hospitals, whose support was necessary for their successful uptake. For example, Metropolitan Life Insurance and Massachusetts' health authorities had conducted a tuberculosis screening demonstration project in Framingham, Massachusetts, in 1916 whose aim was to demonstrate that it was feasible to screen an entire community for tuberculosis and to transform lay, medical, and public health screening beliefs and behaviors.[7] The goal of these projects was to effect immediate change in clinical and public health practice, not to evaluate the efficacy of particular measures. Among the underlying assumptions of such studies were that demonstration was better than exhortation in changing deeply held beliefs and practices, and that medicine's and the lay public's caution about innovation was a barrier to be overcome, rather than an important check on scientific hubris.[8]

The public disclosure of the breast cancer diagnosis of many prominent women in the early 1970s, including Betty Ford, Happy Rockefeller, Shirley Temple Black, and Marvella Bayh, increased public interest in breast cancer prevention. Growing use of chemotherapy and less mutilating breast cancer surgery had also raised women's expectations and decreased fear of treatment, probably contributing to greater lay and medical acceptance of screening mammography.

The plans for BCDDP were ambitious and expensive. The investigators planned to recruit some 290,000 women at 29 mammography centers.[9] In addition to "demonstrating" physical examination and mammography, the project's organizers added thermography, the diagnostic technology that had been championed by Gershon-Cohen. The technology was presumed harmless and BCCDP planners hoped it might ultimately prove a way to "prescreen" women and decide who needed mammography. This was deemed especially important in the under-50 group who had not benefited from screening mammography in the HIP trial and among whom breast cancer incidence was low and mammography more difficult to interpret.

While not a research project per se, the organizers argued that the project could help answer some practical questions: Would large numbers of women get screened? Do women perform self breast examinations (SBE)? Does screening detect many small cancers whose treatment organizers assumed to lead to better outcomes? To answer these questions, BCDDP organizers planned to collect data on cancers detected, surgical survival rates (to be compared to historical controls), and SBEs.

However, in keeping with the reality that BCDDP was launched to change hearts, minds, and routines, not to produce generalizable knowledge, the first substantive planning for data management did not begin until 6 months after the study began. At different times, some NCI officials proposed changes that would make BCDDP more of a research project, but BCDDP organizers did not incorporate them. For example, in 1974, the BCDDP's Protocol Committee rejected a proposal to randomly vary screening intervals in order to study the impact of different periods between mammograms.[10]

From the beginning, NCI insiders were critical of the wasted opportunity to collect useful data. Data from BCDDP's volunteer sample, one person involved with early planning wrote in 1973, "will tell us virtually nothing about the problem of reaching the average woman."[11] "I tend to wonder what any 'demonstration project' is supposed to demonstrate," another NCI official noted in 1973.[12] Biostatistician Marvin Zelen made three site visits to BCDDP projects early on and concluded that "the proposed protocol will not be able to generate data which will help answer questions about the benefit of early detection using mammography, thermography, and a physical examination ... In view of the above difficulties, it would be wise to re-consider the entire protocol ... Why not simply give $100,000 to any institution who wishes to participate with the proviso that these institutions screen some minimum number per year free of charge?"[13]

Concerns were also raised about the use of women under 50 among whom the HIP study was showing that mammography was not effective. Malcolm Pike, a professor of Community Medicine and Pediatrics at the University of Southern California, wrote the chief of NCI's Cancer Biology and Diagnosis division in 1974 that "giving a woman under the age of 50 a mammogram on a routine basis is close to unethical."[14]

BCDDP planners knew about and discussed almost every other flaw in the program that would later elicit severe criticism prior to the program's launch. Such internal criticisms, however, did not divert BCDDP planners from their goal to make screening mammography routine throughout the United States.[15] BCDDP's failings as a research project were beside the point. Holleb voiced his antipathy toward statistician critics of BCDDP who did not understand the clinical realities of cancer and cancer prevention: "The critic draws diagrams which are pure hypotheses and meaningless clinically," Holleb wrote to an NCI official, "yet presented as statistical gospel. This is a fine example of the application of statistical methodology without knowledge of the natural history of a disease process."[16] Holleb observed that had he and other ACS officials paid full attention to the complaints and concerns of researchers, there would never have been the successful ACS push to promote the Pap smear. Holleb depicted BCDDP "biological determinist" critics as hypocritical, publically skeptical about screening programs "yet rush their wives to the physician's office at the first suspicion of possible cancer."[17]

BCDDP implementation thus progressed undeterred by insider criticism. Each center was able to recruit some 5,000 women each year. Altogether, 245,000 women participated in the project in the first year. Approximately half were under 50. Participants made 1,074,019 visits during which program doctors detected 4,443 cancers. Another 886 cancers among BCDDP participants were detected by doctors outside the program.[18] Approximately 50 of every 1,000 visits resulted in a clinical cancer diagnosis, biopsy, or surgery. Approximately one-half of the breast cancers were detected by mammography alone and the other half by mammography in concert with physical examination. This detection rate by mammography alone was much higher than reported in the HIP program, known incidence rates for breast cancer, or from extrapolations from breast cancer death rates.[19] Many of the volunteers must have previously noted lumps or had other reasons to suspect cancer. Not surprisingly, the cancer detection rate declined in subsequent years of BCDDP.

BCDDP organizers and mammography enthusiasts soon celebrated the large number of detected cancers, especially small and noninvasive ones, as signaling the program's success. Its promoters hoped that reports of the large number of detected cancers would lead women throughout the United States to conclude that mammography was effective and to demand mammograms. "The publicity that has accompanied each unit has served to alert women," observed the BCDDP project directors in 1974, during the first year of the program. "Each woman who will be

examined will tell others. This produces a swamping effect. This will create a demand and has done so."[20]

Not So Fast: Critical Insiders Go Public

John Bailar, a physician with epidemiological training who was the NCI
Deputy Associate Director for Cancer Control, was the most persistent
insider critic of the evolving BCDDP program. Although Bailar later
recalled that his main criticism was the rush to implement screening
mammography without good data on its benefits, his warning that mammography might itself induce cancer would soon attract the most public
attention. Bailar had raised the radiation risk danger from repeat mammograms internally. For example, he mentioned it amidst other concerns
about excess biopsies in an internal 1973 NCI memo.[21]

Bailar derived his initial estimates of radiation risk from the recently
released report of the Advisory Committee on the Biological Effects of
Ionizing Radiation, which had reviewed data from the nuclear bombs
dropped on Hiroshima and Nagasaki and estimated the long-term dangers of radiation exposure.[22] Radiation risk from medical x-rays, however, was not newly evident in the mid-1970s.[23] Bailar had simply drawn
attention to this "chronic" concern at a crucial moment in the history of
BCDDP.

Concerns about radiation risk provided a way to raise questions about
the wisdom of rushing to implement a nationwide screening effort,
because radiation risk was necessarily linked to questions about efficacy.
If women under 50 did not benefit from mammography, there could be
no level of acceptable radiation risk. Moreover, the breasts of younger
women might be more vulnerable and their lifetime radiation exposure
would be greater if women began screening at younger ages.[24]

Despite the uncertainty of both benefit and risk, BCDDP planners had
generally assumed that radiation risk was small and trumped by mammography's presumed benefits. On a practical level, BCDDP radiologists had
tried and succeeded to significantly reduce radiation exposure in the first
years of the program.[25]

As he was preparing a critical paper entitled, "Mammography: a contrary view" in 1975, Bailar approached senior NCI officials with his serious reservations about BCDDP and screening mammography in general. In response, NCI director Frank Rauscher appointed three panels

to review what was known from the HIP study and to apply their analysis to the future direction of BCDDP (there was not yet enough data generated from BCDDP to make meaningful inferences).[26] The publication of Bailar's contrary views in 1976 made this hitherto internal controversy publically visible.[27]

In the years since Bailar ignited the radiation controversy, many radiologists have argued that the radiation risk associated with mammography was small and acceptable. One claimed that Bailar had made women afraid of getting mammograms even for diagnostic purposes.[28] Another minimized the absolute risk by comparing it to the risks of everyday life. The presumed absolute risk of mammography (one death per 4 million women screened per year) was later equated by one mammography advocate with the risk of "100 miles traveled by air, 15 miles traveled by car, smoking one quarter of one cigarette, one-third minute of mountain climbing, and 5 minutes of being a man."[29] Phillip Strax wrote that Gershon-Cohen had been following a group of 1,000 women who had periodic mammography for over 10 years and had told him before his death that he had never felt there was any evidence of a breast cancer developing as a result of repeated mammography. "In the HIP study we found no evidence to suggest such a possibility," Strax further argued.[30] Yet cancers caused by mammography would be indistinguishable from other cancers. Such putative mammography-caused cancer could only be known in some probabilistic and statistical sense.

The three working groups released their reports in July 1976. They concluded that radiation risk was small but real. They recommended that BCDDP severely curtail its recruitment of women under 50, among whom the HIP study had found no benefit and who therefore should not be exposed to any risk, however small. They also recommended lower radiation limits for x-rays and urged the NCI to conduct more clinical trials of mammography. Another recommendation was more bureaucratic but in line with the general nascent consumer rights and bioethics movements of the period – a revision of the benefit and risk consent form to include more accurate information about radiation risk.[31]

In response to these reports, BCDDP directors developed new guidelines that would allow only women younger than 50 who were at high risk to participate. Nevertheless, project sites interpreted these guidelines in such a manner that in the first months following the implementation of the new guidelines nearly 80 percent of women under 50 were still eligible to participate.[32] Bailar called the statement that 80 percent of BCDDP participants were at high risk "mathematically absurd."[33] The ACS in official publications generally dismissed any lingering concerns about radiation, noting that the risk of radiation was "small," the level of undetected cancer is "high," and therefore the benefit of mammography was "considerable."[34]

In later publications, Bailar countered some of the more pragmatic arguments offered for screening mammography. "I feel that the use of mammography to counteract cancerphobia is incompatible with caveats to screenees that a negative examination does not rule out cancer." Bailar was distressed by the clinical observation that women underwent mammography because they were attracted to "impressive, expensive, newly developed machinery." "If so," he argued, then "something is fundamentally wrong with the way the program has been promoted to the public."[35]

Bailar argued that mammography promoters zeroed in on the woman who might be prevented from dying from cancer to the near exclusion of the woman who might be harmed from screening. "On other occasions, mammographers have spoken with eloquence of young women with breast cancer found by screening," Bailar conceded. "Their moving descriptions of the corrosive effects of anxiety, as well as the ravages of cancer, contained some truth. But what of the trade-offs? Who speaks with equal eloquence for the many young women, now free of cancer, who will have cancer induced by radiation? We do not know who they are, nor can we ever know. We can, however, estimate their numbers within some margin of error, just as we can estimate the benefits of screening at young ages. Informed but disinterested observers have now made those estimates, and they have recommended that with some very limited exceptions, routine mammographic screening of woman under 50 should be stopped."[36]

The 1977 Consensus Conference

Although their conclusions were clear and their suggestions workable, the three panels that had reviewed the HIP data in 1976 had not resolved the controversy over BCDDP and screening mammography in general. The most contentious issue remained whether women under 50 should be screened. Unlike the era of "do not delay" and its predeterminist critics, there was now a clinical trial of prevention (HIP) and centralized efforts to review and interpret its results. Yet these developments seemed to fuel rather than resolve controversy.

The first ever NIH consensus conference (September 1977) was organized to make recommendations about screening mammography. Unlike the other three panels, which had focused on HIP data, this panel would in addition directly review data from BCDDP itself. The NIH had already launched a fourth review panel, chaired by surgeon Dr. Oliver Beahrs, in January 1977. The final results of this review would not be ready until 1979, but the 1977 consensus conference was supposed to respond to the Beahrs panel's interim findings as well as to the continued widespread controversy over mammography and BCDDP.[37]

Samuel Thier, a respected leader of internal medicine and Chair of Yale's Department of Medicine, was in charge of the conference. The 16 committee members met for 3 days. The diversity and prominence of attendees was unprecedented. Those present included Rose Kushner, who had almost single-handedly invented lay breast cancer advocacy, prominent consumer advocate Sidney Wolfe, mammography innovator Robert Egan, HIP researchers Sam Shapiro and Phillip Strax, clinical trials expert Archie Cochrane (in whose name "evidence-based medicine" would rally itself in the 1990s), and leading epidemiologist David Eddy.

Many of the pitfalls and paradoxes of consensus conferences that would become apparent as such conferences grew in popularity in the next decades were present in this inaugural one. Health policy organizations generally have consensus conferences when there is no consensus among knowledgeable and interested parties about what to do in light of existing data. Gathering experts together does not make the interpretation of discordant and/or ambiguous data easier in any straightforward way. Instead, participants typically hammer out a consensus among themselves via compromise under internal and often external pressure.

The strange situation of this particular consensus panel – it was supposed to make recommendations about the future course of the ongoing BCDDP and mammography policy based on a review of two recent set of reviews, each of which had a similar set of goals – was not lost on conference participants. Controversy had obviously persisted despite these credible reviews of the data. In order to resolve the controversy, panel members would have to grapple with a large set of concerns besides data, such as the skepticism of the NCI–ACS alliance and its rapid push to make mammography a routine medical practice and the assumptions and beliefs that undergirded enthusiasts' support for screening women under 50 despite the HIP study's results. Yet there were even fewer norms or rules for making explicit and evaluating such concerns. Under whose authority could such competing interests and beliefs be balanced? What kinds of credibility, expertise, and legitimacy could justify a synthesis of what doctors and women should actually do?

These unresolved questions were apparent from the onset of the meeting. Donald Friedrickson, then head of NIH, in his opening remarks urged the conference participants to have no pretensions that there was a science of going from data to practice. Instead, Friedrickson argued that the group deliberations should result in some technical consensus about the "state of the art," of what "we know and do not know." With this knowledge, government and society "will lay their own value judgments upon the base we provide them." He also gently warned of the dangers of "self-deception," of elevating the consensus process to anything more than a "frank discussion of the available facts." Nevertheless, such a concentrated frank discussion should allow conference participants "to roll a little faster toward temporary resolution of questions to which many people anxiously need an answer. If we do this, people will be gentle with us for appearing to think we have re-discovered the wheel."[38]

Thier stated that the committee's task was analogous to the way physicians routinely gave advice to patients in situations where there was some uncertainty about what the available data meant. The committee, like a good doctor, should identify the best course of action. Thier's approach was in apparent conflict with NIH director Friedrickson's more modest plea to make sense of facts about risks and benefits upon which others would "lay their own value judgments" and "make decisions." Epidemiologist Brian McMahon seized on this conflict between summarizing data and making recommendations, arguing that it was unscientific to go from analysis of one reliable experiment (HIP) to practice. In response, Thier expressed frustration at what he perceived as an early attempt to abandon the goal of issuing a clear recommendation about mammography for doctors and the public. As the existing review panels had already summarized the facts, Thier argued that medical authority now needed to give guidance to clinicians and ordinary women about what to do with these facts. Thier caricatured McMahon's caution as naive and typical of the way a statistician, rather than a clinician, works. Thier observed that regardless of what the consensus panel concluded, clinicians and patients will do what they want. The panel's job was not to set absolute standards, but to articulate best practices given the available knowledge at that time.

Thier's position was supported by Sidney Wolfe, the prominent Ralph Nader-affiliated consumer advocate. Wolfe noted that the public was confused, especially about the age at which to begin mammography. "I think that we have to try and simplify things as much as possible. If some simple thing such as you suggest could be done, fine."[39] The clinician conference chair and the consumer advocate par excellence were arguing for an authoritative medical pronouncement, while the head of the NIH had called for patients and physicians to negotiate their individual decisions based on a consensus reading of medical evidence.

The credibility of the consensus conference was attacked in advance by mammography critics who believed that the jury had been stacked against them. "I have no interest in participating in any consensus which will serve only to cover up past mistakes," one statistician invitee wrote Thier, "to prolong the operations of the BCDDP, and to restore the cozy relationship between NIH and the health industry it is supposed to regulate."[40]

Some radiologists expressed their annoyance that there was so much controversy over radiation risk, while physicians and patients had long since accepted the risks associated with x-rays in clinical practice. They also argued that caving into radiation fears of screening mammography would inevitably jeopardize diagnostic mammography. While mammography boosters focused on the woman with breast cancer who might potentially be saved by mammography, mammography skeptics focused on the healthy woman who might suffer needless harm from screening mammography. These parallel yet opposite concerns led to the frequent appropriation by one side of the other side's rhetoric. "Instead of iatrogenically producing a breast cancer epidemic by using mammography as suggested by at least one renowned statistician," Strax argued, "we may be iatrogenically producing a serious drop in survival statistics by not using mammography to detect early disease."[41]

During these deliberations, Bailar noted that many radiologists had claimed that radiation risk was merely theoretical. Bailar argued that the risk was not theoretical – it was real enough in many population studies. A more accurate view was that the magnitude of mammography risk and dose–response relationship was indeterminate. The fact that the risk was difficult to quantify precisely did not make it any less real.[42] Bailar "modestly" proposed termination of screening programs until the groups can "develop sensible policies that will result in better selection of which patients to treat and how."[43]

MacMahon wanted to know why there had been such a rush to push mammography into practice. "I know of no large-scale national or medical policy," MacMahon argued, "that has been entered into on such a large scale on the basis of a single study, with the exception of some studies such as the trials of polio vaccine, where the effect was obviously overwhelming."[44] Other conference participants, most notably Archie Cochrane, concurred and in addition to criticizing BCDDP as a step backward in preventing cancer, argued for more randomized controlled trials (RCTs) of screening mammography.[45]

While it was difficult to compare BCDDP results to those of the HIP study because the former was not designed as a research experiment, everyone acknowledged that BCDDP had found many more "minimal" cancers than HIP. Mammography enthusiasts extrapolated from this result many expected benefits, while skeptics argued that finding of so many minimal cancers could lead to increasing amounts of surgery, an apparent improvement in survival statistics, but no mortality decline. Bailar argued that the term minimal cancer was itself problematic because it often "included lesions that are either entirely benign or of dubious malignant potential ... To call them 'minimal cancers' is to confuse doctors, mislead the public and, again, overstate the value of screening."[46]

On the other side, Strax remarked that the very idea of pulling back from mammography was wrong because medicine had no other tool that might give women some control over their cancer destiny. "In the present status of anxiety over breast cancer in this country, can anyone evaluate the benefit or reassurance of a negative breast examination in a frightened woman? We have tens of thousands of such women who now look forward with trepidation and hope to their scheduled breast examination. This is particularly true in the women under 50. Those of us who are involved on a daily basis with women who live in dread of breast cancer can appreciate the great benefit of reassurance for these women."[47]

At the conference, Oliver Beahrs presented the preliminary results of their review of BCDDP. While noting that many more better prognosis minimal tumors were picked up in BCDDP than in HIP, especially in the under-50 cohort, he was circumspect about the meaning of this development. More randomized trials were needed to see what benefit resulted and also to evaluate the continued questions of radiation risk.

One preliminary finding from the Beahrs' panel review that attracted a lot of attention at the conference was that 66 cases diagnosed as minimal cancer by BCDDP pathologists were found on review of a sample of 270 cases to be benign (this was only one of a series of observations made about the accuracy of pathological diagnosis).[48] Rose Kushner asked, "How could these atrocities have happened? I hope somebody is going to tell them they didn't have cancer after all, and that it was just a terrible mistake."[49] And underlining a persistent irony crucial to understanding the appeal of screening, Bailar noted a "funny thing, there have been a substantial number of women with lesions found to be perfectly benign on review, who had mastectomies and feel quite grateful to this project."[50]

To many in the media, the public, and the medical profession, the 66 benign cases misdiagnosed as cancer were scandalous and evidence of the unholy alliance between ACS and NCI, the poor scientific basis upon which BCDDP was based, and the rush to implementation. "In this particular case," a Washington Post journalist reported, "the yen for what looks like progress traces back to the American Cancer Society, which feasts on terrorizing the public about a dread disease ... (BCDDP) aimed at stampeding hundreds of thousands of women into enrolling in long-term x-ray screening projects."[51] BCDDP defenders argued that the misdiagnosed cases were in part inevitable error and reflected the real and problematic continuity between the normal and abnormal, even in such an ontologically secure area as cancer. Arthur Holleb wrote in an official ACS publication that in the focus on misdiagnosis, the public had not taken stock of the 2,000 cancers detected in BCDDP. "To many clinicians who treat breast cancer regularly, that's pretty good news. But it went essentially unreported ... perhaps it has become too fashionable to report only the bad news."[52]

By the end of the conference, participants had generally not moved from their original positions. There was almost no perceptible change to the limited conclusions and recommendations that had been reached by the earlier review panels studying HIP or the ongoing one on BCDDP. Participants did wrangle about changing BCDDP's informed consent form. The indirect relationship between screening and outcomes led some conference participants to argue over whether mammography's risks should be limited to direct effects like radiation, or include risks that were the result of actions triggered by mammography such as the dangers associated with biopsy and surgery.[53]

At the end of the conference, Thier was able to get a large number of participants to agree to support continuing BCDDP and screening mammography, but only for women over 50 and for high-risk younger women. Screening was recommended for women in their 40s only if they had a family history or prior personal history of breast cancer. Screening for women 35–39 was only recommended for women with a personal history of breast cancer. The committee took no issue with diagnostic mammography and saw little value in thermography. The consensus panel acknowledged the different ethical calculus for screening than testing done for evaluation of symptoms and signs by hedging the screening recommendation for women over 50, adding the phrase "if you wished to be screened for breast cancer."[54] However, since patients generally wanted to evade both cancer and unnecessary surgical procedures, and do not generally have some abstract preference for screening or no screening, this hedge did not fully address the ethical complexities. Few participants wanted to end BCDDP outright. Among other factors, repeated examinations had been promised in recruiting materials, and more generally it was feared that canceling BCDDP would be the end of mammography.

Nevertheless, there was considerable dissent over the call to abandon routine screening for women under 50. "I am very much concerned about breast cancer and I detest the fact that you are denying women under 50 access to a modality that can save their lives," one physician complained.[55] There was also continued skepticism about the very nature of the consensus panels' charge. Thier and MacMahon resumed their argument over whether the panel should make specific recommendations about what women and physicians should do and not do, or whether the result of the process should be a statement about what the experimental evidence means without such a recommendation. After Thier concluded at the end of the conference that "I believe we have reached a consensus here," MacMahon interrupted:

> No. We still haven't passed from the fact that there is some evidence for mammography, to going over to say that you would recommend that people have it. There is incontrovertible evidence that people get killed on airplanes. This leads some people not to go on airplanes. It leads

others to accept the risk. I don't think one can pass from the fact that there is some evidence to the recommendation that any single person, or everybody, should have mammography.

Thier retorted: "I guess this is where the physician and the biostatisticians part ways. You can go only so far in staying with the statistical likelihood that says you have a 43 percent chance of being helped, and a 22 percent chance of being injured. Then there needs to be some interpretation of what that means."

Tensions also arose over some suggested minor modifications to the panel's conclusions. In response to one of these suggestions, Thier retorted, "Don't even modify what I am saying. I am going to be like Humpty Dumpty. The words will mean exactly what I mean them to mean, and I won't say anything I don't mean, I hope." And going from nursery rhyme to Alice in Wonderland, Thier later responded to suggestions for language to clarify any misinterpretation, "I am concerned at being put in the position of having to say something that I don't necessarily believe because somebody might not hear what I believe if I say it."[56]

In 1979, the Beahrs review panels (divided into epidemiology, pathology, and clinical review) published their final reports on BCDDP. They noted that many more minimal cancers had been found in BCDDP than in HIP, presumably because of greater image resolution and changed diagnostic norms. The review also found a disturbing amount of variation among sites in the prevalence of cancer and the accuracy of mammography interpretation (features that were noted at the very onset of the study). The final report also noted that the proportion of cancers found by physical examination and/or mammography varied greatly between sites. In over half the centers, for example, there were no cancers that were detected on the basis of physical examination alone, while in others more than 20 percent of cancers were detected in this manner. In two centers, less than 25 percent of cancers were detected by mammography alone, while in seven others more than 60 percent of cancers were detected this way.

Radiation exposure also varied significantly among sites but tended to decrease with time in all sites. The Beahrs' group extrapolated from BCDDP radiation exposure and published estimates of the dose–response relationship between radiation and breast cancer that a 35-year-old woman's risk of cancer might increase due to screening mammography from a "7.58% lifetime risk to 7.59–7.61 or 110 to 240 excess cases of cancer per million women screened. Repeated annually this risk increased to 7.9–8.25% or 3,100 to 6,700 cases per million women."[57] Whether this extrapolated risk was acceptable was and is relative to the putative benefits of mass mammographic screening. Investigators not only called for more randomized controlled trials to answer this question, but urged study designs that could measure the incremental benefit of mammography separate from physical examination, so that it might be weighed against radiation risk.

The Beahrs' committee also concluded that "the informed consent should provide women having routine mammography with a reasonable basis for weighing radiation risks against known benefits or against benefits not established but which the BCDDP's experience suggest might result from including mammography."[58] This vague formulation reflected the very clear difficulty, perhaps even the impossibility, of individual patients, with or without the help of their doctors, understanding and balancing incredibly small and largely unknown benefits and risks, for example, increasing their lifetime risk of developing breast cancer by 1/100 of 1 percent. Although "informed consent" had become standard operating practice, the modern woman deciding about screening was making a much less informed and meaningful decision than Susan Emlen and other women with symptomatic breast cancer in the past.

The final report of the Beahrs review offered a nuanced and cautious interpretation of the misdiagnosis problem that had become a significant public controversy. The pathological review retreated from the initial report that 66 cases of BCDDP-diagnosed minimal cancers were really benign. Upon further review, 11 were put back in the cancer category and 5 were officially noted as borderline. It was also revealed that not all of these 66 minimal cancer diagnoses had led to surgery – 9 of the women so diagnosed only had biopsies. The review concluded that there were many instances in which the pathological diagnosis was in the end equivocal. "Cell change from normal to abnormal (cancer) is a continuum," the pathological review committee explained in language reminiscent of many nineteenth-century formulations, "and exactly where the line is to be drawn between a benign and malignant condition is a matter of opinion." The review panel added that "correctness of therapy must depend on surgical judgment, which is based on a multitude of factors, including an estimate of the magnitude of risk, the degree to which cell change is evident, the personal attitude and desires of the patient, the evaluation of the patient's personal medical background and other factors that indicate increased risk of breast cancer, and the findings on physical examination of the patient. In some instances, after analyzing these various factors, the surgeon may believe that mastectomy is indicated even though the pathologic diagnosis is equivocal; in other circumstances, the same surgeon may prefer to follow the patient carefully without further immediate therapy. Sometimes, the disagreement in diagnosis and the risks are discussed with the patient and the patient herself may elect surgery (which is also considered by the surgeon and which appears to have occurred in at least 6 of the cases)."[59]

Biomedical insights and technological advances had not reduced the central role of clinical judgment that Halsted had articulated and promoted much earlier in the century. BCDDP's minimal cancer problem demonstrated that mass surveillance and the push to define cancer at "earlier" points in its natural history had in many ways increased the uncertainty around diagnosis and treatment. At the end of the twentieth century, individual preference and idiosyncrasy remained central to decision-making. Breast cancer was often an elusive diagnosis and the best course of treatment unclear.

DESPITE ITS MANY FAILURES AND LIMITATIONS, ACS AND NCI SUPPORTers claimed that BCDDP was a success. They were undoubtedly right in terms of BCDDP's original goals. Stripped of the always thin veneer of a research mission, BCDDP had demonstrated that women would come in droves to get screening mammograms, that radiologists would respond to this demand, and that surgeons would accept mammography. Over the next decade, screening mammography would become an annual ritual for many American women and a secure part of American clinical practice. And the increased screening mammography had its own ripple effects. For example, it increased the number of women diagnosed with localized disease, which in turn led to greater use of less mutilating breast surgery.

The rapid diffusion of screening mammography largely was propelled by factors other than clinical experiments. As Gershon-Cohen had predicted in the 1950s and 1960s, different aspects of screening mammography proved appealing to patients and to physicians in private practice. Patients turned out to have more faith in technology-based surveillance than in their own or their physician's physical examination. Physicians found that mammography not only offered a more sensitive and objective way to screen for breast cancer than either clinical or self-breast examination, but it left a material trace – the film – of normality and abnormality that could be reviewed, studied, and passed along among consultants and hospitals. Mammography turned out to be a boon for surgeons rather than an intrusion into their diagnostic supremacy. While physician offices had not become cancer detection centers, generalists in private practice were busier as a result of screening mammography. They could refer patients to radiologists or mammography centers without fear of losing control or fees.

The USPHS sponsorship of radiologist training and the ACS/NCI support of BCDDP catalyzed massive private investment in screening infrastructure by hospitals and radiological practices. The 29 BCDDP centers were the nidus of a nationwide network of facilities that resulted in easy access for patients with insurance. In addition to facilities, other economic and structural changes would sustain screening mammography's initial momentum, including new classes of work (mammographers, technicians), producers of technology (machine manufacturers), professional groups (radiologists specializing in mammography), medical settings (mammography units), and even kinds of research (studies of screening effectiveness). Following the successful Pap smear script, increased patient demand for screening mammography had worked to overcome medical skepticism.

Screening mammography was a larger and more successful effort than the "do not delay" campaign. Individual responsibility had shifted from people with suspicious cancer signs and symptoms to all adult women, who were now implored to get annual screening. Similar to "do not delay," mammography's diffusion was sustained by a positive feedback loop between the perceived efficacy of cancer prevention and treatment and compliance with screening recommendations. Increased numbers of screened women meant more diagnoses, especially of minimal and non-invasive disease. Increased numbers of breast cancer diagnoses, especially "early" ones, were seen as evidence of screening's efficacy in itself as well as by leading to an apparent lowering of the disease's case-fatality ratio. At the same time, greater numbers of mammographic diagnoses led to a dramatic – and for many, frightening – increase in the lifetime prevalence of breast cancer for the "average" women. As Strax pointed out in the conference, mammography promised individuals a way – perhaps the only way – to do something about it. By contributing to the increased fear of cancer, screening mammography had in effect generated its own rationale.

Screening mammography changed the spectrum of diagnosed breast cancer. Mammography innovator Robert Egan claimed that screening mammography had created a new form of breast cancer, one defined by its small size and often in situ pathological description. "An entirely new breast cancer evolved," Egan celebrated, "a cancer clinically occult, detected by mammography with a 95 percent cure rate. Today few of us like to be reminded of the old breast cancer, much less returned to it. The premammography, huge breast mass, often ulcerating, satellite nodules, matted axillary nodes requiring extensive surgery, radiation, chemotherapy for barely a 25-percent salvage rate."[60] Of course small, noninvasive, and in situ cancers were not entirely new things, but they were so much rarer in the era prior to screening mammography. What Egan did not say or believe but which may very well be the case is that this new type of cancer did not so much replace invasive cancer as lived in coexistence with it.

However successful screening mammography has been in these terms, controversy has persisted from the onset of BCDDP to the present (2007), especially for women under 50. Why? It is not for lack of trying to reach consensus. The 1977 consensus panel made the predictable recommendation for further research into mammography. But 30 years of further research and many other attempts have not led to consensus. The first consensus panel foreshadowed the shape and content of almost all future attempts at resolving the controversy and the difficulty of imposing some uniform message from contradictory perspectives and interests on the screening problem.

As was the case at the first NIH consensus panel, the data on screening mammography's benefits and risks have often served more like a Rorschach test than a road map. For decades, mammography enthusiasts have argued that we had entered a new and better world of effective cancer screening while skeptics worried that we had increased the amount of emotional and physical harm and economic costs to women without saving many lives from breast cancer.

The historical record does not reveal a moment in which BCDDP planners *added* the under-50 group to the screening program. Organizers simply assumed that preventing breast cancer meant targeting this group, regardless of the early returns from the HIP study. Ontological and localist assumptions about cancer's natural history and the momentum of the war against time supported screening women at earlier ages. Younger women not only developed and sometimes died from breast cancer, but the cancers of older women were presumably growing in women's bodies for years and possibly detectable by mammography. Mammography promoters also hoped to silence predeterminist critics, so it seemed only logical to screen younger women among whom cancer might be detected before their fate was fixed. The HIP study's results were often dismissed as a problem of inadequate radiological resolution that could be overcome by technological innovation that was just around the corner.

Since the HIP study there have been technological improvements and many more studies in different countries, but there has been no decisive knockout favoring one side or another in the under-50 controversy. Furthermore, debates have not been limited to the question of screening among your women. While most subsequent clinical trials have generally confirmed the HIP study's conclusion that for women over 50 screening mammography can significantly reduce the chance of dying from breast cancer, some skeptics have found problems with these data and have suggested greatly reduced or absent benefit even among older women.[61]

The decentralized and contested nature of medical authority has sustained the mammography controversy. During BCDDP, many questioned the very legitimacy of the NCI–ACS collaboration, noting these organizations and the interests they represented had much to gain in the push to spread screening mammography. ACS and NCI leaders seem to have been genuinely surprised that questions would be raised about the representativeness and self-interest of individuals and institutions who make cancer and other health policies. The inability to fully account for or discipline the local BCDDP practices and the great variation in practices among the sites only provided fuel for the skeptics.

The 1977 consensus conference explicitly raised and debated many questions that have not been subsequently answered and that have often been submerged under the accumulated mountains of data. Does self-interest taint the judgment of groups who stand to gain from particular medical initiatives? How much complexity needs to be swept under the table for the sake of clarity for the nonexpert? How do we balance the perspectives and interests of the laboratory scientist, clinician, researcher, epidemiologist, clinical trial expert, consumer, patient with cancer? The person potentially harmed by screening? Should screening recommendations be a matter of health policy at all or should decisions be made by informed medical consumers one at a time? It is revealing that this first consensus conference in NIH history began and ended with an unsettling and abstract debate over the very meaning and reach of the authority of the NIH-appointed panel.

From an historical perspective, the controversy over screening mammography is the modern iteration of a century-long debate between cancer activists and skeptics. On the one side, there are the inheritors of the activism of the ASCC, who hold new versions of older assumptions about cancer, especially its uniform, orderly, and localized natural history and faith in both individual responsibility and medical progress. And it has not been simply these ideas but the institutional, structural, behavioral, and social realities that have evolved in tandem that has given them their momentum and staying power. On the skeptical side, there has been an equally long continuity among those who have believed in the important role of idiosyncrasy and as yet unknown constitutional factors and who have been wary of medical hubris and positivism.

In the last decades of the twentieth century, it became clear that screening mammography was not by itself leading to a major decline in breast cancer. New ways of preventing and treating breast cancer were developed as well as a new "risk factor" style of understanding the disease's causes and natural history. Older, unresolved tensions continued to shape these developments.

ELEVEN

Breast Cancer Risk

"Waiting for the Axe to Fall"

By the end of the twentieth century, the average American woman faced a frightening 1:8 lifetime odds of being diagnosed with breast cancer. Many American women, with and without the disease, would agree with one breast cancer sufferer that "we are all waiting for the axe to fall."[1] Yet there had been no dramatic increase in the biological devastation directly attributable to cancer that could adequately explain either these greatly increased odds or the greater number of women who fear breast cancer compared to earlier in the century. A better explanation is that our medical and social response to breast cancer had transformed the disease's experiential, clinical, and population-level meaning. Nowhere is this more evident than in the way Americans think about and respond to *breast cancer risk*.

What I am calling *breast cancer risk* is not simply a number or a set of numbers. It is a set of beliefs, practices, and structural elements. Breast cancer risk has become our generation's dominant way of understanding what causes breast cancer and what to do to avoid it. Breast cancer risk has a history within American society. It is a consequence of roads taken and not taken.

Yet the beliefs, practices, and structural elements that constitute breast cancer risk seem such necessary and merely logical responses to epidemiological and biological insights that they are in some sense invisible and not subject to critical inquiry. We nevertheless need to make them more visible and subject to critical inquiry if we are to respond adequately to present challenges. In this chapter, I will consider (1) the construction of risk statistics and the meanings attached to them; (2) the way efforts to assert control over the frightening increase in risk have perpetuated fear; (3) the problematic blurring of the experience of risk and disease; (4) the often troubling uses to which breast cancer risk factors are put; (5) the marketing of risk reducing medications; and (6) doctor–patient relations in the age of risk.

"The Numbers Scream Out" – But What Do They Say?

Given the astounding 1:8 lifetime risk statistic, it may seem absurd to ask why more Americans fear breast cancer than in earlier eras or whether our individual, medical, and public health efforts to reduce this risk are in any way an overreaction. As one prominent breast cancer advocate observed, "the numbers scream out."[2] But what do the numbers actually say? Not only are there alternative ways to frame the aggregate impact of breast cancer that are less frightening, but the high lifetime risk is not simply the result of more disease. 1:8 is a set of odds with its own social as well as biological history.

In absolute terms, large numbers of American women currently die from breast cancer and many more are diagnosed with it. In 2003, there were almost 40,000 deaths and some 213,000 new cases of breast cancer diagnosed in the United States.[3] However tragic and shocking this high number of deaths is, when expressed as a proportion of the population (mortality rate) and adjusted for the aging of the population, it has been remarkably constant during most of the twentieth century. Breast cancer mortality in the United States has been essentially the same from 1930, when minimally accurate mortality statistics were first collected, to about 1990, after which it has declined. In contrast, breast cancer's *incidence*, the number of new cases diagnosed yearly, has steadily increased, accelerating in the last quarter of the twentieth century.[4]

Putting aside for the moment whether this rising incidence reflects more disease in the bodies of American women or greater surveillance, these trends could plausibly be interpreted by a twenty-first-century American woman in very different ways. She could infer from the dramatically increased incidence, compared to her grandmother's era, that there are frightening, new physico-environmental causes that required urgent study, societal intervention, and individual life style modification. As a science writer explained, "the mystery of what lies behind in the inexorable rise in risk over the past half-century seems to have deepened and grown more complex. And, to millions of women confronted by the bleak statistics and wondering how they can reduce their own chances of getting breast cancer, the mystery is unsettling."[5] Alternatively, she might find comfort in the knowledge that her chances of surviving breast cancer if she were to develop it are much better than in earlier eras.

Looking at the figures in yet another way, the twenty-first-century American woman could focus on the higher likelihood compared to her grandmother that she will die of breast or another cancer relative to other diseases. It might make little difference to her fears that this increased likelihood is the result of greater life expectancy and reduced odds of dying from other causes. Finally, she could examine the near constant age-adjusted mortality from breast cancer for most of the century and its more recent decline and decide that there is not much new to be concerned about, either in terms of individual danger or in terms of some unseen physical or environmental determinants.

None of these interpretations is wrong, and none excludes the others. They underscore that aggregate trends in breast cancer incidence and mortality do not determine in any absolute sense why breast cancer is feared more or by more people nor why breast cancer risk has become a central cultural and medical concern.

If we distinguish between different types of breast cancer, then the overall picture becomes open to even more diverse interpretations, some of which run directly against conventional views of the disease's aggregate impact. I will consider the changing incidence of *noninvasive* (the in situ cancers) and *invasive* breast cancer separately, because the former has risen at a much faster rate and this increase reflects different influences. In 1975, the incidence rate of noninvasive cancers among American women was 11.3 new cases per 100,000 women per year. By 2002, this rate had risen to 91.2 per 100,000. During the same interval, there was much less of a relative increase in invasive cancers. Their frequency had risen from 274 to 371 new cases per 100,000 women per year, increasing by a third rather than almost an order of magnitude.[6] But because diagnoses of invasive cancers are still much more common than noninvasive ones, their increase is responsible for a slightly greater share of the absolute increase in overall breast cancer incidence (97 vs. 80 cases per 100,000 women).

These numbers tell us that a significant proportion of the rise in breast cancer incidence in the last quarter of the twentieth century was almost certainly due to increased diagnosis of disease that would not have led to serious problems or death if not detected by screening. This phenomenon is sometimes labeled overdiagnosis and in sum, an "epidemic of diagnosis." Overdiagnosis is most evident in the more than eightfold rise in noninvasive cancers in the last quarter of the twentieth century. Almost all these cases (since they are typically too small to be palpated) were diagnosed after abnormal screening mammograms triggered biopsies.[7] If excising these "early" cancers were really preventing "later" disease, then one would have expected that their removal by surgery would have been followed by a declining incidence of invasive cancer diagnoses in subsequent years. The "epidemic of diagnosis" explanation is compelling because this decline has not happened. As we just observed, invasive diagnoses in American women have actually *increased* during the last quarter of the twentieth century.

Some of this increased incidence of *invasive* breast cancer may also be due to increased detection of disease not destined to seriously harm or kill women if it were treated later or remained undetected. This overdiagnosis interpretation is consistent with the near constant age-adjusted mortality rate during most of the period that invasive cancer incidence was rising. If more destined-to-harm disease was appearing in the bodies of more American women, we might have expected a rise in the death rate from breast cancer.

Complicating this overdiagnosis interpretation of incidence trends is the possibility that improved treatment might have offset a "real" increase in breast cancer incidence, resulting in rising incidence while mortality was constant or declining.[8] My own interpretation of these data is that there has been some increase in destined-to-harm disease (especially apparent in the rise in invasive disease incidence) and some improvements in, and greater access to, treatment. The increased incidence of destined-to-harm disease is likely due to delayed childbearing and increased estrogen exposure (as in wider use of hormone replacement therapy). The best candidates for improved treatment are the much wider use of antiestrogens and adjuvant chemotherapy that began in the 1980s. These treatments have been proven effective in clinical trials and have probably contributed to the *declining* age-adjusted mortality rate since 1990. A role for improved treatment is especially plausible when one understands that "delaying" a death from breast cancer has the result of lowering the age-adjusted mortality of a population.

But it is implausible that these treatment improvements have been enough to offset the expected mortality increase from the eightfold increase in noninvasive cancer and the 35-percent increase in invasive breast cancer incidence that occurred in the 1975–2003 period. In other words, while some of the increased incidence, especially of invasive disease, is likely to be "real," some portion of the rise in invasive disease as well as much of the rise of noninvasive disease is almost certainly due to over-diagnosis. This pattern of overdiagnosis corresponds chronologically with the wide diffusion of screening mammography after BCDDP's success in the mid-1970s.

My imprecision over the exact magnitude of overdiagnosis is not simply due to my own interpretive limitations. While the reality of the phenomenon of screening-induced overdiagnosis is accepted by nearly all observers, its magnitude is not. To give some sense of the possible magnitude of over-diagnosis, a recent analysis of a carefully implemented Swedish clinical trial of screening mammography used a narrow definition of overdiagnosis and estimated the rate was 10 percent.[9] However, the authors of a series of "rapid" online responses to this article used the same data and arrived at estimates of 18 and 30 percent.[10]

Another way to frame the potential dimensions of the problem would be to figure out the percentage of women dying from causes other than breast cancer who have undiagnosed disease in their bodies. The difference between cancer detected by unselected autopsy series and current incidence and mortality figures could yield a rough estimate of the potential dimensions of the overdiagnosis problem. Similar kinds of data have been very useful in framing the overdiagnosis problem in prostate cancer, but there are surprisingly few data to answer this question in breast cancer. Welch reviewed existing, limited autopsy studies, finding estimates among middle-aged women (the likely screened population) of breast cancer prevalence ranging from 7 to 39 percent, compared to a less than 4-percent lifetime risk of dying from breast cancer.[11]

Whatever its magnitude, overdiagnosis has had a major societal impact and has been troubling to individuals. The most challenging clinical problem is how to respond to the increased number of in situ carcinomas, lobular carcinoma in situ (LCIS) and ductal carcinoma in situ (DCIS). In the introduction, I discussed the case of Janet, whose doctors had laid out a series of options, from "watchful waiting" to prophylactic mastectomies as treatment for her LCIS, which was detected as a result of her screening mammogram. In earlier eras, LCIS was routinely treated by radical surgery but as the years passed most doctors increasingly understood

LCIS as a marker of breast cancer risk present throughout both breasts rather than as a localized pathological process. As a result, treatment has generally become much less aggressive and focused on reducing risk. The situation with DCIS is somewhat different. DCIS has generally been considered to be more of a localized, precursor lesion than LCIS, while also serving, like LCIS, as a "risk factor" for future disease in other parts of the same or opposite breast.[12] As a result, DCIS has been generally treated similarly to invasive breast cancer, despite its better prognosis.[13]

Unfortunately, pathologists do not have a reliable way to distinguish DCIS cases that might be helped by surgery, hormonal therapy, and radiation from those that will not. As we have seen, this is not a new problem in the history of breast cancer. Mass screening with increasingly sensitive diagnostic technology has made this problem that much bigger and more important to solve.

It is very difficult to balance screening mammography's inherent risks (e.g., radiation) plus the considerable costs and health and psychological harm associated with overdiagnosis with its positive contribution to saving the lives of some women otherwise destined to die from breast cancer. As indicated in the previous chapter, ever since the onset of BCDDP in the early 1970s, there have been intense but unsuccessful efforts at reaching consensus. As mentioned earlier, some reviewers of clinical trial data are not only skeptical of screening mammography's efficacy for women under 50 but for older women as well.[14] While there is general but not universal acceptance of some role for screening mammography in the recent decline in breast cancer mortality, there is no agreement on the magnitude of the effect. A recent "thought experiment" by different decision-analytic groups, using the same assumptions and data on treatment and mortality, produced estimates of screening mammography's contribution varying from 7 to 23 percent of the mortality decline.[15]

While in my own practice I do not urge my under fifty patients to get screening mammography but include it on the list of preventive practices for older patients, it would be a mistake to understand what I and my clinical colleagues do as a direct result of our individual or collective interpretation of the medical evidence. Evidence of course plays a role, but the momentum of breast cancer's social history in American society, especially the fear of cancer and the resulting need to control this fear, has been equally or more important.

Wages of Fear

Many overlapping factors are at work in shaping modern fears of breast cancer. The fact that many breast cancer patients will not be cured by modern treatments and that we have failed to identify specific products or behaviors to avoid (as in the role played by cigarettes in lung cancer) has contributed to both breast cancer fears and the magnified interest in those aggregate associations which have some plausibility and might suggest some effective means of prevention.

Perhaps the most accepted macrolevel association has been the link between breast cancer and affluence, whether one is comparing societies or individuals within a society. One observer noted that cancer generally "represents the major health problem for which private wealth cannot purchase solutions."[16] While affluence is associated with some other cancers (e.g., colon cancer), breast cancer is both the most prevalent cancer to show this effect and its association with affluence one of the strongest. This epidemiological association is not simply problematic, but the felt reality of Americans who cannot hope that economic or other kinds of progress will lead to reduced risk of the disease.

In Chapter 1, I mentioned the many largely positive changes in the material and social conditions of life over the last two centuries that are generally evoked to explain the association of breast cancer with affluent societies and individuals. Better nutrition and greater reproductive freedom have led to fewer children, later age of first childbirth, earlier menarche, and later menopause; in turn these changes have led to an increase in the number of lifetime menstrual cycles and thus greater estrogen exposure, resulting in more breast cancer. This knowledge, however, does not immediately suggest evasive action for either societies or individuals. As a society, we would not and could not set back the clock on better nutrition and greater control over reproduction. Individual "choice" in the timing and number of children is influenced by many other factors besides the putative consequences for breast cancer risk.

There are also other plausible explanations for the association between breast cancer and affluence. Many people prefer to invoke the material basis of modern affluent life, especially what we eat and encounter in the environment. For example, there has been considerable lay activism for investigating and responding to putative links between pollution and breast cancer at the local level – even when apparent "cancer clusters" can be explained by the risk factor profiles of individuals who live in particular places.[17] Many environmental activists and residents, and the politicians who supported them, were angered by a Federal study of breast cancer in Nassau County, New York during the 1990s that concluded that the higher breast cancer rates were better explained by the demographic characteristics of its citizens than by environmental toxins.[18] Others have attempted to recast breast cancer as a disease of overconsumption, providing yet another rationale for interventions already considered in relation to obesity.

Historians have speculated on other kinds of links among cancer, affluence, and demand for control. Some have wondered whether twentieth-century Americans had come to fear cancer more and increasingly embraced preventive ideas and programs because increased affluence had led them to place more value on the length and quality of life.[19] At the same time, the declining importance of religion in daily life associated with affluence and modernity has led people to be more bereft of spiritual resources with which to deal with fears of illness and death. Allan Brandt has seen in Americans' embrace of the risk paradigm in cancer and other diseases a "subtle psychological defense against the reality that human vulnerabilities and, indeed, mortality ultimately may lie beyond these efforts of individual reform."[20]

While these ideas have provided a fertile soil for cancer fears, the seed in the specific case of breast cancer has undoubtedly been screening mammography. Following the pattern of the "do not delay" campaign, screening mammography has led to many more breast cancer diagnoses, increased individual risk, greater demand for some means of control, more screening, more diagnoses, etc. Everything about screening mammography's impact has been on an even larger scale than the earlier "delay" campaign – greater investments in technology and personnel, higher expectations about efficacy, bigger controversy, and greater numbers of Americans fearing breast cancer.

Screening mammography has been promoted as the best if only modern means to reduce one's individual risk of breast cancer. One doctor argued for screening mammography despite controversy over its efficacy because women did not "want to go back to the days of thinking that there's absolutely nothing they can do to detect breast cancer early."[21] This comment unintentionally emphasizes the fundamental importance, more than efficacy and effectiveness, of the historical accomplishment, however illusory, of women gaining some control over their future risk of developing breast cancer. "They've made us scared of the disease, and it's understandable that women want to believe that there's something they can do," noted a breast cancer activist.[22]

One might imagine that growing awareness of the limited benefits of screening and its high individual and societal costs might have significantly derailed this interaction between greater cancer prevalence, more fear of cancer, heightened need for control, and increased utilization of screening mammography. The limited specificity of mammography and its annual use mean that many women will have an abnormal mammogram at one or more times in their lifetime. They may be told or infer from the situation that they are likely to have breast cancer. After a breast biopsy, they might live with a possible diagnosis of cancer for days or weeks until they learn that their pathology is benign. Not only do such women suffer a loss of well being and the morbidity of diagnostic procedures, but some will learn that the finding of a "benign biopsy" puts them at higher risk for breast cancer than the average woman, necessitating even greater vigilance and increased surveillance.

But the harms of false positive tests have not served as a brake to the cycle of fear and increased uptake of screening. One convincing explanation can be gleaned from a 2002 survey of cancer screening beliefs and attitudes. Thirty-eight percent of this sample of 500 U.S. adults reported they had experienced at least one false positive result on one of three cancer screening tests (mammography, Pap smear, or PSA). Thirty-five percent of the female respondents had experienced a false positive screening mammogram. Some of those respondents with false positives waited over a month before finding out they did not have cancer and many reported that this was "very scary" or the "scariest time" of their lives. But before we jump to the conclusion that all we need is some "tipping point" agitation to create a mass movement of cancer detection skeptics, some 98 percent of this sample reported that they were glad they had been screened. The experience of a cancer diagnosis and its subsequent removal appeared to only strengthen already positive attitudes about cancer screening.[23]

Many such people probably believe that they had a significant and meaningful life experience, having had a brush with their mortality and yet having escaped. This confrontation and seeming victory over risk might even make many Americans feel healthier. The fact that "false positive" tests might only encourage more screening is another bit of evidence that the cycle of fear and the demand for control has an autonomous quality, beyond the rational calculation of cost and benefit in "objective" terms such as financial cost or even physical and mental health. Aided by the significant economic and structural investments in screening (discussed in the previous chapter), we have created a momentum from which it has been difficult to pull back, change direction, or even question.

The Problematic Blurring of the Experience of Breast Cancer and Breast Cancer Risk

What was formerly limited to the experience of a small number of women with symptomatic disease, has now become a mass phenomenon, extending to the much larger pool of women *at risk for* breast cancer. This idea that breast cancer risk is a mass phenomenon with a blurred boundary with symptomatic breast cancer is a mainstream scientific notion. Bernard Fisher, who directed many of the clinical trials of breast cancer treatment, including those that demonstrated that less extensive surgery could accomplish results similar to those of radical surgery, offered a personal reflection on scientific progress in breast cancer in which he presented the clinical spectrum of breast cancer as a multilevel phenomenon with a pyramidal distribution (see Figure 11.1).[24]

At the top of the pyramid are women with invasive breast cancer whose disease could be detected by clinical examination or mammography. Below them are a larger group of women whose disease could only be diagnosed by mammography, often with in situ cancers. The next level down is an even larger group of women, who have pathological changes of breast cancer (in situ cancers but also hyperplasia and other entities) but that are undetectable by present screening methods. Below these women are others with presumed genetic damage that represents the biological precursors to the observed pathological damage seen at the higher levels. Finally, at the bottom of the model, are women with no biological changes but who possess lifestyle and demographic risk factors for the genetic damage that produces breast cancer.

Fisher estimated that "below" the 175,000 new cases of invasive cancer each year in the United States are a million women with undetected but real disease. He did not specify the number of women in the "at risk for breast cancer" category, but it is not a big leap from the bottom of Fisher's

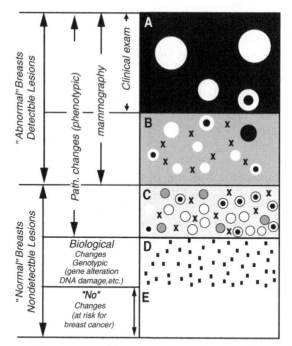

Figure 11.1. Spectrum of breast cancer: from undetectable risk to disease apparent by clinical examination. ●, invasive cancers; ○, *in situ* cancers; ◉, hyperplasia, atypical hyperplasia, sclerosing adenosis; **X**, fibroadenomas, simple cysts, adenosis, duct ectasia; ■, biological cancers. (Adapted from B. Fisher, "The evolution of paradigms for the management of breast cancer: A personal perspective," *Cancer Research*, 52 (1992): 2371–2382. Reproduced with permission of the author and the American Association for Cancer Research.)

model to the idea that an astounding number of American women are at risk for breast cancer on the basis of the putative lifestyle and demographic influences on breast cancer development.

Fisher's model provides a scientific rationale for the existence of so many American women who are waiting for the "axe to fall" as well as for the indistinct boundary between risk and disease. This boundary is further blurred by clinical responses to breast cancer. The majority of American women with breast cancer are currently diagnosed with localized disease.[25] Almost all will not have any symptoms and signs of cancer after initial treatment. Their problem is largely with the future – how best to avoid breast cancer recurrence.

Women who are "merely" at high risk on the basis of one or more risk factors often live in remarkably similar ways to women who have had a pathological diagnosis and have received medical treatment. They also face decisions and consequences that derive from their desire to lower their future risk of breast cancer. They must, for example, decide whether or not to take preventive hormonal treatment (which, as illustrated in the Tamoxifen advertisement in Chapter 1, has been marketed directly to consumers) and consent to more intensive surveillance. They must manage fear and uncertainty, assessing the credibility of different experts and their often competing claims about the disease and best practices to prevent and treat it.

Even women of "average risk," who nevertheless face a 1:8 lifetime odds of developing breast cancer, can share aspects of this "life at risk." In addition to complying with recommendations for yearly screening mammography, with attending concerns about being diagnosed with breast cancer and the high likelihood of false alarms, they must also make sense of a constant and often bewildering barrage of journalistic, medical, proprietary, and public health reports about new surveillance technologies, preventive treatments, and risk-reducing lifestyle modifications. Like others further up the pyramid, they may participate in advocacy groups and, in other venues, connect with women who have, or are at high risk for, breast cancer. Looked at from a broad perspective, changes in the way we have named, diagnosed, treated, and attempted to prevent breast cancer have transformed the experience of symptomatic or detectable breast cancer and breast cancer risk, resulting in many points of convergence.

Some women, of course, live and die with breast cancer in ways relatively untouched by the processes considered here, but they represent an increasingly smaller proportion of breast cancer patients, and their experience has been profoundly affected by being in this minority. The dominant perception of, and societal reaction to, breast cancer risk has had the unfortunate effect of distorting the complexity and diversity of disease experience, sometimes adding to the isolation and suffering of women with very aggressive disease. With or without medical intervention, in our present era or in the past, some women have died quickly and often young. I have observed breast cancer patients live from the period after surgery to death in ways similar to Mary Cope, whose experiences were described in Chapter 3. I suspect that better prevention and treatment have not made a profound difference in the life course of many women who suffer extremely aggressive disease. Rather, their experience has been overwhelmed by the transformed twenty-first-century disease experience, especially that of many women diagnosed with localized disease after screening mammography. The well-intentioned public displays of optimism, progress, and group solidarity may be especially difficult for women whose intense suffering may not even allow them a chance to relate to or meaningfully participate in races for cures, recovery programs, advocacy, and the like.[26]

In addition to the converging *experience* of disease and risk, there has been a parallel historical development in which the underlying assumptions and logic of breast cancer *decision-making* have become part of the lay and medical response to breast cancer risk. We previously observed that Susan Emlen ultimately decided to consent to unimaginably painful surgery of questionable efficacy (as she and her surgeons understood the situation) because she did not want to later be in the position of dying from cancer and regretting not having done everything possible to avert this end. Almost 200 years later, a breast cancer patient similarly chose the more extreme of different medical options because "I wanted to know that, if some time down the road I have a recurrence, I could be certain that I had done everything possible."[27] Emlen and other early-nineteenth-century women with symptomatic breast cancer also consented to breast amputations because they believed that one should fight fire with fire, one large evil with another. A similar logic underlies the difficult and even desperate decisions of many women suffering breast cancer today. "I will offer my breasts and save my own stupid life," Annette Jaffee explained in 1999 about why she consented to bilateral, prophylactic mastectomies.[28]

After surgery had failed to cure them, Emlen submitted to compression therapy and Rachel Carson to radioactive ablation of her pituitary gland at the end of her life because they and their physicians wanted to "do something," sustain hope, and reassert some degree of control against a feared and advancing disease. When faced with bad options and advancing terminal disease, even the most spiritually oriented patient skeptical of the progress touted by her physicians (Emlen) or the assertive lay critic of science and public policy and her skeptical surgeon (Carson and Crile) have found this logic compelling.

At a more cognitive level, the choice of surgery in the nineteenth century when physicians and patients were very pessimistic that it ever cured cancer was not necessarily an illogical clinical decision for individuals who had breast masses. Many women and their doctors have decided to try dangerous, mutilating, and painful treatments that were not believed to be curative on average, because of the small chance that in the particular case such treatment might prove effective. As they often had only one chance to wage a bet, individuals have typically made decisions using the law of small numbers. With little to lose and so much to gain from a treatment that works, it sometimes makes sense to gamble on treatments that on average offer no benefit.[29]

The strong constituency both within and outside medicine for practices like screening mammography for women in their 40s, despite the lack of evidence that the putative aggregate benefit outweighs risks, reflects a decision-making calculus more appropriate for the symptomatic cancer patient facing a terminal disease than for a person "merely" at risk. Women and their physicians may feel the need to "do something" vis-à-vis screening or other risk interventions, even if on average there is no mortality benefit. Like the cancer patient, persons at risk may feel compelled to assert some control over a feared outcome and find a small dose of hope. Women under 50 and their physicians may also want to avoid "anticipated regret" by erring on the side of "too much screening." Cancer is so greatly feared that the decision-making around risk intervention feels like a gamble worth taking even if the overall odds are against you.

It is easy to understand how norms and beliefs from clinical decision-making in symptomatic cancer have become operative in decisions and policies about screening, prevention, and mass communication about risk.[30] The lines between symptomatic cancer, precancer, and risk as well as between prevention and treatment have been blurred, sometimes quite consciously. Decision-making has relied on persistent but unsubstantiated assumptions about the uniformity and ontological stability of cancer. As individuals and as a society, Americans have accepted the expensive, intrusive, and at best marginally effective risk factor screening and prevention paradigm because in the presence of a feared, deadly disease we similarly want to leave no stone unturned if there is even a remote chance of averting a future breast cancer death. Senator Thomas Harkin, a fervent and important supporter of screening younger women as a matter of *health policy*, explained that he was convinced "that had my two sisters had access to mammography they would not have died so young because of this terrible disease."[31] Americans have also heavily discounted the burdens of screening – iatrogenic harm, disturbance to peace of mind, and financial costs – believing that they were necessary to fight the evil of cancer. Our clinical and public health "system" must not just sit there, according to this logic, but needs to offer something to reassert control and sustain hope.

While I do not want to suggest that *all* modern risk intervention practices are inherently wrong or misguided, these extrapolations from symptomatic disease to risk are troubling because they involve shifting decision-making styles which are defensible in one context to another where there should be less fear, more sensitivity to the average and aggregate outcomes, and less attention to the law of small numbers. In deciding about screening mammography at age 40 or whether to take Tamoxifen because of such risk factors as being postmenopausal and childless, the unaffected individual is not in a desperate situation. Availing or not availing oneself of some risk interventions is likely to have little effect on one's health and life expectancy. There is more reason for asymptomatic women to believe in the laws of large numbers and to map their individual decision-making onto what is known at the aggregate level.

The Risk Factor Way of Understanding Causality and Prevention

Breast cancer risk is not equal for everyone. Its magnitude depends on individual *risk factors* for breast cancer. Such putative risk factors include older age, older age at first pregnancy, young age at first menses, mutations in the breast cancer genes *BRCA1* or *BRCA2*, close family relatives with breast cancer, history of a previous benign breast biopsy, oral contraceptive and hormone replacement therapy use, overweight, tall stature, high socioeconomic status, and Ashkenazic Jewish family background. These risk factors and the high lifetime risk are not simply objective epidemiological facts. Like earlier aggregate perspectives on breast cancer, they have been shaped by clinical and public health responses, behavioral routines, ways of making decisions and evaluating efficacy, and assumptions about health and the body.

Breast cancer risk has been marketed as useful for making individual clinical decisions, giving legs to risk ideas and practices. The National Cancer Institute, for example, has developed a website in which American women can plug in some of their risk factors – present age, age at menarche, number of prior breast biopsies, age at first live birth and number of first degree relatives affected with breast cancer – and find out their relative risk of developing breast cancer.[32] The web site explains in relatively simple language what one's 5-year and lifetime risk of breast cancer is and how that compares with someone of "average" risk.

The NCI "Breast Cancer Risk Assessment Test" and most other quantitative risk formulas are based on the Gail formula, itself derived from BCDDP data. This formula is a mathematical equation that predicts an individual's risk, relative to someone at average risk, on the basis of individual factors such as those mentioned above. This is an ironic development, given the 1970s consensus that data from the project would never serve any useful purpose. Even though BCDDP was not set up as an experiment, the data are useful for modern risk factor analysis because they contain large numbers of diverse people with and without breast cancer. Nevertheless, there are some problems with the Gail formula whether considered as a technology for individual prediction, clinical decision-making, or public health policy. As was noted by critics at the onset of the program, the BCDDP population was drawn from volunteers fearful of cancer and therefore not representative of the general population. BCDDP lumped invasive cancers with in situ cancers, and despite the large size of its population, there were small numbers of women who had specific clusters of risk factors.

Yet what is most problematic are not these acknowledged technical limitations, but rather the reification of breast cancer risk as an individual and societal health problem akin to symptomatic disease. For example, there has often been a misleading pseudoprecision attached to breast cancer risk formulations. Derived empirically rather than by etiological theory, the breast cancer risk equations are equivalent to offering precise odds of producing bread from the presence or absence of different ingredients on the shopping lists of bread makers. Not only does an idealized and incomplete list of ingredients (constituted from hundreds of thousands of self-reported shopping lists of people who bake or do not bake bread) masquerade as a recipe, but many of the purported ingredients could very well be items bought by people who bake bread although they are not actually used as ingredients. The idealized list of ingredients may also leave out the most important ones either because they are on the shopping lists of people who do and do not make bread (flour, sugar) or because they are never or infrequently purchased (water, yeast).

In addition to the way risk factors are problematic reflections of causality and are often only pseudoprecise, nonexperts generally misunderstand published assertions about their magnitude. In one study, lay respondents to a questionnaire about breast cancer risk overestimated their probability of dying from breast cancer by more than 20-fold and the benefit from screening (in terms of absolute risk reduction) by more than 100-fold.[33] As a consequence, the use of risk factors may not lead to better individual decision-making.

In so many risk interventions, a number of practices have evolved to make the clinical interaction feel familiar and meaningful, closer to traditional diagnosis, treatment, and prognosis of evident disease, for example, the way precise cut-offs defining high cholesterol (say a serum value of 300 mg/dl) lead to both a diagnosis of hyperlipidemia and a cholesterol-lowering pill. Within breast cancer risk, promoters of Tamoxifen as a preventive medication, as discussed in Chapter 1, have used a 1.7 relative risk threshold above which Tamoxifen might be initiated. The familiar sequence of clinical visit, laboratory test, diagnosis, and pill helps elide the difference between disease and risk factor diagnosis and intervention.

The quantitative character of the risk knowledge we have constructed does facilitate decision-making by allowing quick comparison of alternative choices. Yet I frequently have ambivalent feelings about this use of risk knowledge because often neither doctor nor patient fully understands the assumptions and imprecision behind risk estimates. This ambivalence is heightened because quantitative risk comparisons are most typically evoked for decisions in which there are very small differences in known consequences. To take one example at the blurred boundary of disease and risk, one of my patients had a very small invasive breast cancer and had to decide whether to add adjuvant chemotherapy to her existing regimen of surgery, radiation, and Tamoxifen. Her oncologist had suggested this course, but she was torn between the impulse to "do everything" now to lower the chances of cancer recurrence and her suspicion that there might be little benefit and some harm to adding chemotherapy to her other treatments. This skepticism arose partly from the hedged way her oncologist framed his advice: "I would do it, but since the data are unclear it is up to you to decide." She had also read conflicting advice on web sites and lay-oriented magazines and books.

I referred her to a breast cancer expert who was active in clinical trials. He told my patient that based on stage and grade and receptor status of her particular tumor and previous treatment that her risk of a breast cancer recurrence in the next 10 years was 12 percent. If she added adjunctive chemotherapy, her risk would be reduced by one tenth – that is

10.8 percent. But such adjunctive chemotherapy carried its own risks. In addition to side effects such as fatigue and nausea, my patient also faced very low odds, less than 1 percent, of serious complications such as heart failure, a second cancer, and major infection. Based on this information, my patient agreed to undergo adjunctive chemotherapy.

The expert's numbers proved very helpful to my patient. They were certainly more useful, in the sense of allowing her to measure risks and benefits of alternative decisions, than the more subjective language of "low" risks and "small" benefits. On the other hand, these numbers potentially presented a falsely solid picture of what was known and not known, since they were extrapolated from a small number of studies, which, while well designed, were not without problems and were not designed to answer this particular question for women just like my patient. There is also some degree of imprecision in any quantitative estimate which is difficult, but not impossible, to convey to someone unfamiliar with different types of error, probability, and tests of significance. I suspect that my patient – and some of my medical colleagues – do not understand the large amount of uncertainty that surrounds these extrapolations and invest these numbers with more certainty and precision than they merit.

In the end, the consultation was helpful and the use of imperfect evidence reasonable, but I was left with the feeling that the quantified risk estimates mostly performed symbolic work, giving the veneer of rationality and objectivity to a decision that was, given current ignorance and the range of most people's preferences, a coin toss. Although we often crave control over randomness and uncertainty, in some situations it might be better or at least more honest to recognize that we just do not have enough information to make a rational decision. Such recognition would at least allow us to acknowledge more openly and to evaluate the not-strictly-logical ways (the anticipated regret and fighting-evil-with-evil heuristics discussed earlier) that are often used to make decisions under great uncertainty.

Breast cancer risk factors and risk are not only quantified, but they are frequently embodied, giving them a corporeal identity, often resulting in a tangled blend of pathology and probability. The embodied nature of the risk factor may influence both clinician and patient to understand risk as more frightening and determinative of the future than the very same information constituted in another way. Diagnoses such as LCIS are at one moment real and material pathological processes that can be excised from the body and examined under the microscope. At another moment, their meaning is mainly or perhaps exclusively as a marker of the individual's location on a physiological continuum, one which signifies an increased probability of developing cancer in the future.

Similarly, we have reframed our understanding of the dangers of hereditary predisposition from knowledge of family history to possession of a mutation in either the BRCA1 or BRCA2 gene. Although the presence of these mutations is much more predictive than family history, the information is still probabilistic and difficult to utilize. The concrete nature of the breast cancer gene has profoundly shaped the clinical encounter, from the need for blood tests to the involvement of family members in counseling and testing. Such embodied risk also carries more determinist connotations than probabilities drawn from aspects of one's clinical history.

Even some well-established clinical routines, such as the practice of surgically removing involved axillary lymph nodes (commonly done since the nineteenth century), have sometimes been reformulated in terms of risk. The rationale for lymph node exploration and excision has become ambiguous – is the surgeon excising dangerous disease or gleaning information about future risk? Clinical trials that have compared removing or leaving lymph nodes in the body have been interpreted to mean that involved lymph nodes signify advanced disease but in themselves possess no special danger to the patient. According to Bernard Fisher, "positive nodes indicate an interrelationship between host and tumor that permits the development of distant metastasis."[34] In other words, it is not the danger posed by cancerous lymph nodes that is the rationale for excising them. Rather lymph nodes must be excised from the body so that they can be analyzed for prognostic information and better clinical decisions can be made.

A similar understanding has become accepted wisdom about the meaning of local recurrences following surgery and radiation for breast cancer. While surgery and radiation effectively reduce the probability of such a recurrence, from the vantage point of ultimate survival such treatment seems to have merely eliminated the ability to divine a sign of a deeper underlying problem. An "ipsilateral breast tumor recurrence" (IBTR) – a recurrence of cancer on the same side of the chest as the original breast tumor – has thus become a marker of risk rather than a physical danger in itself (thus taking something away from the rationale for treatments that most effectively prevent local recurrences). "The relationship of an IBTR to distant disease," Fisher explained, "is analogous to that of a woman without breast cancer who learns on one day that her sister has been diagnosed with disease. On that day, the "normal" sister becomes at greater risk for developing breast cancer than she was the day before, even though her increased risk existed before her sister's diagnosis."[35]

This embodiment of risk has led not only to misunderstanding between doctors and patients as well as among doctors with different degrees of epidemiological and epistemological sophistication, but problems for the patient who has an accurate understanding of the ambiguity surrounding embodied risk markers. Prominent breast cancer activist Rose Kushner, who used her own experiences as a breast cancer patient to significantly change practices and policies, recalled her shock years after surgery when she and her doctors found cancerous tissue in the skin near her sternum (breastbone). She knew that if the disease was categorized as a late local recurrence, her overall survival would not be affected. If it was instead categorized as a stage IV subdermal metastasis, then she had incurable disease.[36] Such boundary problems expose how even small degrees of ambiguity or imprecision, given the important consequences of being in one risk category or another, can have major implications.

Pills Against Risk

As illustrated by the direct-to-consumer Tamoxifen advertisement in Chapter 1, we have already arrived in the era of pills for breast cancer risk reduction. The appeal of a safe pill that could prevent breast cancer is obvious. However, there are reasons to believe that such preventive use may be premature. First, on the data side, studies testing different types of antiestrogen prevention have not been consistently positive and have used incidence rather than mortality as the primary endpoint.[37] While using incidence data may be the only feasible way to conduct a clinical experiment (because of the huge number of women and great amount of time needed to prove a mortality difference), especially at the initial stages of knowledge generation, the positive incidence studies may not be evidence of a substantial overall mortality benefit. The antiestrogens might very well be delaying the onset of otherwise treatable disease and/or curing nonfatal "pseudodisease" in some people, so when applied at a population level there might not be a net saving of lives (especially since the medicines themselves carry mortality risks).[38] This caution and skepticism may sound arbitrary, but in the history of cancer prevention and therapeutics, from Halsted through the evaluation of the "do not delay" education campaign and BCDDP, there has been a repeated pattern of promise that arose from initial experience or trials with limited endpoints, which has delivered much less than was expected.[39]

It is also relevant to draw attention to the substantial market rewards for developing risk-reducing drugs in breast cancer and to place this breast cancer risk within the larger context of risk-reducing products in American medicine and economic life. Pharmaceutical firms understand there may be only limited economic rewards for developing effective and successful drugs that cure or modify disease. There is a limited number of sufferers of any given disease, and often people are sick for only a limited length of time because treatment works, the disease is self-limiting, or the patient dies. In contrast, everyone is potentially "at risk" for a disease that only affects a minority of people. A risk-reducing drug for a feared disease might have as its market the entire population. Such a drug might need to be taken over one's entire lifespan. So it is not surprising that we live in an era of almost daily health risk discoveries and claims, endless tinkering with and promotion of new screening technologies, and the development and marketing of risk-reducing drugs, products, and services.[40]

This phenomenon does not simply derive from the economic self-interest of drug companies. There are also other historically contingent and culturally specific trends in the history of breast cancer – exaggerated claims of disease impact, resulting in a greatly increased sense of personal risk; the promise of effective prevention to restore a sense of control against random and feared disease; and the constant fanning of fears of breast and other cancers by public education campaigns and clinical practices, catalyzed both by self-interested and altruistic cancer entrepreneurs, and propelled by an autocatalytic process of aggregate perception and changed behavior.

Perhaps the most public controversy arena in which breast cancer risk and pills have figured in recent years has been one over the use of hormone replacement therapy (HRT). This controversy, in large measure because it has been resolved in favor of the once minority position of medical skepticism, has already been well analyzed as a rich precautionary tale about hubris, for-profit interests, sexism, and the limitations of observational data.[41] But it is also important to read the HRT controversy for what it reveals about the idealized view of the medical consumer. In the idealized world of some decision analysts, medical market enthusiasts, and consumer advocates, patients or medical consumers are viewed as making medical decisions that lead to the greatest utility.

Throughout the 1990s there was a consensus that individual women, with the help of their doctors, should decide on the basis of personal preference and data on efficacy and risks whether to take HRT to prevent both heart disease and osteoporosis. The most controversial aspect of this problem for the consumer and doctor was whether the putative benefits of HRT outweighed the known dangers, most prominently, the risk of breast cancer. There was a consensus that for most women the benefits outweighed the risks, derived largely from analysis of large observational trials.[42] Both the uncertainty of the estimate and the very individual nature of deciding a reasonable trade-off between possible benefit and harm, however, led to the frequent recommendation for patient/consumer choice. This consensus, with its tilt toward HRT use hedged by shared decision-making, was actively promoted by professional medical groups, in the hope of doing something in the here and now to reduce women's heart disease and damage from brittle bones in addition to treating them for symptoms associated with menopause.

Unfortunately, the evidence base supporting this consensus turned out to be wrong.[43] Starting in 2000, analysis of data from the Women's Health Initiative (WHI), a large, randomized, controlled trial (RCT) of HRT for chronic disease prevention, began to show increased risk of heart disease, stroke, blood clots, and breast cancer in women taking the drugs as compared to the placebo group, eventually resulting in a premature ending of the trial in July 2002.[44] Along with the coincident reporting of data from other randomized clinical trials, the results of the WHI led to many policy statements recommending caution or discontinuation of HRT use to prevent chronic disease. This has led to a very rapid decline in the use of these drugs for this indication as well as for treatment of menopausal symptoms, rationales which in practice were often combined. No one was now recommending women *choose* for themselves whether to take HRT or not for disease prevention.

The evident moral of the HRT saga for many observers was skepticism towards any data except those from RCTs. But this is a shortsighted view of how risk is constructed and used in decision-making. The earlier pro-HRT consensus reflected not only the heavy influence of the immensely powerful pharmaceutical industry, but also priorities familiar from the larger history of breast cancer interventions, especially (1) "doing something" over clinical and feminist skepticism toward medical adventurism and (2) individual responsibility to reduce risk over population interventions (in this case, interventions that might reduce the danger of heart disease and injuries among the elderly).

The HRT saga also reveals some limits of the idealized consumer ethos. Why did we expect in the 1990s that patient/consumers could make their own individual judgment about the meaning of complex evidence about risk? The average consumer simply did not have the knowledge or skill to make an informed judgment about such small risks. The average physician in practice also had neither the time nor the skill to present the kinds of medical evidence and sociological analysis that underlie the uncertainty in this decision. Invoking individual choice when there is controversy and ignorance has become almost reflexive, but it is hardly market neutral in the context of buying and consuming a pill or undergoing a screening test or medical procedure. There is a difference between having no policy and actively promoting shared decision-making. The latter focuses a great deal of attention on a decision about risk that might better be simply ignored. In these cases, "choice" often means scientific legitimation for particular market players and commodities.

In this special context of risk interventions, where one is dealing with aggregate, probabilistic benefits and harms, there is often no reason to privilege or evoke individual idiosyncrasy or personal preference. One may want to respect the individual's belief that zinc brings relief to his or her cold, but there is much less individual authority to say that zinc safely reduces the probabilities of heart disease or cancer. That is something only known in aggregate. Instead of actively promoting discussion and shared decision-making about using HRT for prevention, organized medicine would have had less egg on its face, and women would have been less harmed, if there had no active policy at all and a more disciplined fidelity to the traditional medical ethos of "first, do no harm."

Crucial to understanding the significance of pills for breast cancer and other risks is recognizing that we are currently in the midst of a profound shift in the way the efficacy of therapy and definitions of health more generally are understood in medicine and the larger culture. Modern therapeutics is dominated in a very material sense by health risk interventions. A significant proportion of prescribed medications as well as the meaning and purpose of many clinical interactions is devoted to the management of risk. Risk interventions constitute a large fraction of medical expenses, and these expenses represent a significant part of our whole economy.[45]

Risk intervention in breast cancer and other diseases has depended on a new way of understanding efficacy.[46] Knowing what works has never been straightforward or self-evident. American women and their physicians have decided what is efficacious from different kinds of empirical evidence, beliefs about health and the body, and judgments about the credibility of experts. At the beginning of the nineteenth century, Susan Emlen and her English physicians believed that changes in climate and diet, as well as local applications, could influence the growth and character of a breast tumor. Emlen carefully observed her body for signs that compression therapy might reduce the size of her tumor. Emlen and her family and friends exchanged stories and books, as well as materia medica, between England and America, and negotiated the credibility of different healers and their techniques.

By the end of the twentieth century, women were similarly motivated to maintain health and make the best possible decisions, but the kinds of data available, the reigning body metaphors, and the tools for deciding what was credible had changed. Women had learned from their doctors, medical advertising, and peers the probabilities of breast cancer diagnosis, survival, and death under different scenarios. They had shared in a culture that has increasingly understood the body as accumulating and reducing risk depending on genes, lifestyle choice, and the use (or not) of screening tests and preventive drugs. And they have had to make sense of a constant barrage of often contradictory health reports on things that are risk producing or averting, relying not only on their doctors and friends, but also on lay advocacy groups and websites for information. Sometimes efficacy is seemingly undermined in one stroke, as happened when the results from the WHI dealt a blow to the preventive rationales for HRT use. At other times, there has been a prolonged war of attrition along relatively fixed battle lines, as has been the case with judging the efficacy of mammography, especially for women in their 40s.

It is difficult to fully understand the implications of this shift in the underlying assumptions about what constitutes efficacy, but the implications can be unsettling. There is a considerable distance between taking a pill because one believes it will reduce one's risk of a bad outcome and taking it because it leads to a change in symptoms. Probabilistic risk assertions are difficult to evaluate and understand and not just for the lay person. Speaking of clinician confusion in the face of assertions and counterassertions about the statistical risk of breast cancer, one researcher wrote that "the new concepts challenging his position are based on evidence at times so esoteric that, being often unable to comprehend it, he may subconsciously tend to distrust it. To his further dismay, clinicians and investigators of equal caliber and repute in this field disagree so widely and on so many important issues that he can no longer refer to an authoritative source for guidance; his horizons are therefore blurred and the stage is set for confusion."[47]

Doctor–Patient Relations in the Age of Risk

It would be difficult to make a case for ethical *progress* in the doctor–patient relationship from the experiences of Susan Emlen, Mary Cope, many of Halsted's patients, and Rachel Carson. Emlen's impossible dilemma – whether or not to consent to conscious breast amputation – was ultimately hers alone to make, although she relied on the support and advice of her husband and Quaker friends and relatives. Her doctors worked hard to apply their knowledge and experience to Emlen's particular case. Early-nineteenth-century surgeons, including her brother-in-law Physick, were deeply pessimistic that a real cancer could be cured by surgery or anything else. But they understood and empathized with the terrible dilemma faced by the patient, and sometimes reluctantly concluded that in the face of a rapidly advancing deadly disease, an otherwise healthy middle-aged woman with many years of life ahead of her might want to bear a lot of suffering for a very small chance of survival. So on the one hand, Emlen's doctors stressed her uncertain prognosis with or without surgery ("until the parts are laid open...," etc.). On the other hand, they ultimately shouldered some responsibility by making a clear recommendation for surgery. Emlen ultimately found a timeless logic with which to make and live with her decision – it was better to go to her death knowing that she had tried everything.

In the "middle course" of her disease, Emlen navigated through a series of ever more difficult options, weighing, with her family and friends, the credibility of healers and their tools, and monitoring her body for fleeting signs of success and more frequently recognizing disease progression. At each juncture there was not only a collective effort to sustain hope but also to redefine it, from cure, to arrest of tumor progression, for less suffering than imagined, and finally to greater spiritual awareness and acceptance. At the end of her life, medical intervention was there but backgrounded, and family and friends made sure that Emlen was not alone.

Breast cancer surgery and other aspects of medicine and society changed radically in the 100 years after Emlen's death in 1819. Halsted's patients were not given much choice about the less painful but more extensive surgery they were to undergo, the cancer diagnosis was now not typically mentioned, and Halsted's pessimism about surgery's effect on the ultimate course of metastatic disease was either not mentioned or left ambiguous. After patients underwent "complete operations" and had their one reasonable shot at disease control, Halsted urged them to somehow get on with their lives and discouraged medical surveillance and follow-up (except for his own research needs).

While much of Halsted's style of managing uncertainty was callous and paternalistic, his appreciation of the dilemmas surrounding truth, fear, and medical surveillance and his efforts to balance them with individual patients have not aged that badly. His 1907 published plea that medical professionals avoid adding to cancer fears and acknowledge medical impotence in the face of advancing disease still retains a good deal of wisdom: "Shall we let women know that a dangerous process may be going on which they cannot detect, and keep them in a constant state of apprehension, or shall we encourage them to seek 'expert' advice which may be insufficiently expert, and expose them to the annoyance of repeated and useless examinations, each of which for only a brief period, if at all, would bring a measure of reassurance?"[48]

Halsted claimed his "complete operation" was efficacious in controlling local recurrence. Most of his patients, however, sooner or later progressed to regional and metastatic disease while hoping for medical responses that worked. "Completeness" thus proved illusory. A web of more aggressive and effective (in the short run at least) salvage therapies and cancer specialists sprouted up to respond to this stage of disease and raised patient expectations. Compared to earlier eras, patients generally invested more hope for cure and control in these salvage therapies and believed more in the value of self- and medical surveillance. They lived a "life at risk." For women fortunate enough to live for years in this highly intervened state, there was reason to construct more hope for survival, even though there is little evidence that, in aggregate, death was forestalled by medical intervention and lots of evidence for the harms and costs of such intervention. Life and death with breast cancer had become much more medicalized.

By the time of Rachel Carson's life and death from breast cancer in the early 1960s, there was a small but influential medical backlash against Halstedian certainties and practices and the decades of an ultimately ineffective "war against time" happening in the public arena. In the course of her own disease, Carson understood and rejected the role of the compliant patient to medical authority. She found her iconoclastic equal in Barney Crile, who, while influenced by the statistical and ideological objections to the clinical status quo of the predeterminists and others, had a more personal and clinical "common sense" critique of reigning cancer ideas and practices. Using the skills and knowledge derived from her analysis of the harm done by modern societies to the environment, Carson questioned the wisdom of standard clinical approaches (often not presented to her as a choice) and tried treatments not in the mainstream medical canon.

However, Carson's relationship with Crile was not simply that between a consumer advocate and a medical provider. Nor did their shared critique of medical hubris and aggressiveness lead Crile and Carson to eschew treatments that might in retrospect seem futile and without "common sense." Crile and Carson demonstrated a joint construction of hope for cure and, when that became increasingly impossible, hope for prolonged survival. This involved a deft and delicate avoidance of grim prognostic statements, an acceptance of the need to always keep "doing something," and at the end of Carson's life, a more conventional grasping for hope in the form of aggressive medical treatment. Crile never abandoned Carson, and her friends supported her with loving and encouraging letters and displays of affection. But the realities of late-twentieth-century American secular life and medical intervention foreclosed the crowded deathbed social scene and spiritual epiphany that Emlen and others routinely experienced a century and a half earlier.

From Emlen, to Halsted's patients, to Carson, to our present era of breast cancer risk, there have been dramatic changes in the experience, treatment, and understanding of breast cancer. For most of the last 200 years, these transformations have resulted from our societal and medical response to breast cancer without significantly influencing the disease's deadliness. Alongside change, there have been significant continuities in the ways that affected women, their doctors and family members, and ordinary people have made decisions and made sense of the disease. At some point in the course of illness, patients and family members have often reached their particular perfect storm of uncertainty, where the limits of extant medical knowledge and available treatments become evident. Patients, physicians, and family members have often had to draw on a small set of existential, pre-empirical ways of thinking about cancer and things to say to oneself and others on the way to making impossible decisions (such as Emlen's "anticipated regret" and Burney's "evil against evil" heuristics). Truth and objective perception of clinical reality have not only often been elusive, but they have also frequently been in a necessary tension with a near universal desire to maintain hope. While the substance of hope has been historically contingent and specific to the clinical circumstances and individual spiritual resources, a more timeless observation is that individuals continuously redefine hope during the course of their illness. At the same time, hope has often remained in an unavoidable tension with the limits of biological life, clinical realities, and truth, however defined and constructed.

These many historical continuities in the breast cancer experience of both healers and sufferers lead me to a sober assessment of the necessarily tragic and unsatisfying situation in which patients with cancer, especially those with aggressive disease, often find themselves. They necessarily have to balance competing goods, without one trumping the other.

Americans live in an era that celebrates the historical progression to honesty in the naming and diagnosis of cancer, informed patient consent, and shared decision-making. But closely examining the felt experience of breast cancer patients and their doctors, especially how they have actually made decisions, suggests an alternative history.[49] In this less positivist history, there has been more continuity than progress in the ways in which doctors and patients have actively worked together, often colluded with one another, to balance hope, despair, and the existential demands and consequences of clinical decisions.

Breast cancer, like almost all other diseases, has been and will continue to be transformed by what we believe about it and how we respond to it. Breast cancer risk, our generation's most prominent way of bringing order to the idiosyncrasy associated with breast cancer, is a composite and often contradictory set of ideas and practices drawn from scientific understandings, the imperatives and limitations of new diagnostic technologies and preventive treatments, and our historically conditioned fears and hopes. Breast cancer risk ideas and practices are not "wrong" but have both good and bad consequences, depending on where one is situated. Certainly they need more critical analysis and subtler application.

Past choices, beliefs, and modes of response to breast and other cancers have cast long shadows. Fear of cancer has reached so intensely and intimately into our lives and the allure of control has been so incessantly promoted that the experience of cancer risk in American society has a unique, self-sustaining existence. We may have oversold cancer fears, the effectiveness of treatment and prevention, and the degree to which decision-making is more ethical and "evidence-based" than in earlier eras. But just as breast cancer's present meaning and impact have resulted from its contingent history within society, its future meanings and impact are not inevitable.

Notes

1. INTRODUCTION

1. See P.A. Wingo, T. Tong, and S. Bolden, "Cancer statistics, 1995," *CA Cancer Journal for Clinicians*, 45 (1995): 8–30; and L. A. G. Ries, B. A. Miller, and B. F. Hankey, et al., eds., *SEER Cancer Statistics Review, 1973–1991: Tables and Graphs* (Bethesda: National Cancer Institute, 1994). The frequently quoted stability as far back as 1930 usually derives from the U.S. Mortality Volumes from the CDC's National Center for Health Statistics (see, for example, http://www.cancer.org/downloads/ PRO(Cancer%20Statistics%202004.ppt#277,7, Cancer Death Rates*, for Women, U.S., 1930–2000, accessed in March 2006).

2. I will also make frequent reference to European (especially British) developments, especially when they have played a role in North American ones. I will occasionally draw on, and switch back and forth between, citations about breast cancer and cancer in general. This follows from the fact that most medical and lay beliefs and practices during the nineteenth century and for much of the twentieth century were focused on cancer in general, not site-specific cancers. The gradual emergence of breast cancer as a specific disease is traced in Chapters 3–5.

3. See, for example, G. Wyshak and R. Frisch, "Evidence for a secular trend in age of menarche," *New England Journal of Medicine*, 306 (1982a): 1033–1035. The authors reviewed 218 statistical reports in Europe and the United States and concluded that between 1800 and 1945 the average age of menarche dropped from 17.5 years to less than 13 years. These and other similar data suggest that American and European women in the early nineteenth century had many fewer lifetime menstrual cycles than 150 years later. It seems a plausible extrapolation from present belief in the causative role played by lifetime menstrual cycles and estrogen exposure that disease incidence was rising for most of this period. The wide consensus today that estrogen exposure and lifetime menstrual cycles play causal roles in breast cancer is underscored by the most dramatic epidemiological observation about breast cancer (whose implications I think are generally underappreciated): women have roughly 100 times more breast cancer than men. Men and women both have breasts. The postpuberty anatomic divergence happens largely under the influence of sex hormones.

4. American Cancer Society, *Cancer Facts and Figures 2002* (Atlanta: ACS, 2002). The jury is still out on the best explanation for this decline. See my analysis in Chapter 11.

5. To cite only a few of the most influential studies, see Alvan Feinstein's criticisms of the contemporary failure to incorporate clinical perspectives and categories in epidemiological research in cancer and other diseases, *Clinimetrics* (New Haven and London: Yale University Press, 1987); Leon Eisenberg's criticisms of the overly individualistic focus of prevention practices ("The perils of prevention: a cautionary note," *New England Journal of Medicine*, 197 (1977): 1230–1232); and Louise Russell's skeptical policy analysis of screening practices, *Educated Guesses: Making Policy About Screening Tests* (Berkeley: University of California Press, 1994). For a clear presentation, written for patients but important for all audiences, of the dilemmas posed by current cancer screening, see H. G. Welch, *Should I Be Tested for Cancer? Maybe Not and Here's Why* (Berkeley, University of California Press, 2004).

6. See, for example, M. Douglas, *Risk and Blame: Essays in Cultural Theory* (London and New York: Routledge, 1992).

7. Y. Miki, J. Swensen, D. Shattuck-Eidens, P. A. Futreal, K. Harshman, S. Tactigian, et al., "A strong candidate for the breast and ovarian cancer susceptibility gene BRCA1," *Science*, 266 (1994): 66–71. R. Wooster, S. L. Neuhasen, J. Mangion, Y. Quirk, D. Ford, N. Collins, et al., "Localization of a breast cancer susceptibility gene, BRCA2, to chromosome 13q12–13," *Science*, 265 (1994): 2088–2090. J. P. Struewing, D. Abeliovich, T. Peretz, N. Avisai, M. M. Kaback, F. S. Collins, et al., "The carrier frequency of the BRCA1 185dekAG mutation is approximately 1 percent in Ashkenazi Jewish individuals," *Nature Genetics*, 11 (1995): 198–200.

8. I and many others have discussed this and other related dichotomies in the history of medicine. See my *Making Sense of Illness: Science, Society and Disease* (New York and Cambridge, U.K.: Cambridge University Press, 1998): 7–10, especially endnote 3.

9. A. S. Ketcham and F. L. Moffat, "Vexed surgeons, perplexed patients, and breast cancers which may not be cancer," *Cancer*, 65 (1990): 387–393.

10. This moralistic twist has its echoes in earlier public health campaigns that blamed unnecessary deaths from cancer on women's "false modesty," that is, their unwillingness to examine their breasts or report breast problems.

2. CANCER IN THE BREAST, 1813

1. The term "breast cancer" was rarely used in the nineteenth century. Cancer was generally thought of as a unitary disease that might affect different parts of the body under particular conditions.

2. Obituary by Hannah Logan Smith, reprinted in Thomas Gilpin's *Memorials and Reminiscences in Private Life* (Philadelphia: Thomas Gilpin, 1839). This collection is kept at the Historical Society of Pennsylvania.

3. I learned of the Emlen case from Susan Garfinkle's essay "'This trial was sent in love and mercy for my refinement': A Quaker woman's experience of breast cancer surgery in 1814," *New Jersey Folklife*, 15 (1990): 18–31. Garfinkle carefully and persuasively analyzed the way gender norms, Quaker beliefs and practices (especially as regards the nature of suffering and women's social roles), and medical knowledge and practice shaped the experience and recollections of events leading up to and surrounding Emlen's breast amputation. Garfinkle also contrasted Emlen's narrative as revealed in letters among Quaker friends and family with the more literary account of Fanny Burney, revealing how the function and constraints of different types of narratives shaped the representation of the cancer experience. My analysis, which covers a longer time period (Garfinkle's account essentially ends with Emlen's surgery and recuperation) and a greater variety of correspondents and archival sources, is put to other ends, especially to establish a "baseline" for later changes in the way patients and doctors made treatment decisions and generally understood cancer in the breast.

4. The Emlens and correspondents frequently noted that they were retelling the same narrative and monitored the dates when prior accounts were sent off to England because of the hazards of intercontinental correspondence.

5. The relatively large size of tumors, when brought to medical attention, was frequently noted by nineteenth-century physicians. For a collection of such observations, see J. E. Lane-Claypon, "Cancer of the breast and its surgical treatment," *Reports on Public Health and Medical Subjects*, 28 (1924): 50–58.

6. Susan Emlen to William Dillwyn, November 5, 1814. Folder 25, Vol. 5, Dillwyn Papers, Historical Society of Pennsylvania (hereafter, Dillwyn Papers).

7. See note 3, Chapter 1.

8. W. Buchan, *Domestic Medicine*, 2nd edition (London: Balfour, Auld, and Smellie, 1785) accessed on May 2004 via http://www.americanrevolution.org/med45.html. See P. Jasen, "Breast cancer and the language of risk, 1750–1950," *Social History of Medicine*, 15 (2002): 17–43, for a careful sampling of such ideas in medical texts.

9. J. Rodman, *Cancer in the Female Breast With the Method of Cure and Cases of Illustration* (London; Glasgow; and Edinburgh: Paisley, 1815), 60. As for local causes of cancer in the breast, Rodman speculated that some poison might later be discovered but for the present he noted that the breast was subject to all kinds of engorgements and releases and that cancer was evidently caused by tight lacing.

10. J. Rodman, *Cancer in the Female Breast With the Method of Cure and Cases of Illustration*, 28.

11. Jasen speculates that the many reports of trauma preceding cancer in the breast reflected the high prevalence of domestic abuse in this period. P. Jasen, "Breast cancer and the language of risk, 1750–1950."

12. J. Rodman, *Cancer in the Female Breast With the Method of Cure and Cases of Illustration*, 65–69.

13. Ibid., 56–57.

14. W. Buchan, *Domestic Medicine*, Chapter 45, "Of Scirrhus and cancer."

15. Philip Syng Physick (1768–1837) was at one time a pupil of British surgical innovator John Hunter. Physick was appointed surgeon to Pennsylvania Hospital in 1794 and the first chair of surgery at the University of Pennsylvania. He was famous for removing bladder stones from Chief Justice John Marshall in 1831.

16. Samuel Emlen to William Dillwyn, June 15, 1814, Dillwyn Papers.

17. Susan Emlen to William Dillwyn, November 5, 1814, Dillwyn Papers.

18. J. Hemlow, ed., *The Journals and Letters of Fanny Burney (Madame D'Arblay)* (Oxford: Oxford University Press, 1975), 598. Burney wrote her account in a letter to her sister. Many historians and others have analyzed this account for what it says about the disease itself, treatments, gender, literature, and other important issues. See, for example, J. L. Epstein, "Writing the unspeakable: Fanny Burney's mastectomy and the fictive body," *Representations*, 16 (1986): 131–66.

19. J. Hemlow, ed., *The Journals and Letters of Fanny Burney*, 598.

20. From Hippocrates' Aphorisms, VI, 38. W. H. S. Jones, ed., *Hippocrates*, Vol. 4 (Cambridge, MA: Harvard University Press, 1953), 189. As quoted in D. De Moulin, *A Short History of Breast Cancer* (Boston: Martinus Nijhoff, 1983), 2.

21. As quoted in D. De Moulin, *A Short History of Breast Cancer*, 14. De Moulin also noted (p. 5) that Archigenes and Leonides, Alexandrian school physicians from the first century A.D., wrote that patients with cancer in the breasts are to be regarded as lost.

22. As quoted in M. Yalom, *A History of the Breast* (New York: Ballantine Books, 1997), 217.

23. L. J. Rather offered a careful description of seventeenth-century iatrochemical ideas about cancer such as Stahl's that were evidently shaped by operative experiences with cancer. G. E. Stahl, "Theoria medica vera," edited and translated by. L. Choulant (Leipzig: Sumptibus Vossii, 1831), 291, as quoted in L. J. Rather, *The Genesis of Cancer: A Study in the History of Ideas* (Baltimore and London: Johns Hopkins University Press, 1978), 33. Stahl believed that cancer often existed "beyond the apparent extent of the breast" making it impossible to surgically remove. Stahl also understood that even if these "seeds of cancer" could somehow be found in the breast that contained the tumor, the patient would likely develop cancer in the second breast (Rather, 34).

24. *The Lectures of Sir Astley Cooper on the Principles and Practices of Surgery* (Philadelphia: Haswell, Barrington, and Haswell, 1839), 386. As cited in W. R. Williams, *The Natural History of Cancer, with Special Reference to its Causation and Prevention* (New York: William Wood and Company, 1908), 402.

25. W. Buchan, *Domestic Medicine*. For those who failed surgery or progressed without it, Buchan recommended hemlock. Foul and sordid ulcers were best treated by "an obstinate performance of antisepsis" and application of a carrot poultice.

26. Susan Emlen to William Dillwyn, June 15, 1814. Dillwyn Papers.

27. Susan Emlen to William Dillwyn, November 5, 1814. Dillwyn Papers.

28. Samuel Emlen to William Dillwyn, March 11, 1814. Dillwyn Papers.

29. According to Samuel Emlen, the earlier nonsurgical measures had resulted in "a tendency to increase the tumor in Susan's breast" and by the time of the Physick consultation, "she began to experience some pain from it." Samuel Emlen to William Dillwyn, June 15, 1814, Dillwyn Papers.

30. Samuel Emlen to William Dillwyn, June 15, 1814, Dillwyn Papers.

31. Knowledge of the bad prognosis of axillary swellings was also associated with surgical approaches that included axillary dissection. Haagensen, for example, noted in his 1932 museum exhibit on the history of cancer that Hildanus (1560–1634) performed axillary dissections as part of breast cancer surgery. C. D. Haagensen, "An exhibit of important books, papers, and memorabilia illustrating the evolution of the knowledge of cancer, for the Graduate Fortnight on Tumors at the New York Academy of Medicine, October 17 to 28, 1932," *American Journal of Cancer*, 18 (1933): 42–126.

32. But as we saw earlier, Rodman was also a great enthusiast for the role of fear as both cause and vector of cancer. Rodman may have understood that individual constitution controlled the appearance of growths while the transformation to malignancy was a local process. J. Rodman, *Cancer in the Female Breast with the Method of Cure and Cases of Illustration*, v.

33. Some scholars have urged a reconceptualization of the history of surgery in which surgery and surgeons are not depicted as the handmaiden of more elite and scientific medicine and physicians. A key insight motivating this point of view is that surgery should not be distinguished from medicine solely on the basis of surgical practice but also on intellectual grounds. Christopher Lawrence, for example, has argued that surgery should not be defined primarily as practice – barbarian or barber-like – but as that field of medicine/physic that has been motivated by localistic, platonic ideas. In Lawrence's view, "high" surgery was often based on theory and physiological insights. C. Lawrence, *Medical Theory, Surgical Practice: Studies in the History of Surgery* (New York and London: Routledge, 1992). Oswei Temkin argued that surgeons were not in need of a "specific disease" revolution; they had already assimilated many aspects of the disease specificity idea in both their theories and practices. See O. Temkin, "The role of surgery in the rise of modern medical thought" in *The Double Face of Janus and Other Essays in the History of Medicine* (Baltimore: Johns Hopkins University Press, 1977), 487–496.

34. See D. De Moulin, *A Short History of Breast Cancer*, especially 17–30 and 66–71, for a comprehensive and lively treatment of the history of localist, mechanistic, and solidistic ideas and assumptions that surgeons used to understand and rationalize cancer practices since antiquity. In the early Renaissance period, for example, De Moulin noted how the idea that cancer resulted from blocked pores was refashioned as arising from blocked blood vessels and lymphatics. Other mechanical and local explanatory concepts were used by Renaissance physicians to explain the origins of breast cancer and crucial transformations. So stagnation could produce scirrhus, but if acid came into play, carcinoma might result.

35. The association of menopause with breast cancer has often been attributed to Galen. Demaitre noted: "This process conveniently explained the occurrence of

cancer in the breast due to insufficient cleansing, by menstruation, of the blood from the dregs of spoiled black bile." See L. E. Demaitre, "Medieval notions of cancer: Malignancy and metaphor," *Bulletin of the History of Medicine*, 72 (1998): 609–637, 618.

36. Samuel Emlen to William Dillwyn, June 15, 1814, Dillwyn Papers.

37. Joseph Parrish to John Cox, May 7, 1814. Folder January-June 1814, Box 7, Cox, Parrish, and Wharton Papers, Historical Society of Pennsylvania (hereafter, Cox, Parrish, and Wharton Papers).

38. Susan Emlen to William Dillwyn, November 5, 1814, Dillwyn Papers.

39. Humoral explanations of cancer date from antiquity. Most prominent was Galen's conception of breast tumors in which a flux of black bile mixed with blood gave rise to a kind of inflammation called scirrhus, "one form was related to, or capable of converting into, cancer." L. J. Rather, *The Genesis of Cancer: A Study in the History of Ideas*, 13. Rather's detailed history of elite medical ideas and practices emphasized, however, that Galenic humoral explanations of cancer had long since lost their cache among elite physicians and scientists by the early eighteenth century, having been admixed with and supplanted by a variety of chemical (especially notions of fermentation), inflammatory, and protocellular notions.

40. Susan Emlen to "Dear Aunt" (probably G. M. Smith), not dated. Folder Emlen, Susanna D, Box 3, Howland Collection, Magill Library Special Collections, Haverford College (hereafter, Howland Collection).

41. Susan Emlen to William Dillwyn, November 5, 1814, Dillwyn Papers.

42. "Watchful waiting" rather than surgery was the most frequent approach. In his case notes from 1842, George Washington Norris recorded this typical case of waiting over 2 years before surgery (time was not yet the enemy): "September 30th. Extirpated an ulcerated cancerous tumor from the right breast of Mrs. Williamson aged about 45. Very slight enlargement of the axillary glands. One or two parts of breast only extirpated the tumor being small. I had been consulted two years previously and advised against its removed and to watch it. Her health being bad. Cicatrisation was perfect in about 8 weeks, and cicatrix perfectly healthy." George Washington Norris, Record of private surgical practice and operations (1835–1843). Philadelphia, College of Physicians of Philadelphia.

43. All these references are from an unnumbered box labeled "Shipley and Bringhurst Family and Religious Materials, Tracts, Spiritual Pamphlets and Diaries." Rockwood Collection, Delaware Historical Society, Wilmington, DE.

44. It is worth noting that Burney consulted surgeons whose experience and reputation derived from the Napoleonic wars. The quick and brutal extirpation of a diseased breast was probably understood in relation to wartime amputations of mutilated and gangrenous limbs.

45. J. Hemlow, ed., *The Journals and Letters of Fanny Burney*, 611, 603.

46. Ibid., 607.

47. Ibid., 605.

48. Susan Emlen to William Dillwyn, November 5, 1814, Dillwyn Papers.

49. Samuel Emlen to William Dillwyn, June 15, 1814, Dillwyn Papers.

50. Susan Emlen to William Dillwyn, November 5, 1814, Dillwyn Papers.

51. Susan Parrish to Joseph Parrish, May 23, 1814. Folder January–June 1814, Box 7, Cox, Parrish, Wharton Papers.

52. Susan Emlen to William Dillwyn, November 5, 1814, Dillwyn Papers.

53. Deborah Logan to Susan Emlen, May 29, 1814. Folder Logan, Deborah, Box 6, Howland collection.

54. The title of a frequently republished American domestic medicine manual by John Tennent, *Every Man his own Doctor: or, the Poor Planter's Physician*, 3rd edition (Williamsburg: William Parks, 1736). See Charles Rosenberg and William Helfand's catalogue essay "The Book in the Sickroom: A Tradition of Print and Practice" written for the exhibit hosted by the Library Company entitled "'Every Man His Own Doctor': Popular Medicine in Early America" and viewable online at http://www.librarycompany.org/doctor/intro.html, accessed on February 14, 2005.

55. Susan Emlen to William Dillwyn, November 5, 1814, Dillwyn Papers.

56. J. Hemlow, ed., *The Journals and Letters of Fanny Burney*, 604–605.

57. Ibid., 611.

58. Susan Emlen to William Dillwyn, November 5, 1814, Dillwyn Papers.

59. Samuel Emlen to William Dillwyn, June 6, 1814, Dillwyn Papers.

60. Margaret Allinson to Unknown, undated (sometime immediately after surgery). Folder Allinson, Margaret, Box 1, Howland Collection.

61. Susan Emlen to William Dillwyn, November 5, 1814, Dillwyn Papers.

62. Samuel Emlen to William Dillwyn, June 6, 1814, Dillwyn Papers.

63. Susan Emlen to William Dillwyn, November 5, 1814, Dillwyn Papers.

64. Susan Emlen to William Dillwyn, July 24, 1814, Dillwyn Papers.

65. Samuel Emlen to William Dillwyn, August 4, 1814, Dillwyn Papers.

66. Samuel Emlen to Robert Vaux, June 13, 1814. Folder "Correspondence 1814–1820," Box 2, Vaux Papers, Historical Society of Pennsylvania (hereafter, Vaux Papers).

67. Susan Emlen to William Dillwyn, November 5, 1814, Dillwyn Papers.

68. Samuel Emlen to Robert Vaux, September 19, 1817. Folder "Correspondence 1814–1820," Box 2, Vaux Papers.

69. Susan Emlen to Sally Norris Dickinson, January 19, 1817. Folder 44, Vol. 9, Logan Papers, Historical Society of Philadelphia (hereafter, Logan Papers).

70. Quoted in E. F. Lewison and J. G. Lyons, Jr., "Relationship between benign breast disease and cancer," AMA *Archives of Surgery*, 66 (1953): 94–114, 96.

71. E. Gelles, *Portia: The World of Abigail Adams* (Bloomington and Indianapolis: Indiana University Press, 1992), especially 156–169.

72. K. M. Roof, *Colonel William Smith and the Lady* (Boston: Houghton Mifflin Co., 1929), 304.

73. E. Gelles, *Portia: The World of Abigail Adams*. Original letter is from William Smith to Abigail Adams, August 19, 1811, DeWindt Collection, Massachusetts Historical Society.

74. E. Gelles, *Portia: The World of Abigail Adams*. Original letter is from William Smith to Abigail Adams, September 15, 1811, Adams Papers, Microfilm edition, reel 412.

75. E. Gelles, *Portia: The World of Abigail Adams*, 156–169.

76. Susan Emlen to Sally Norris Dickinson, January 19, 1817. Folder 44, Vol. 9, Logan Papers.

77. Susan Emlen to Sally Norris Dickinson, July 14, 1817. Folder 44, Vol. 9, Logan Papers.

78. She died the next month – August 25, 1789 – in her home in Fredericksburg, VA, presumably of cancer at age 81 (her exact date of birth is unknown, sometime late 1708 or early 1709).

79. Benjamin Rush, Letter to Dr. Elisha Hall, Fredericksburg, VA, with report on the condition of Mary Washington, suffering from breast cancer, Philadelphia July 6, 1789, College of Physicians of Philadelphia.

80. George Birkbeck (1776–1841) was a physician in London who later went on to establish the London Mechanics Institute, which is now (as Birkbeck College) part of London University.

81. Mary Stacey and George Birkbeck to Susanna Emlen, November 13, 1816. Folder Stacey, Mary and Rachel, Box 12, Howland Collection.

82. George Birckbeck and John Pearson (?), undated. Folder Birkbeck, George, Box 1, Howland Collection.

83. Susan Emlen to Aunt G. M. Smith, February 5, 1817. Folder Emlen, Susanna, Box 3, Howland Collection.

84. Samuel Emlen to Thomas Stewardson, March 29, 1817, Folder Sam Emlen Letters, 1795–1819, Box 10 Cox, Parrish, Wharton Papers.

85. Susan Emlen to Sally Norris Dickinson, April 7, 1817. Folder 46, Vol. 9, Logan Papers.

86. Philip Physick to Sam Emlen, April 11, 1817. Folder Physick, Philip S, Sally and Susan D., Box 10, Howland Collection.

87. L. J. Rather, *The Genesis of Cancer: A Study in the History of Ideas*, 33.

88. Samuel Emlen to Robert Vaux, September 19, 1817. Folder "Correspondence 1817," Box 2, Vaux Papers.

89. Samuel Emlen to Joseph Bringhurst, February 7, 1818. Folder Sam Emlen Letters, 1795–1819, Box 10, Cox, Parrish, Wharton Papers.

90. See G. T. Haneveld, "Compression as a treatment of cancer, a historical survey," *Archivum Chirurgicum Neerlandicum*, 31 (1979): 1–8. Compression was first used in Imperial Rome on young women's breasts to influence their adult shape. Some Renaissance physicians used leaden plates to treat ulcerating cancers. British surgeon John Hunter (1728–1793) advocated compression for tumors, believing it compressed tumors' blood supply. Young's work received considerable attention as well as skepticism, fueled by reports of the therapy's harmful consequences for some patients.

91. S. Young, *Minutes of Cases of Cancer and Cancerous Tendency, Successfully Treated by Samuel Young; With a Prefatory Letter, Addressed to the Governors of the Middlesex Hospital, by Samuel Whitbread* (London : Cox, 1815), xiv, 5.

92. Ibid., 29.

93. Ibid., 33. Also included was a letter from the Matron of the Bedford House of Industry, S. Smith, dated May 16, 1815 (35–36), in which she wrote that "The size of Wildman's cancer at the time of her death, I suppose to be about a fifth part of what it was when Dr. Young took it in hand. It evidently appeared, that Wildman's breast would have become ulcerated, in a very short time, had it not undergone Mr. Young's treatment, which had every appearance of cure, provided she had a stronger constitution."

94. Samuel Emlen to Robert Vaux, September 19, 1817. Folder "Correspondence, 1817," Box 2, Vaux Papers.

95. Susan Emlen to Aunt G. M. Smith, June 13, 1817. Folder Emlen, Susanna, Box 3, Howland Collection.

96. This theme is especially well developed in Susan Garfinkle's essay "'This trial was sent in love and mercy for my refinement.'"

97. John Cox to Samuel Emlen, October 1, 1817. Folder Cox, John and Ann, Box 2, Howland Collection.

98. Box labeled "Shipley and Bringhurst Family and Religious Materials, Tracts, Spiritual Pamphlets and Diaries." Rockwood Collection, Delaware Historical Society, Wilmington.

99. Samuel Emlen to Robert Vaux, September 19, 1817. Folder "Correspondence, 1817," Box 2, Vaux Papers.

100. Susan Emlen to Sally Norris Dickinson, September 24, 1817. Folder 47, Vol. 9, Logan Papers.

101. John Cox to Richard Mott, August 18, 1817. Folder Cox, John, Box 2, Richard Mott Papers, Magill Library Special Collections, Haverford College (hereafter, Richard Mott Papers).

102. Ann Cox to Samuel Emlen, March 31, 1818. Folder Cox, John and Ann, Box 2, Howland Collection.

103. Samuel Emlen to Robert Vaux, September 19, 1817. Folder "Correspondence, 1817," Box 2, Vaux Papers.

104. Philip Syng Physick to Sam Emlen, November 1, 1817. Folder Physick, Philip S, Sally and Susan D, Box 10, Howland Collection. Later, Physick would write directly to Emlen about compression therapy and told her, honestly and directly, about a recent case in which he tried the bandages in Pearson's style for 3 months but "hitherto with no benefit than a slight diminution of the tumor." Physick to Susan Emlen, March 30, 1818. Folder Physick, Philip S, Sally and Susan D, Box 10, Howland Collection.

105. "English Diary of Samuel Emlen, Jr., of West Hill, Burlington, N.J.," September 29, 1817. Howland Collection.

106. Ann Cox to Susanna Emlen, November 13, 1817. Folder Cox, John and Ann, Box 2, Howland Collection.

107. Samuel Emlen to Joseph Bringhurst, February 7, 1818. Folder Sam Emlen Letters, 1795–1819, Box 10, Cox, Parrish, Wharton Papers.

108. Ann Cox continued to write the Emlens about herbal treatments such as pyrole (which she was arranging to be sent to England for their use) as well as positive

reports on compression therapy in America. See Ann Cox to Samuel Emlen, September 17, 1817, Folder Cox, John and Ann, Box 2, Howland Collection.

109. "English Diary of Samuel Emlen, Jr., of West Hill, Burlington, N.J.," October 3, 1817, Howland Collection.

110. "English Diary of Samuel Emlen, Jr., of West Hill, Burlington, N.J.," November 19, 1817. Howland Collection.

111. "English Diary of Samuel Emlen, Jr. of West Hill, Burlington, N.J.," October 8, 1817, Howland Collection.

112. Susan Emlen to G. M. Smith, December 12, 1817. Folder Emlen, Susanna, Box 3, Howland Collection.

113. John and Ann Cox to Samuel and Susan Emlen, February 1, 1818. Folder Cox, John and Ann, Box 2, Howland Collection.

114. Samuel Emlen to Robert Vaux, September 6, 1818. Folder "Correspondence August–September, 1818," Box 2, Vaux Papers.

115. Richard Lawrence to Samuel Emlen, August 30, 1818. Folder Emlen, Samuel, Box 3, Howland Collection.

116. Susan Emlen to Deborah Bringhurst, January 26, 1819. Folder Susanna Emlen, 1819, Box 10, Cox-Parrish-Wharton Papers.

117. John Cox to Richard Mott, October 4, 1819. Folder Cox, John, Box 2, Richard Mott Papers.

118. Sally N. Dickinson to cousin, October 7, 1819. Folder Dickinson, Sarah N, Box 2, Howland Collection.

119. Samuel Emlen to Joseph Bringhurst, November 11, 1819. Folder Samuel Emlen Letter, 1795–1819, Box 10, Cox, Parrish, Wharton Papers.

120. "Notes of some of the expressions of our dear Susanna Emlen, taken by Sally Sharpless and Margaret H. Smith during the few last weeks of her life, 1819." Folder Susan Emlen, 1819, Box 10, Cox, Parrish, Wharton Papers.

3. PESSIMISM AND PROMISE

1. Thomas Newlin to Joseph Shipley, January 26, April 15, August 19, September 13, October 14, and October 30, 1844; Sally Bringhurst to Joseph Shipley, March 28, 1844. Joseph Shipley collection, Hagley Museum Archives. Mary Shipley's married name was Mary Shipley Dixon.

2. Up until the late nineteenth century, for example, old and new partial insights into cholera's nature and causes intermingled, such as contingent contagionism, portability, animacularity, and fermentation. See C. E. Rosenberg, *Cholera Years* (Chicago: University of Chicago Press, 1987).

3. Walshe's major contributions were in heart and lung diseases and cancer. Born and raised in Dublin, he attended Trinity College, and between 1832 and 1835 studied medicine at the Hotel Dieu, La Charité and La Pitié; among his teachers were the surgeon Baron Guillaume Dupuytren and the master clinician Phillipe Charles Alexandre Louis. In Paris, Walshe was exposed to the new scientific and numerical approach to disease. After an additional year of medical

studies in Edinburgh, Walshe graduated in 1836. He held increasingly important positions at University College and became a Fellow of the Royal College of Physicians. With a few colleagues, he founded the London Medical Society of Observation, a private society that met at Walshe's house. In his clinical practice, Walshe closely followed the scheme for clinical observations proposed by the society, and he took extensive notes on every case.

4. See W. H. Walshe, *The Nature and Treatment of Cancer* (London: Taylor and Walton, 1846), 6. "Whatever was the motive in thus naming it," Walshe also noted about cancer's archaic classification and naming, "the affection itself was at first presumed to be peculiar to the breast; but, in proportion as morbid states of similar character were found to occur in other parts, they were included under the same general title."

5. Ibid., 55.

6. Ibid., vi.

7. In Walshe's view, the different levels "agree *anatomically*, for they are all composed of elements forming a combination without its counterpart, either in other adventitious products or in the natural structures; they agree *chemically* for they are all distinguished by the vast predominance of protein-compounds in their fabric; they agree *physiologically*, for they all possess in themselves the power of growth and of extending by infiltrating surrounding tissues, they agree *pathologically*, for they all tend to affect simultaneously or consecutively various organs in the body, and produce that depraved state of the constitution known as the cancerous cachexia." Ibid., 8.

8. Ibid., 154.

9. Ibid., 141.

10. D. Hayes Agnew, *The Principles and Practice of Surgery, Being a Treatise on Surgical Diseases and Injuries*, Vol. 3 (London: J. B. Lippincott and Co., 1881), 655.

11. J. Paget. "The distribution of secondary growths in cancer of the breast," *Lancet*, I (1889): 571–573. Sir James Paget (1814–1899) was an illustrious British surgeon, known to many doctors today by numerous eponyms, including some attached to cancer of the nipple (Paget's (breast) disease, Paget's sign). One of his sons, Stephen Paget (1855–1926), was a surgeon who has been widely credited for fully articulating the "seed and soil" explanation of the selective pattern of cancer metastasis. See "International symposium. Critical determinants in cancer progression and metastasis. A centennial celebration of Dr. Stephen Paget's 'seed and soil' hypothesis. March 6–10, 1989, Houston, TX," *Cancer Metastasis Review*, 8 (1989): 93–197.

12. Parker (1800–1884) graduated from Harvard Medical School in 1830. In 1839, he was appointed Professor of Surgery at the College of Physicians and Surgeons at Columbia University, a post he held for 30 years. In addition to consulting at other New York hospitals, Parker took an active interest in public health issues, serving as a commissioner to the Metropolitan Board of Health in New York in 1866 and supporting the creation of a hospital for infectious diseases, which eventually was named after him.

13. Clinical record book 1830–1880, 1. Parker Papers, Downstate Medical Center, Brooklyn, NY (hereafter Parker Papers).

14. See case of Mrs. Dickerson, seen at age 65 by Parker in September of 1852. Clinical record book 1830–1880, 3. Parker Papers.

15. Testimony of Mr. Payne [PathSocLondon], "Discussion on cancer," *Transactions of the Pathological Society of London*, 25 (1874): 339.

16. J. Paget, "The Morton lecture on cancer and cancerous disease," *British Medical Journal*, ii (1887): 1091–1094, 1091.

17. See DeMorgan's explanation of why cancer is not necessarily malignant [PathSocLondon], "Discussion on cancer," 288.

18. See J. Paget, "The Morton lecture on cancer and cancerous disease," 1091.

19. [PathSocLondon], "Discussion on cancer," 289.

20. Ibid., 291.

21. Ibid., 294.

22. Ibid., 293.

23. D. Hayes Agnew, *The Principles and Practice of Surgery*, Vol. 3, 583.

24. [PathSocLondon], "Discussion on cancer," 343–351, quote is 343.

25. Ibid., 310–313.

26. Ibid., 382.

27. Ibid., 328.

28. See discussion in Jacob Wolff, *The Science of Cancerous Disease from Earliest Times to the Present* (New York: Science History Publications, 1989), 197–198. This is an English translation (by Barbara Ayoub) of Vol. 1 of Wolff's four volumes *Die Lehre von der Krebskrankheit* (Gustav Fischer: Jena, 1907).

29. See M. Nicolson, "The metastatic theory of pathogenesis and the professional interests of the eighteenth-century physician," *Medical History*, xxxii (1988): 277–300.

30. J. C. A. Recamier, *Recherches sur le traitment du cancer* (Paris: Gabon, 1829). C. D. Haagensen ("An exhibit of important books, papers, and memorabilia illustrating the evolution of the knowledge of cancer, for the Graduate Fortnight on Tumors at the New York Academy of Medicine, October 17 to 28, 1932," *American Journal of Cancer*, 18 (1933): 42–126) claimed that Recamier discovered metastases and coined the term in 1829. The context was the spread of breast cancer to the brain. L. Weiss ("Concepts of metastasis," *Cancer and Metastasis Reviews*, 19 (2000): 221) suggested that Recamier believed that the physical spread of cancer material was only one way that primary cancers were related to secondary ones; "nervous consensus," via presumed nervous connections among organs, was another method. De Moulin (*A Short History of Breast Cancer* (Boston: Martinus Nijhoff, 1983), 31–41) argued that although the word metastasis appeared before Recamier in the late eighteenth century, the meaning was bound up to older notions of sympathy between different parts of the body.

31. W. H. Walshe, *The Cyclopedia of Practical Surgery*, Vol. 1 (London, 1841), 620. Quoted in W. I. B. Onuigbo, "A history of the cell theory of cancer," *Gesnerus*, 20 (1963): 92. Onuigbo also gives many examples of the halting progression from humoral to solidistic (cells) understandings of metastasis in the eighteenth and nineteenth century.

32. D. Hayes Agnew, *The Principles and Practice of Surgery*, Vol. 3, 654.

33. Ibid., Vol. 3, 706. See next chapter for discussion of parallels between embolism and metastases.

34. For example, Paget compared the latency of cancer with similar phenomena in infectious diseases: "Syphilis may reappear after years in which no sign of it could be found; or malarial fever may be for some years dormant till, with some accidental disturbance of the health, it may be renewed with its specific characters unchanged. In both cases we must believe that some morbid material remained inactive and apparently harmless in the body." J. Paget, "The Morton lecture on cancer and cancerous disease," 1093.

35. [PathSocLondon], "Discussion on cancer," 299.

36. Herbert Lumley Snow specialized in cancer, tumors, and gynecology. In addition to his publications on cancer, he also was prominent for his antivivisection and antivaccination positions.

37. H. Snow, *The Proclivity of Women to Cancerous Diseases* (London: J&A Churchill, 1891), 27.

38. "What is ability worth?" *New York Times*, April 29, 1894, 22.

39. Clinical record book 1830–1880, Parker Papers, and W. Parker, *Cancer: A Study of Three Hundred and Ninety-Seven Cases of Cancer of the Female Breast; With Clinical Observations* (New York: G. P. Putnam, 1885). Parker saw enough breast cases and apparently had a large enough reputation in this area that even a few male cases are recorded in the case book.

40. W. Parker, *Cancer*, 3–4.

41. D. Hayes Agnew, *The Principles and Practice of Surgery*, Vol. 3, 584.

42. Agnew, for example, agreed with Billroth and others that all epithelial cancers derived from normal epithelium. Ibid., Vol. 3, 650.

43. [PathSocLondon], "Discussion on cancer," 289.

44. W. Parker, *Cancer*, 36.

45. Ibid., 56 (italics in original).

46. Ibid., 22.

47. Ibid., 27. See also the case of Mrs. Allen who consulted Parker on August 24, 1867. She had a long history of cancer, had prior surgery, and now had a recurrence. There were "very great and depressing influences on account of her son-in-laws conduct. And this I regard as the cause of the return." Clinical record book 1830–1880, 97. Parker Papers.

48. See Clinical record book 1830–1880, 55. Parker Papers.

49. W. Parker, *Cancer*, 61.

50. Ibid., 3.

51. J. Paget, *Lectures on Surgical Pathology* (Philadelphia: Lindsay & Blakiston, 1860), 300.

52. Walshe at mid-century was highly skeptical of this received clinical (and lay) wisdom (he felt it had "spread from the schools to the vulgar"), attributing "this prejudice" to the patients' discovery of tumors at the time of injury. W. H. Walshe, *The Nature and Treatment of Cancer*, 95.

53. George Washington Norris, Record of private surgical practice and operations (1835–1843), case histories, "cancerous tumor of breast," 27, College of Physicians of Philadelphia.

54. First case is Mrs. A. Biggs, seen in 1863 and second case is Mrs. D., age 70 with date unknown. Clinical record book 1830–1880, 63 and 69, Parker Papers.

55. "It is safe to say that in the greater number of cases not included in blows and inflammations," Parker extrapolated, "more or less injury is caused by habitual pressure produced in this manner." W. Parker, *Cancer*, 11.

56. H. Snow, *The Proclivity of Women to Cancerous Diseases* (London: J&A Churchill, 1891), 11–12.

57. He continued, "What, then, have the localists to offer us in explanation of the rebellion of cells? Nothing but local irritation. Our minds contain a saturated solution of cases of cancer arising from local irritations. We are all familiar with the epitheliomas of lips and tongue arising from the irritation of pipes and teeth, chimney-sweeps' cancer from the constant contact of soot, cancer arising from the worry of old ulcers and the fretted scars of old burns, and we might almost extend the list indefinitely." [PathSocLondon], "Discussion on cancer," 374.

58. While generally skeptical, this statistical review also noted six cases in which there were multiple family members of the index case with cancer (134). "The last quoted case by itself forms as strong an argument in favour of the hereditary nature of the disease as an individual case possibly could, and taken in connexion with other facts, it constitutes all but conclusive evidence that cancer is, to a certain extent at least, hereditary." S. W. Sibley, "A contribution to the statistics of cancer, collected from the cancer records of the Middlesex Hospital," *Medico-Chirurgical Transactions*, 24 (1859): 111–152.

59. J. Paget, "The Morton lecture on cancer and cancerous disease," 1094.

60. At the London conference on cancer, Dr. Crisp noted the depressing increase in cancer mortality – 2448 in 1838 and 9508 in 1870, enormous "even taking into account the increase in the population." [PathSocLondon], "Discussion on cancer," 356. There were dissenters. For example, as discussed earlier, Walshe speculated that these trends were artifactual.

61. Parker shared nineteenth-century environmental and Lamarckian assumptions such as that individuals' mental states throughout their lifetime shaped their underlying constitution and cancer diathesis. "This case goes to increase the number of those which, in my opinion, indicate that cancerous tumors have their origin in injuries or seats of irritation in constitutions prepared for the development of the disease, the constitutional condition being acquired by certain habits of living." W. Parker, *Cancer*, 32. C.f., C. E. Rosenberg, "The bitter fruit: heredity, disease, and social thought in nineteenth century America," *Perspectives in American History*, 8 (1974): 189–235.

62. W. Parker, *Cancer*, 36.

63. H. Snow, *The Proclivity of Women to Cancerous Diseases*, 13–14.

64. J. Scotto and J. C. Bailar, "Rigoni–Stern and medical statistics: A nineteenth-century approach to cancer research," *Journal of the History of Medicine*, 24 (1969): 65–75. Rignoni Stern also noted that "cancer is at least eight times more

frequent in females as compared to males." Cancer in males had been known since antiquity.

65. H. Snow, *The Proclivity of Women to Cancerous Diseases*, 41.

66. Ibid., 36.

67. Ibid., 38.

68. Ibid., 9.

69. Ibid., 42.

70. "In the numerous cases of fibromata in the mammae of young unmarried women," Snow wrote of the benign breast condition that was believed to be a precursor to cancer, "which we see at this hospital, the presence of undue compression by stays, is always sufficiently conspicuous; and is generally associated with other manifest results of the same, such as anemia, fainting-fits, and the like – all of which are almost unheard of in males the same age." Ibid., 38.

71. Ibid., 43.

72. L. Edel, ed., *The Diary of Alice James* (New York: Penguin, 1987), 207. Diary entry is for May 31, 1891.

73. J. Paget, "The Morton lecture on cancer and cancerous disease," 1094.

74. D. Hayes Agnew, *The Principles and Practice of Surgery*, Vol. 3, 715.

75. "Death from lock jaw," *New York Times*, Nov. 24, 1883, 2.

76. Sibley reported an operative mortality of 4.8 percent among patients at the Middlesex Hospital who underwent cancer surgery (at any site). S. W. Sibley, "A contribution to the statistics of cancer, collected from the cancer records of the Middlesex Hospital."

77. D. Hayes Agnew, *The Principles and Practice of Surgery*, Vol. 1, 713.

78. Photograph of A. N. R. Photographs of patients operated on by Addinell Hewson, Philadelphia, 1861–1865, College of Physicians of Philadelphia.

79. J. Wolff, *The Science of Cancerous Disease from Earliest Times to the Present*, 174.

80. D. Hayes Agnew, *The Principles and Practice of Surgery*, Vol. 3, 654.

81. Ibid., 704.

82. J. Paget, "The Morton lecture on cancer and cancerous disease," 1094.

83. D. Hayes Agnew, *The Principles and Practice of Surgery*, Vol. 3, 710.

84. Ibid., 710–714.

85. Ibid., 711.

86. Ibid., 712.

87. Ibid., 714.

88. W. Parker, *Cancer*, 1.

89. Ibid., 10. Other statistical reports from mid to late century reported similar modest survival gains among operated cases. Sibley reported an average life expectancy of 53 months in operated versus 32 months in cases that did not have surgery (among cases of cancer in the breast). S. W. Sibley, "A contribution to the statistics of cancer, collected from the cancer records of the Middlesex Hospital."

90. S. W. Gross, *A Practical Treatise of Tumors of the Mammary Gland* (New York: Appleton, 1880), vi.

91. W. Parker, *Cancer*, 60.

92. Clinical record book 1830–1880, 49. Parker Papers.

93. Clinical record book 1830–1880, 61. Parker Papers.

94. Parker's book of cancer cases contained many examples of women who presented with very large breast masses. One patient presented to Parker with a 2-pound breast mass (p. 5) and another patient presented with tumor with which she had lived for 17 years (p. 43). See Clinical record book 1830–1880. Parker Papers.

95. The decision-making calculus was not that different from earlier in the century when amputations were rarer. In 1837, a 23-year-old woman consulted Philadelphia physician George Washington Norris. Norris recorded clinical details that suggested a good prognosis such as that her "skin and nipple [were] natural" and that there was "no enlargement of the axilla." Despite these signs and the patient's youth and vigor, surgery was not offered nor carried out. Norris recorded in his casebook, "Treat. App. of leeches, sling and soap plaster." (George Washington Norris, Record of private surgical practice and operations, Philadelphia, 1835–1843. College of Physicians of Philadelphia, 17.) If bad prognostic signs were present, the decision not to operate was that much easier. In 1841, Norris examined a 45-year-old woman with a breast tumor who had "a very slight enlargement of one or two glands below the clavicle and in the arm pit." Although he noted that her "general health [was] good," he recorded in his case book that he "recommended her to avoid an operation," presumably because of this bad prognostic sign (27).

96. Samuel Gross to John Ashurst, n. d. Ashurst collection. John Ashurst Correspondence. College of Physicians of Philadelphia.

97. For example, Parker recorded the case of a woman who had three prior breast surgeries and whose tumor had over the previous 6 months "changed in character and began to grow rapidly." Clinical record book 1830–1880, 11. Parker Papers.

98. W. Parker, Cancer, 13–14.

99. S. W. Gross, A Practical Treatise on Tumors of the Mammary Glands, v.

100. Nineteenth-century aggregate perceptions of cancer and other diseases typically followed from observations of clinical practice rather than population-based samples. Busy surgeon Willard Parker observed the following age distribution in cancer in the breast from his practice in the latter half of the nineteenth century: 93 cases under 40, 165 under 45, with only 147 over 45. W. Parker, Cancer, 22. Similarly, the average age of the 192 cases of cancer in the breast treated at the Middlesex Hospital in London during 1853–1856 was 48.6. S. W. Sibley, "A contribution to the statistics of cancer, collected from the cancer records of the Middlesex Hospital."

101. Jonathan Evans to Rachel Reeve Evans, June 22, 1887. Folder 4 "Letters June–July, 1887," Box 13, Cope-Evans Family Papers, Quaker Collection, Magill Library, Haverford College (hereafter Cope-Evans Family Papers).

102. Jonathan Evans to Rachel Reeve Evans, July 18, 1887. Folder 4 "Letters June–July, 1887," Cope-Evans Family Papers.

103. Jonathan Evans to Rachel Reeve Evans, August 22, 1887. Folder 5 "Letters August–November 1887," Cope-Evans Family Papers.

104. Jonathan Evans to Rachel Reeve Evans, September 24, 1887. Folder 5 "Letters August–November 1887," Box 13, Cope-Evans Family Papers.

105. Jonathan Evans to Rachel Reeve Evans, September 29, 1887. Folder 5 "Letters August–November 1887," Box 13, Cope-Evans Family Papers.

106. Jonathan Evans to Rachel Reeve Evans, September 22, 1887. Folder 5 "Letters August–November 1887," Box 13, Cope-Evans Family Papers.

107. Hetty Newlin Stokes to Katherine Wistar Stokes, September 27, 1887. Folder "Hetty Newlin-Stokes, 1838–1899," Box 4, Stokes-Evans-Cope Family Papers, Quaker Collection, Magill Library, Haverford College (hereafter, Stokes-Evans-Cope Family Papers).

108. Of course, cancer surgery was and still is feared because of its inherent dangers, pain, and resulting disfigurement. As a result, mass marketed cancer "specifics" were frequently pitched as ways to avoid surgery. For example, an advertisement for "Holloway's Pills And Ointment," began "dispense with the necessity of surgical operations for cancer." See "Important surgical operation with nitrous oxide," *New York Times*, April 3, 1860, 8.

109. Jonathan Evans to Rachel Reeve Evans, September 22, 1887. Folder 5 "Letters August–November 1887," Box 13, Cope-Evans Family Papers.

110. Hetty Newlin Stokes to Katherine Wistar Stokes, September 27, 1887. Folder "Hetty Newlin-Stokes,1838–1899," Box 4, Stokes-Evans-Cope Family Papers.

111. Jonathan Evans to Rachel Reeve Evans, September 26, 1887. Folder 5 "Letters August–November 1887," Box 13, Cope-Evans Family Papers.

112. Hetty Newlin Stokes to Katherine Wistar Stokes, September 27, 1887. Folder "Hetty Newlin-Stokes, 1838–1899," Box 4, Stokes-Evans-Cope Family Papers.

113. Jonathan Evans to Rachel Reeve Evans, September 29, 1887. Folder 5 "Letters August–November 1887," Box 13, Cope-Evans Family Papers.

114. Margaret Cope (Mary's younger sister, 1856–1948) to Katherine Wistar Stokes (Evans), September 29, 1887. Folder "Correspondence, diaries, etc: Stokes, Francis Joseph," Box 4, Stokes-Evans-Cope Family Papers.

115. Hetty Newlin Stokes to Katherine Wistar Stokes, September 27, 1887. Folder "Hetty Newlin-Stokes, 1838–1899," Box 4, Stokes-Evans-Cope Family Papers.

116. The Friend, presumably January 1888, in Box 4, Cope-Evans Family Papers.

117. See note in H. Snow, *The Proclivity of Women to Cancerous Diseases*, 29.

118. See B. L. Goodbody, "'The present opprobrium of surgery': *The Agnew Clinic* and nineteenth-century representations of cancerous female breasts," *American Art*, 8 (1994): 32–51.

119. D. H. Agnew, *Principles and Practice of Surgery*, Vol. 2, 711, as quoted in D. E. Long, "The medical world of *The Agnew Clinic*: A world we have lost?" *Prospects*, 11 (1987): 185–198, 190.

4. TAKING RESPONSIBILITY FOR CANCER

1. See for instance, S. B. Nuland, "Medical Science comes to America: William Stewart Halsted of Johns Hopkins," *Doctors: A Biography of Medicine* (New York: Alfred A Knopf Press, 1988), 386–421. D. A. Power, "The history of the amputation of the breast to 1904," *Liverpool Medico-Chirugical Journal*, 52 (1934): 49–56. J. L. Cameron, "William Stewart Halsted: Our surgical heritage," *Annals of Surgery*, 225 (1997): 445–458.

2. W. G. MacCallum, *William Stewart Halsted, Surgeon* (Baltimore: Johns Hopkins University Press, 1930), 84–102.

3. See E. Leopold, *A Darker Ribbon: Breast Cancer, Women, and Their Doctors in the Twentieth Century* (Boston: Beacon Press, 1999). C. Bland, "The Halsted Mastectomy: Present illness and past history," *Western Journal of Medicine*, 134 (1981): 549–555.

4. D. A. Power's, "The history of the amputation of the breast to 1904" gave a particularly rich account of incremental surgical innovations. Power cited the pathological work of Trother Heidenhain in Berlin who in 1889 was removing part of the pectoralis major muscle and lymphatics. C. H. Moore in 1859 was incising and draining the lattissimus dorsi muscles. In 1880, Samuel Gross in Philadelphia urged dissecting off the fascia of the pectoral muscles as did the surgeon Richard von Volkmann in Germany, with whom Halsted had studied during his early 1880s European tour. Other observers have noted that Halsted created in his own career and status something akin to the prestige and authority of elite German surgeons of that period.

5. J. C. Bloodgood, "Halsted thirty-six years ago," *American Journal of Surgery*, 14 (1931): 89–148, 143.

6. See G. H. Brieger, "From conservative to radical surgery in late nineteenth-century America," in C. Lawrence, ed., *Medical Theory, Surgical Practice: Studies in the History of Surgery* (New York: Routledge, 1992), 216–231. Brieger thoughtfully dissects what the terms "radical" and "conservative" denoted and connoted in nineteenth century American surgical practice and why these terms were often applied to the same surgical practices. To simplify, "conservative" gradually shifted its meaning from as little as needed to help the patient to practices necessary to save or conserve the patient. Extensive cancer surgery could be both "radical" and "conservative" if it saved the patient.

7. From W. S. Halsted, "A clinical and histological study of certain adenocarcinomas of the breast – and a brief consideration of the superclavicular operations and of the results of operation for cancer of the breast form 1889 to 1898 at the Johns Hopkins Hospital," *Transactions of the American Surgical Association*, 16 (1898): 144–181; Cited by Cordelia Bland in "The Halsted mastectomy: Present illness and past history." Matas was responding to Halsted's presentation.

8. "The original conception to the complete operation for cancer of the breast." Abstracted from a letter from Halsted to William Welch, dated August 26, 1922,

and published in *Surgical Papers by William S. Halsted*, Vol. 2 (Baltimore: Johns Hopkins University Press, 1924), 101.

9. D. A. Power "The history of the amputation of the breast to 1904." Banks' quote is from p. 55, the other is from p. 54. Power attributed the contemporary shift away from radical surgery to the "delay" campaign (Chapter 6) and innovations like radium and x-rays. See also B. Lerner, *The Breast Cancer Wars* (New York: Oxford University Press, 2003) for a detailed and compelling account of the controversies over the radical mastectomy that began almost immediately after Halsted's death and continued through the 1980s.

10. Sigerist also captured the continuing pessimism surrounding cancer by quoting what Berlin surgeon August Bier once said to him, "If a great scientist at the end of a brilliant career wants to make a fool of himself, he takes up the problem of cancer." H. Sigerist, "The historical development of the pathology and therapy of cancer," *Bulletin of the New York Academy of Medicine*, 8 (1932): 642–653.

11. C. P. Childe, *The Control of a Scourge, or How Cancer Is Curable* (London: Methuen and Co., 1906), 87–89.

12. The Halsted correspondence contains many letters from surgeons about patients who had repeated, less-than-complete operations and often radiation treatments, asking Halsted for advice. See, for example, Walter P. Steiner to W. S. Halsted (hereafter Halsted), January 25, 1912. Folder 21, Box 23, Halsted Papers, Alan Mason Chesney Medical Archives, Johns Hopkins University (hereafter Halsted Papers).

13. J. Frank Small to Halsted, March 14, 1897. Folder 4, Box 23, Halsted Papers.

14. In Halsted's era, the shift in women's behavior toward earlier presentation to medical care was perceptible but by no means complete. Halsted recognized that the spectrum of disease was changing and these changes made his ideal of diagnosis by the surgeon based on clinical and gross operative findings more difficult. W. S. Halsted, "The results of radical operations for the cure of carcinoma of the breast," *Annals of Surgery*, 46 (1907): 1–19.

15. W. S. Halsted, "The results of operations for the cure of cancer of the breast performed at the Johns Hopkins Hospital from June 1889 to January 1894," see reprint in *Surgical Papers by William S. Halsted*, Vol. 2 (Baltimore: Johns Hopkins University Press, 1924), 3–50, 13. Original article appeared in *John Hopkins Hospital Report*, Baltimore, IV (1984–1985): -297–350.

16. W. S. Halsted, "The results of radical operations for the cure of carcinoma of the breast."

17. See, for instance, a report by J. E. Lane Claypon, *Cancer of the Breast and Its Surgical Treatment: Ministry of Health Reports on Public Health and Medical Subjects* (London: Ministry of Health, 1923), which summarizes these comparisons from surgical practice.

18. J. C. Bloodgood, "Halsted thirty-six years ago," 105–107.

19. W. L. Rodman, "Carcinoma," in *Diseases of the Breast with Special Reference to Cancer* (Philadelphia: P. Blakiston's Son & Co., 1908), 172–371, 241.

20. J. C. Bloodgood, "The diagnosis of early breast tumors, based on the clinical history and pathology at the exploratory incision," *Journal of the American Medical Association*, 81 (1923): 875–882, 882 (Dr. Rodman made this point in the discussion following Bloodgood's paper).

21. Anecdote recalled in A. McGee Harvey, "The Influence of William Stewart Halsted's Concepts of Surgical Training," in *Research and Discovery in Medicine: Contributions from Johns Hopkins* (Baltimore: Johns Hopkins University Press, 1981), 61.

22. Handley argued, "embolism (metastasis, spread of physical pieces of cancer from original site to distal ones via blood) is necessarily an impartial process, to which all the organs are liable. But the distribution of cancerous metastasis in the various organs is by no means impartial. Some organs are very frequently invaded, others only rarely." Handley made an analogy (p. 17) between the spread of cancer via "lymphatic permeation" to the spread of erysipelas, a bacterial infection, through the tissue planes of the skin. See W. S. Handley, *Cancer of the Breast and Its Operative Treatment* (London: John Murray, 1906).

23. "Although it undoubtedly occurs, I am not sure that I have observed from breast cancer, metastasis which seem definitely to have been conveyed by way of the blood vessels; and my views as to the dissemination of carcinoma of the breast accord so fully with Handley's." W. S. Halsted, "The results of radical operations for the cure of carcinoma of the breast," 9.

24. See W. S. Halsted, "The results of radical operations for the cure of carcinoma of the breast." Handley called spread by the blood system "embolization," the term now reserved for spread of atherosclerotic blood clots or physical fragments of infection, whose spread is understood in very physical terms and whose distribution would expect to include, even be predominated by, spread to the smallest and most distal vessels (unlike the drawings of breast cancer). Handley noted that cancer's spread in the body was dictated by physical pathways such as the lymphatic system and the spaces in between and around muscles (fascial planes). W. S. Handley, *Cancer of the Breast and Its Operative Treatment*.

25. W. S. Halsted, "The results of radical operations for the cure of carcinoma of the breast," 16.

26. Not all turn-of-the-century American surgeons understood and accepted the consensus about metastasis and cancer's natural history. Cancer's slow and orderly progression were after all deduced rather than directly observed. Cancer's appearance in noncontiguous time and space was still puzzling. Rodman speculated, for example, "that nearly all such reported last recurrences are really not recurrences at all, but fresh outbreaks in subjects with a demonstrated susceptibility to the disease. . . . It is difficult to understand how cancer cells could lie dormant in internal organs for so many years without giving trouble." W. L. Rodman, *Diseases of the Breast with Special Reference to Cancer*, 256.

27. W. S. Halsted, "The results of operations for the cure of cancer of the breast performed at the Johns Hopkins Hospital from June 1889 to January 1894," 7.

28. The late twentieth-century recognition that limited breast surgery and radiation were as equally (in)effective as radical mastectomies in terms of saving lives, that is, intervening in metastatic disease, has led to a rediscovery of this independence.

29. Halsted claimed a 6-percent local recurrence rate and produced a table comparing this very low rate with those of published case series of great European and American surgeons, all of whom had local recurrence rates 60 percent or greater. Halsted was clear that this rate measured the efficiency of the operation, not its effectiveness in saving lives. W. S. Halsted, "The results of radical operations for the cure of carcinoma of the breast."

30. W. Halsted, "The results of operations for the cure of cancer of the breast performed at the Johns Hopkins hospital from June 1889 to January 1894," 17.

31. W. S. Halsted, "The results of radical operations for the cure of carcinoma of the breast."

32. Most of the paper's discussion concerned other issues, such as the problem of patients with neck involvement and whether dissection of glands at the base of the neck should be a routine part of the complete operation, the question of blood-borne metastasis, and need for surgeons to diagnose cancer using clinical rather than microscopic criteria.

33. W. S. Halsted, "The results of radical operations for the cure of carcinoma of the breast."

34. Ibid., 12.

35. W. G. MacCallum, *William Stewart Halsted, Surgeon*.

36. W. S. Halsted, "The results of operations for the cure of cancer of the breast performed at the Johns Hopkins Hospital from June 1889 to January 1894," 13.

37. W. S. Halsted, "The results of radical operations for the cure of carcinoma of the breast," 6.

38. J. C. Bloodgood, "Halsted thirty-six years ago," 145.

39. H. B. Walter to Halsted, not dated. Folder 13, Box 25, Halsted Papers.

40. John Whitehead to Halsted, October 3, 1908. Folder 11, Box 26, Halsted Papers. Whitehead describes a case of adenoma, mistaken initially for a lipoma.

41. W. S. Halsted, "A clinical and histological study of certain adenocarcinomata of the breast and a brief consideration of the supraclavicular operation and of the results of operations for cancer of the breast from 1889 to 1898 at the Johns Hopkins Hospital," see reprint in *Surgical Papers by William S. Halsted*, Vol. 2 (Baltimore: Johns Hopkins University Press, 1924), 51–65, 52. Original article appeared in *Transactions of the American Surgical Association, Philadelphia*, XVI (1898): 144–181. Cited in D. A. Power, "The history of the amputation of the breast to 1904," 53.

42. J. C. Bloodgood, "Halsted thirty-six years ago," 104.

43. W. H. Halsted, "A clinical and histological study of certain adenocarcinomata of the breast," 51.

44. Ibid., 53 Halsted had never been much interested in pathology. As a young surgeon rounding out his education with an obligatory tour of Europe, he recalled

that "tumors proved an uninteresting theme without patients or clinical histories." Quoted in W. G. MacCallum, *William Stewart Halsted, Surgeon*, 25.

45. Halsted divided his existing cases into the following categories: cancer cysts (6), adenocarcinoma (32), medullary carcinoma (25), circumscribed scirrhus (28), small infiltrating scirrhus (80), and large infiltrating scirrhus (39). W. S. Halsted, "The results of radical operations for the cure of carcinoma of the breast."

46. Dr. William Ely to Halsted, March 26, 1907. Folder 19, Box 7, Halsted Papers.

47. Dr. William Ely to Halsted, April 19, 1907. Folder 19, Box 7, Halsted Papers.

48. Mrs. Crumb to Halsted, December 18, 1916. Folder 9, Box 10, Halsted Papers. All patient names are pseudonyms.

49. Pathologist from NY Skin and Cancer Hospital (name unclear) to T. Raymond Biggs, November 10, 1916. Folder 9, Box 10, Halsted Papers.

50. Biggs to Halsted, November 15, 1916. Folder 9, Box 10, Halsted Papers.

51. Halsted to Biggs, November 18, 1916. Folder 9, Box 10, Halsted Papers.

52. Biggs to Halsted, November 15, 1916. Folder 9, Box 10, Halsted Papers.

53. Halsted to Bloodgood, December 4, 1916, Folder 9, Box 10, Halsted Papers.

54. A poultice is defined in the *Oxford English Dictionary* (2nd edition, 1989) as "a soft mass of some substance (as bread, meal, bran, linseed, various herbs, etc.), usually made with boiling water, and spread upon muslin, linen, or other material, applied to the skin to supply moisture or warmth, as an emollient for a sore or inflamed part, or as a counter-irritant (e.g. a mustard-poultice); a cataplasm."

55. Dr. J. C. Wysor to Halsted, May 4, 1900. Folder 39, Box 26, Halsted Papers.

56. Representative replies include (1) Edwin I. Bartlett to Bloodgood, 12 May, 1927, who wrote that "in my work I never resort to frozen sections except when my gross impression is doubtful. I find that rarely am I mistaken in my gross impression and if still in doubt after making frozen sections I always act on my gross impression"; (2) Dr. A. H. Braden wrote to Bloodgood, 19 April 1927 that "as to making micro-scopists out of surgeons I think it is, like Aristotle's Ideal State, a beautiful Utopia but as yet not likely to develop into fruition"; (3) George R. Callendar, unlike most of the other doctors Bloodgood surveyed, wrote to Bloodgood, 28 April 1927 that "while I see tumors that I am quite convinced are benign, I am never satisfied with-out microscopic examination. Some 75 per cent of the malignant breast tumors, however, it seems to me are so evidently malignant that although we always confirm microscopically it is certainly not necessary for the surgeon to await his operation for such confirmation"; (4) Dr. S. F. Hoge, a pathologist working in Little Rock, Alabama, wrote Bloodgood on 23 May, 1927, describing his enthusiasm for rapid pathological diagnosis, the cooperation of some local surgeons, but the skepticism of most surgeons who do not want to "pause a moment in their haste to consider the importance of a tissue diagnosis of the structures removed at operation"; (5) Dr. C. N. Callander of Fargo, North Dakota, wrote Bloodgood on 15 June, 1927, about the dearth of competent and available pathological competence to "pass upon tissues removed at biopsy"; (6) Dr. John McDill of Waukesha, Wisconsin, wrote Blood-good on 16 March, 1927 that he doubted "if any of the Veteran's Hospitals, 51 in

number, unless the Speedway (Chicago) is an exception, have facilities for immediate tissue diagnosis. All from Joseph Colt Bloodgood letters, Folder 2, Box 22, Howard Atwood Kelly Papers, Alan Mason Chesney Medical Archives, Johns Hopkins University.

57. In Chapter 6, I document the rising number of patients in the first decades of the twentieth century presenting to surgeons for evaluation of breast lumps. Apparently responding to James Murphy's inability to accept a new breast cancer referral in 1917, Halsted wrote back, "even if one had nothing else to do he would be swamped with patients should he undertake to treat all the incurable as well as curable cases of cancer of the breast. They would be like the sands of the seashore." Halsted to James Murphy, November 13, 1917, folder entitled "Halsted," James B. Murphy Papers, American Philosophical Society.

58. J. C. Bloodgood, "Halsted thirty-six years ago," 146.

59. J. R. Wright, Jr., "The development of the frozen section technique, the evolution of surgical biopsy, and the origins of surgical pathology," *Bulletin of the History of Medicine*, 59 (1985): 295–326. Wright showed that although frozen sections were described in 1890 textbooks they were rarely used. Wright stated that prior to 1925, no textbook featured the frozen section as an important technique.

60. J. C. Bloodgood, "Halsted thirty-six years ago," 143–144.

61. J. R. Wright, Jr., "The development of the frozen section technique, the evolution of surgical biopsy, and the origins of surgical pathology."

62. Of course, pathologists in the absence of frozen sections hoped to influence surgical practice. For example, one pathologist in 1917 attached to his microscopic description of a breast tumor the advice to perform "a radical amputation." See note from the "Laboratory of Dr. Allen H. Bunce" Atlanta, Georgia, to Drs. Little and Griffin dated January 19, 1917 in the letter from A. G. Little to Halsted, January 22, 1917. Folder 19, Box 20, Halsted Papers.

63. Hilda Martin to Halsted, March 16, 1914. Folder 8, Box 1, Halsted Papers.

64. Halsted to Hilda Martin, June 9, 1914. Folder 8, Box 1, Halsted Papers. Halsted thanked Mrs. Martin in advance for her offer to send photographs.

65. Halsted to Miss Anna Stokes, August 30, 1921. Folder 28, Box 23, Halsted Papers.

66. W. H. Halsted, "The swelling of the arm after operations for cancer of the breast – *Elephantiasis Chirurgica* – its cause and prevention," see reprint in *Surgical Papers by William S. Halsted*, Vol. 2 (Baltimore: Johns Hopkins University Press, 1924), 90–100, 96. Originally published in *Johns Hopkins Hospital Bulletin*, 32 (1921): 309–313.

67. Ibid., 93.

68. Ibid., 92.

69. W. S. Halsted, "The results of operations for the cure of cancer of the breast performed at the Johns Hopkins Hospital from June 1889 to January 1894," 15.

70. Halsted to John B. Deaver, January 26, 1922. Folder 24, Box 6, Halsted Papers.

71. W. H. Halsted, "The swelling of the arm after operations for cancer of the breast. – *Elephantiasis Chirurgica* – its cause and prevention."

72. For example, in 1921, a general surgeon wrote to Halsted for information about a patient he had previously operated on who now had an abdominal metastasis on x-ray. Halsted attached a note to the information the surgeon had requested, slipping in – insensitively given the context of the patient's newly diagnosed metastatic disease – a query about arm swelling. Halsted to Dr. John K. Train, January 24, 1921. Folder 26, Box, 24, Halsted Papers.

73. Halsted to James Murphy, April 5, 1917. Folder 4, Box 19, Halsted Papers.

74. Halsted's obsession with responsibility for arm swelling has also created interpretive problems for historians. Ellen Leopold (A Darker Ribbon) analyzed Halsted's relationship with a patient she called Barbara Mueller, who died 5 years after a complete operation. Leopold faulted Halsted for his inability to see in this case and many others that the complete operation failed. In Leopold's view, Halsted often denied that his patients had developed metastatic cancer after surgery. Contrary to Leopold's assertions, however, there is no evidence in this correspondence that Halsted denied that Mueller died of metastatic breast cancer. When Halsted wrote Mueller's brother after her death that it was satisfying to him that "there was no local recurrence of the growth," Halsted meant, as we have seen repeatedly, that surgery and surgeons had succeeded in Halsted's admittedly myopic terms – no local return of the disease. Leopold misunderstood Halsted's admittedly obsessive interest in building a case that Mueller's longstanding lymphedema was precipitated by an infectious illness as denial that she died of metastatic cancer. Halsted was not denying the reality of cancer spread by distal metastasis. He was trying to pin the blame for her arm complications on something other than her surgery.

75. See, for example, Susan Reverby, "Stealing the golden egg: Ernest Amory Codman and the science and management of medicine," Bulletin of the History of Medicine, 55 (1981): 156–171. See Christopher Crenner, Private Practice: In the Early Twentieth-Century Medical Office of Dr. Richard Cabot (Baltimore: Johns Hopkins, 2005) for a biography of one of the leading voices for acknowledging diagnostic and other errors in American Medicine.

76. The moralism surrounding surgical practice had its correlate in Halsted's severe treatment of trainees whom he believed had committed "moral errors." Halsted's student and biographer Dr. W. G. MacCallum recalled that "the slightest departure from honesty brought down even more prompt and complete disaster. One young man, when asked how a certain patient was that morning, replied that she was doing very well, but when a little later Dr. Halsted went to that ward and found the patient very ill the assistant had to admit that he had not visited her that morning. The service is heavy and the assistants so busy that the mere failure to see this patient during those hours might readily have been forgiven, but this young man left the staff at once." W. G. MacCallum, William Stewart Halsted, Surgeon, 132. See also C. L. Bosk, Forgive and Remember: Managing Medical Failure (Chicago: University of Chicago Press, 1979).

77. Halsted was sometimes praised for his "conservatism" despite being so closely associated with "radical" surgery. One way to understand the use of contradictory political terms is that these modifiers can be appended to either surgical norms or to the

description of surgery itself. The surgeon performing the complete operation might be conservative in the sense that he closely followed the highest surgical ideals at the same time the surgery itself was radical in its extensiveness. See also my note above in which I describe how historian Gert Brieger resolved these apparent contradictions ("From conservative to radical surgery in late nineteenth-century America").

78. W. H. Halsted, "The results of radical operations for the cure of carcinoma of the breast," 7.

79. J. C. Bloodgood, "Halsted thirty-six years ago," 113.

80. Halsted to Mr. Bangs, November 1, 1915, Box 1, Folder 29, Halsted Papers.

81. J. C. Bloodgood, "The diagnosis of early breast tumors based on the clinical history and pathology at the exploratory incision," *Journal of the American Medical Association*, 81 (1923): 875–882, 879.

82. W. W. Duke to Halsted, November 20, 1912. Folder 10, Box 7, Halsted Papers.

83. W. W. Duke to Halsted, February 6, 1913. Folder 10, Box 7, Halsted Papers.

84. Duke's ambivalence suggests more general conflicts and parallels between contemporary beliefs about individual, especially female, psychology and cancer. In the same era in which the physical and emotional stress of modern civilization was seen as making women neurasthenic, women were being told to be more vigilant about their bodies – a double bind if we assume that neurasthenia, despite the protests of some physicians, was a stigmatized diagnosis. Second, cancer was viewed as something happening under the surface of the body yet relentlessly looking for expression just as neurotic drives were always finding physical manifestations. Both occurred more in women and were made worse by civilizing forces.

85. W. W. Duke to Halsted, February 17, 1913. Folder 10, Box 7, Halsted Papers.

86. W. W. Duke to Halsted, March 6, 1913. Folder 10, Box 7, Halsted Papers. Hopelessness about cancer was not eradicated in the twentieth century so much as it was often moved forward in time – there was a time to be hopeful and apply big guns (early cancer) but when it reappeared (as it does so many times in these letters very shortly after surgery) then the older attitudes and reactions were appropriate.

87. W. W. Duke to Halsted, March 6, 1913. Folder 10, Box 7, Halsted Papers. This letter signaled the kinds of experiences that were leading to increased demand for exploratory incision. As physicians saw more cancer and at earlier stages, they increasingly wrestled with proper diagnosis just as they held themselves, like Duke, increasingly responsible for catching it early.

88. W. W. Duke to Halsted, April 16, 1913. Folder 10, Box 7, Halsted Papers.

5. LIVING AT RISK

1. "Smith" folder (undated but sometime Spring 1916), James B. Murphy Papers, American Philosophical Society.

2. General Smith to William S. Halsted, November 28, 1914. Folder 3, Box 14, Halsted Papers, Alan Mason Chesney Medical Archives, Johns Hopkins University (hereafter, Halsted Papers).

3. Halsted to General Smith, December 1, 1914. Folder 3, Box 14, Halsted Papers.

4. General Smith to Halsted, December 5, 1914. Folder 3, Box 14, Halsted Papers.

5. General Smith to Halsted, December 18, 1914, Folder 3, Box 14, Halsted Papers. Smith, like many of Halsted's breast patients, was reticent and indirect in her descriptions of the functional limitations following breast amputations (her husband here is less reticent).

6. Mary Thomas to Halsted, December 22, 1914. Folder 3, Box 14, Halsted Papers.

7. Elizabeth Smith to Halsted, undated. Folder 3, Box 14, Halsted Papers.

8. Halsted to Elizabeth Smith, June 2, 1915. Folder 4, Box 14, Halsted Papers.

9. Elizabeth Smith to Halsted, August 6, 1915. Folder 4, Box 14, Halsted Papers.

10. Elizabeth Smith to Halsted, September 4, 1915. Folder 4, Box 14, Halsted Papers.

11. Elizabeth Smith to Halsted, undated. Folder 4, Box 14, Halsted Papers.

12. Curtis T. Burnham to Halsted, November 16, 1915. Folder 4, Box 14, Halsted Papers.

13. Elizabeth Smith to Halsted, December 23, 1915. Folder 4, Box 14, Halsted Papers.

14. Elizabeth Smith to Halsted, May 13, 1916. Folder 5, Box 14, Halsted Papers.

15. James Murphy did his medical training at Hopkins and later moved to the Rockefeller Institute where he did research into animal and human cancer. His work inducing tumor rejection by irradiated mice had received a great deal of publicity. His treatment of Halsted's breast cancer patients was an apparent extrapolation from his mice studies in which he hoped that radiation would induce a similar lymphocyte-mediated attack on human cancer – a promising research program that he ultimately abandoned in 1925 because it did not work. See I. Lowy, *Between Bench and Bedside: Science, Healing, and Interleukin-II in a Cancer Ward* (Cambridge and London: Harvard University Press, 1997), especially 40, 41, 89–92.

16. Halsted to Murphy, November 1, 1916. Folder Smith, James B. Murphy Papers, American Philosophical Society.

17. Halsted to Murphy, May 16, 1916. Folder 5, Box 14, Halsted Papers.

18. Halsted to Murphy, May 17, 1916. Folder 5, Box 14, Halsted Papers.

19. Elizabeth Smith to Halsted, June 3, 1916. Folder 5, Box 14, Halsted Papers.

20. When Halsted's clinical research program was explicitly discussed with patients, they were invariably enthusiastic about their potential contributions to science. Feelings such as respect and dependence were in part transferred from Halsted as surgeon to Halsted as researcher. One patient's husband in 1914 characteristically wrote Halsted that "if however you wish to make an examination for the sake of science, Mrs. Elias would be willing to let you do so any time you are in New York City." Hugo Elias to Halsted, December 9, 1914. Folder 16, Box 7, Halsted Papers.

21. Halsted to Elizabeth Smith, June 6, 1916. Folder 5, Box 14, Halsted Papers.

22. Halsted to Murphy, June 12, 1917. Folder 4, Box 19, Halsted Papers.

23. Elizabeth Smith to Halsted, April 30, 1918. Folder 5, Box 14, Halsted Papers.

24. Elizabeth Smith to Halsted, May 13, 1918. Folder 6, Box 14, Halsted Papers.

25. Elizabeth Smith to Halsted, July 17, 1917. Folder 5, Box 14, Halsted Papers.

26. Elizabeth Smith to Halsted, June 2, 1919. Folder 6, Box 14, Halsted Papers.

27. Elizabeth Smith to Halsted, February 21, 1920. Folder 6, Box 14, Halsted Papers.

28. Follis to Halsted, July 6, 1920. Folder 6, Box 14, Halsted Papers.

29. Elizabeth Smith related this in a letter to Halsted, July 17, 1920. Folder 5, Box 14, Halsted Papers.

30. Follis to Halsted, January 8, 1921. Folder 6, Box 14, Halsted Papers.

31. Halsted to Follis, January 8, 1921. Folder 6, Box 14, Halsted Papers.

32. General Smith to Halsted, June 2, 1921. Folder 6, Box 14, Halsted Papers.

33. While Halsted did not routinely ask his patients for special permission to conduct his follow-up studies, there was a kind of implied consent since patients could simply not respond to Halsted's queries.

34. Hilda Martin to Halsted, February 27, 1914 and March 6, 1914. Folder 8, Box 1, Halsted Papers.

35. Halsted to Hilda Martin, March 2, 1914. Folder 8, Box 1, Halsted Papers.

36. Hilda Martin to Halsted, March 6, 1914. Folder 8, Box 1, Halsted Papers.

37. Warwick Evans to Halsted, May 31, 1908. Folder 23, Box 7, Halsted Papers.

38. Florence E. Miller to Halsted, not dated but apparently mid-December 1918. Folder 21, Box 21, Halsted Papers.

39. Florence E. Miller to Halsted, October 11, 1919. Folder 21, Box 21, Halsted Papers.

40. W. S. Halsted, "The results of radical operations for the cure of carcinoma of the breast," *Annals of Surgery*, 46 (1907): 1–19, 15–16.

41. It is difficult to make historical comparisons about truth telling, because such behavior is difficult to define and is highly context dependent. American newspaper obituaries avoided naming cancer well into the late-twentieth century yet during much of the same period they published sensationalist accounts of the cancer deaths of prominent citizens. See James Patterson's treatment of, for example, newspaper accounts of Ulysses S. Grant's agonizing cancer death in 1885 in the prologue of *The Dread Disease: Cancer and Modern American Culture* (Cambridge and London: Harvard University Press, 1987). British surgeon C.P. Childe, in his progressivist, popular account of cancer *Control of a Scourge* (London: Methuen and Co., 1906) presented a forceful argument for removing the stigma surrounding cancer, including the evasion of the cancer diagnosis, yet the publishers of the book initially insisted that the word "cancer" not be in the book's title.

42. Ruth Francis to Halsted, October 2, 1915. Folder 5, Box 16, Halsted Papers.

43. Halsted to Ruth Francis, October 16, 1915. Folder 6, Box 16, Halsted Papers.

44. Halsted to Burnham, November 6, 1915. Folder 5, Box 16, Halsted Papers.

45. Ruth Francis to Halsted, December 8, 1915. Folder 6, Box 16, Halsted Papers.

46. Halsted to Ruth Francis, December 14, 1915, Folder 8, Box 16, Halsted Papers.

47. Dr. A. Peskind to Halsted, December 7, 1908. Folder 14, Box 20, Halsted Papers.

48. Akira Kurosawa's film *Ikuru* begins with a dramatic example of such indirection and inference. The lead character suffers from abdominal pain and waits for an appointment in a crowded clinic. He overhears other patients say that when the doctor tells you that you have a minor problem for which there is nothing to do and you can eat whatever you want, they know that you have cancer. After some young physicians examine the patient and the x-rays of his stomach, they exchange knowing glances among themselves and tell him verbatim the circumlocutions he

heard about in the waiting room, to which he understandably reacts with horror and dread.

49. Halsted to James G. Kiernan, December 4, 1921. Folder 21, Box 22, Halsted Papers.

50. James G. Kiernan to Halsted, December 13, 1921 (telegram). Folder 21, Box 22, Halsted Papers. Halsted also bought flowers for the patient with monies that Kiernan had wired from Chicago.

51. Halsted to James G. Kiernan, January 5, 1922. Folder 21, Box 22, Halsted Papers.

52. Walter A. Price to Halsted, December 31, 1921. Folder 21, Box 22, Halsted Papers.

53. Halsted to Walter A. Price, January 5, 1922. Folder 21, Box 22, Halsted Papers.

54. Ida Price to Halsted, May 8, 1922. Folder 21, Box 22, Halsted Papers.

55. Judith Wheaton to Halsted, not dated but probably February 1914. Folder 16, Box 26, Halsted Papers.

56. Ruth Green to Halsted, not dated but probably prior to May 1914. Folder 16, Box 26, Halsted Papers. It is worth noting how few women wrote Halsted about the complications from cancer per se rather than surgery. In part, this was because of Halsted's research interest but it also reflects the fact that the metastatic and constitutional aspects of cancer did not matter that much to Halsted, except that they sometimes triggered referrals for salvage treatment and occasional interventions to alleviate pain.

57. Judith Wheaton (sister-in-law) to Halsted, May 7, 1915. Folder 17, Box 3, Halsted Papers.

58. Halsted to James Ewing, April 23, 1915. Folder 14, Box 3, Halsted Papers.

59. Halsted to James Ewing, May 18, 1915. Folder 14, Box 3, Halsted Papers.

60. Halsted to Judith Wheaton, May 12, 1915. Folder 14, Box 3, Halsted Papers.

61. See E. Leopold, *A Darker Ribbon: Breast Cancer, Women, and their Doctors in The Twentieth Century* (Boston: Beacon Press, 1999), 91. Leopold observed increasing degrees of honesty around the diagnosis and treatment of cancer and in medical care more generally as the century wore on, attributing change to many social influences, especially the rise of feminism. Leopold's fall and rise narrative of ethical progress contrasts sharply to the analysis in this and later chapters.

62. J. Peebles Proctor to Halsted, January 12, 1912. Folder 27, Box 20, Halsted Papers.

63. H. A. Miller to Halsted, February 9, 1920. Folder 21, Box 21, Halsted Papers.

64. For details of Handley's radium implants, see W. S. Handley, "Parasternal invasion of the thorax in breast cancer and its suppression by the use of radium tubes as an operative precaution," *Surgery, Gynecology, and Obstetrics*, 45 (1927): 721. Handley's personal papers also reveal additional variation in how these modalities were actually used in the early-twentieth-century clinical management of breast tumors: against suspicious benign tumors instead of surgery, as a presurgical "adjuvant" treatment for suspected cancer, and as a postsurgical treatment. For example, Dr. Arthur Holt wrote Handley on March 19, 1908 (placed in p. 49 in Handley's clinical notebook) about a 46-year-old woman who had chronic mastitis whom Holt had treated with x-ray treatments to "soften the way" toward more "drastic measures" that Handley might consider. On p. 93 of this notebook, Handley noted a woman who had eight applications of x-rays in 1908 for a "dangerous variety of

chronic mastitis" that he was now "advising operation." On p. 121, Handley wrote about a woman whose lump he excised in January 15, 1909 that "proved to be a carcinoma," whom he irradiated after surgery. Handley Papers, GC/152, Box 2, notebook from Middlesex and Samaratin Hospitals, Wellcome Historical Library, London, U.K.

65. Halsted to Abraham Flexner, April 27, 1915. Folder 5, Box 16, Halsted Papers.

66. Murphy to Halsted, April 12, 1917. Folder 7, Box 16, Halsted Papers.

67. Ruth Francis to Halsted, October 27, 1915. Folder 6, Box 16, Halsted Papers.

68. Janet Fleming to Halsted, April 26, 1915. Folder 33, Box 24, Halsted Papers.

69. Halsted to Janet Fleming, May 4, 1915. Folder 33, Box 24, Halsted Papers.

70. Halsted to Janet Fleming, December 22, 1915. Folder 33, Box 24, Halsted Papers.

71. Janet Fleming to Halsted, January 14, 1916. Folder 33, Box 24, Halsted Papers.

72. Halsted to Janet Fleming, January 22, 1916. Folder 33, Box 24, Halsted Papers.

73. Halsted to Murphy, June 12, 1917. Folder 4, Box 19, Halsted Papers. But Halsted's optimism was a small respite from his overall skepticism about these salvage treatments that was continually reinforced by the inevitable death of breast cancer patients. Halsted wrote Murphy in January 1921 that he recently learned of Francis's death. Revealing once again Halsted's obsession with surgical responsibility, he wrote Murphy that he was "glad to know that there was no local recurrence of the carcinoma." Halsted to Murphy, February 12, 1921. Folder 4, Box 19, Halsted papers.

74. Halsted to Mott D. Cannon, May 17, 1915. Folder 5, Box 16, Halsted Papers. In the first few decades of the twentieth century, general practitioners directed x-rays at a variety of cancerous and noncancerous conditions. Unlike their often dramatic effects on growths and inflammation, the dangers of x-rays took longer to observe and become widely known.

75. Halsted was unusually attuned to problems of pain control at the end of life (an issue which many people today think of as a neglected aspect of medical care in need of reform). A prominent theme of Halsted chroniclers has been his addiction to cocaine and morphine. While I am skeptical about the many attempts to see this as a major influence on Halsted's life, it may very well have contributed to Halsted's sensitivity toward cancer pain.

76. Halsted to Rosalie Dattwyler, March 28, 1914. Folder 34, Box 24, Halsted Papers.

77. Rosalie Dattwyler to Halsted, April 22, 1914. Folder 34, Box 24, Halsted Papers.

78. Halsted to H. H. Young, May 7, 1914. Folder 34, Box 24, Halsted Papers.

79. W. E. Burgess to Halsted, December 13, 1914. Folder 4, Box 17, Halsted Papers.

80. Halsted to W. E. Burgess, December 15, 1914. Folder 4, Box 17, Halsted Papers.

81. W. B. Coley's work has been seen by some modern cancer researchers as the inspiration and prototype of modern cancer immunotherapy such as BCG (similarly made from bacterial material) treatment in bladder cancer. For more detail on Coley, see I. Lowy, *Between Bench and Bedside: Science, Healing, and Interleukin-II in a Cancer Ward* (Cambridge and London: Harvard University Press, 1997), 102–104.

82. W. E. Burgess to Halsted, December 17, 1914. Folder 4, Box 17, Halsted Papers.

83. Halsted to W. E. Burgess, January 5, 1914. Folder 4, Box 17, Halsted Papers.

84. Coley to Halsted, January 12, 1915. Folder 4, Box 17, Halsted Papers. As further evidence, Coley sent Halsted copies of testaments of this case from Dr. Greenleaf in Olean NY (see G. A. Greenleaf to Coley, December 8, 1914), Charles Frazier in Philadelphia (see C. N. Frazier to Coley, October 21, 1914, who calls it Coley's fluid), and William Bott in Buffalo (see W. J. Bott to Coley, October 20, 1914).
85. Coley to Halsted, January 18, 1915. Folder 4, Box 17, Halsted Papers.
86. Halsted to W. B. Coley, January 14, 1915. Folder 4, Box 17, Halsted Papers.
87. Coley to Halsted, January 18, 1915. Folder 4, Box 17, Halsted Papers.
88. Halsted to W. E. Burgess, January 22, 1915. Folder 4, Box 17, Halsted Papers.
89. William Welch to Murphy, March 26, 1931. Folder Welch, William Henry, James B. Murphy Papers, American Philosophical Society.
90. All these points are made in J. Patterson, *The Dread Disease*.

6. "DO NOT DELAY": THE WAR AGAINST TIME

1. This quote was attributed to Thomas Aquinas and displayed in a 1920 exhibit on cancer control at the American Museum of Natural History, reproduced in E.H. Rigney, *History of the American Society for the Control of Cancer 1913–1943* (New York: American Society for the Control of Cancer, 1944).
2. The internal history of this campaign – its funding, ideology, organizational structure, successes and failures – has been well documented by others. See J. Patterson, *The Dread Disease: Cancer and Modern American Culture* (Cambridge, MA: Harvard University Press, 1987), for an account of the founding of the American Association for the Control of Cancer. See also E. H. Rigney, *History of the American Society for the Control of Cancer 1913–1943* and W. Ross, *Crusade: The Official History of the American Cancer Society* (New York: Arbor House, 1987).
3. C. P. Childe, *The Control of a Scourge, or How Cancer is Curable* (London: Methuen and Co., 1906), especially Chapter 14. Quotes are from pp. 143–144 ("Cancer itself is not incurable") and p. 9 ("involuntary suicide").
4. When I refer to cancer activists, unless otherwise specified, I am referring to the leaders of these organizations. The ASCC was started in 1913. Male surgeons and gynecologists dominated its initial leadership. Its renaming as the American Cancer Society in the middle 1940s was one small part of a radical transformation of the organization's style, leadership, budget, and priorities. See J. Patterson, *The Dread Disease*, especially Chapters 3 and 7.
5. See, for example, American Society for Control of Cancer, *Catalog of Education Material* (New York: American Society for the Control of Cancer, early 1940s).
6. A. L. Goodman, "Is cancer curable?" *Quarterly Review*, 2 (1937): 40–43.
7. M. A. Richards, A. M. Westcombe, S. B. Love, P. Littlejohns, and A. J. Ramirez, "Influence of delay on survival in patients with breast cancer: a systematic review," *Lancet*, 353 (1999): 1119–1126, 1119.
8. While some of the early-twentieth-century epidemiological evidence was remarkably sophisticated from our contemporary perspective (see my discussion below of

Janet Lane-Claypon's research), the great majority of quantitative claims about "delay" and "outcomes" were either not substantiated by data or based on data that suffered from the absence of controls, inadequate endpoints, and selection and lead time biases.

9. J. C. Bloodgood, "The diagnosis of early breast tumors, based on the clinical history and pathology at the exploratory incision," *Journal of the American Medical Association*, 81 (1923): 875–882.

10. Miss Sara Johnson to Halsted, May 1 [n.d.], Folder 14, Box 21, Halsted Papers, Alan Mason Chesney Medical Archives, Johns Hopkins University (hereafter Halsted Papers).

11. See, for example, Alice Pickert to William Stewart Halsted, n.d. but mid-April 1912, Folder 20, Box 1, Halsted Papers.

12. E. M. Daland, "Untreated cancer of the breast," *Surgery, Gynecology, and Obstetrics*, 44 (1927): 264–268.

13. James G. Kiernan to Halsted, December 4, 1921, Folder 21, Box 22, Halsted Papers.

14. J. Frank Small to Halsted, March 14, 1897, Folder 3, Box 23, Halsted Papers.

15. "Lump on breast" (undated clipping), found in Frederick Hoffman's 1913 bound volume of correspondence and clippings relating to American Society for the Control of Cancer, Frederick Hoffman Papers, Modern Manuscripts Collection, History of Medicine Division, National Library of Medicine.

16. Charles C. Harrold to Halsted, March 22, 1912, Folder 20, Box 10, Halsted Papers.

17. Dr. William Brady, "Cancer, treated in time, is curable," *The World Magazine*, April 13, 1913.

18. Leonard Keene Hirshberg, "How cancer may be prevented" undated clipping, "Clippings on Cancer [Scrapbook]," Frederick Hoffman Papers, 27–29, College of Physicians of Philadelphia.

19. John P. Deaver Papers, 9, College of Physicians of Philadelphia.

20. The naming and recognition of the precancerous stages in breast cancer has been gradual, ambiguous, and contested. Many observers cite Foote and Stewart's 1941 description of lobular carcinoma in situ as the first pathological description of breast precancer (F. W. Foote, Jr., and F. W. Stewart, "Lobular carcinoma in situ: A rare form of mammary cancer [Classics in Oncology]," *CA: A Cancer Journal for Clinicians*, 32 (1982 [orig. publ. 1941]): 234–237).

21. Henry C. Coe to Joseph C. Bloodgood, March 17, 1927, "Bloodgood letter collection: Letters concerning biopsy" Folder, Box 22, Howard Kelly Papers, Alan Mason Chesney Archives, Johns Hopkins University.

22. Bloodgood was noting the radically changed presentation of women with breast problems in the preceding few years. In more than half of the last 100 women he had examined, he had advised against surgery. J. C. Bloodgood, "Benign lesions of female breast for which operation is not indicated," *Journal of the American Medical Association*, 78 (1922): 859–863.

23. J. E. Lane-Claypon, *Cancer of the Breast and Its Surgical Treatment* (London: Ministry of Health, 1924); Charles Bell is cited on p. 58. The 43.1 percent observation is

on p. 73 and the overall conclusion about the advantages of the operation is from p. 78.

24. "Will you help save 5,000,000 Americans? [Editorial]," *Better Homes and Gardens*, April 1945: 7.

25. American Cancer Society, *Cancer: The Problem of Early Diagnosis, For Professional Audiences* (New York: American Cancer Society, 1949) (pamphlet prepared to accompany 1949 film of the same name), found in "Publicity" Folder, Box 95, Mary Lasker Papers, Columbia University [hereafter "Lasker Papers"]).

26. I. F. Marcosson, "Worry can save your life," *Woman's Home Companion*, May 1944: 36–38, 36.

27. New York City Cancer Committee, *Can We Save the Other Three?* [Pamphlet] (New York: New York City Cancer Committee, 1956), found in "New York City Cancer Committee, 1956" Folder, Box 121, Lasker Papers.

28. B. R. Shore, "The education of the public," *Quarterly Review*, 1 (1936): 53–57, 55.

29. Attributed to Ewing by F. E. Adair, "The doctor looks at women and their problem of cancer of the breast," *Quarterly Review*, 8 (1943): 9–11, 10.

30. Hayworth to Halsted, March 7, 1907, Folder 28, Box 10, Halsted Papers.

31. C. H. Horst to Halsted, March 3, 1914, Folder 13, Box 12, Halsted Papers.

32. "The Right Way" and "The Wrong Way" posters by R. Philips Ward were first shown at the 1920 AMA meeting in New Orleans, and reproduced in E. H. Rigney, *History of the American Society for the Control of Cancer*.

33. C. C. Little, "Education" chapter in his edited *Cancer: A Study for Laymen, Prepared for the Women's Field Army of the American Society for the Control of Cancer, Inc.* (New York and Toronto: Farrar and Rinehart, 1944), 108. See also p. 107: "The first duty of a Field Army worker is to face cancer unafraid and to maintain an attitude of intelligent, rational judgment concerning it."

34. O. Marshino, "Breast cancer," *Hygeia*, 23 (1945): 176–177, 177.

35. G. Palmer, "'I had a cancer': Novelist Mary Roberts Rinehart was cured," *Ladies Home Journal*, July 1947: 143–152, 152.

36. J. Holmes, "I didn't have cancer," *Woman's Home Companion*, June 1948: 10.

37. On the "little red door" campaign, see "Behind the 'little red door' lies cancer help," *New York Post*, June 28, 1951. For an example of "dependent on new discoveries" see "What happens to people who get cancer [Chart]," *Statistics on Cancer* [Pamphlet] (1952), 7, found in "ACS-New York – 1952" Folder, Box 96, Lasker Papers. For the breast cancer story contest, see "Contest is open to cancer stories," *ACS Bulletin*, April 21, 1952: 1.

38. Copy in E. H. Rigney, *History of the American Society for the Control of Cancer*.

39. M. Fishbein, "Cancer [Editorial]," *Hygeia*, 25 (1947): 259.

40. *Man Alive* (United Productions of American for the American Cancer Society), 1952.

41. See "By the Way" cartoon by Francis J. Rigney ("You will carefully get rid of the smallest weed in your flower garden but – How about helping root out the most devastating growth in the human system?"), reprinted in E. H. Rigney, "Cancer

publicity – ten years of growth," *Quarterly Review*, 1 (1936): 47. The "By the Way" cartoons were reprinted in pamphlets funded by the Prudential Life Insurance Company and formed part of one of the New York City Cancer Committee's traveling exhibits. The NYCCC also distributed a cancer pamphlet entitled "Destroy the Weed" to New York schoolchildren in 1927 (E. H. Rigney, "*History of the American Society for the Control of Cancer 1913–1943.*").

42. J. Patterson, *The Dread Disease.*

43. See, for example, the winning posters reprinted in "To fight cancer," *New York Times Magazine*, April 9, 1948: 15.

44. James S. Hauck to Mary R. Lasker, December 15, 1948, "ACS 1949, January through April" Folder, Box 95, Lasker Papers.

45. S. M. Spencer, "Where are we now on cancer?" *Saturday Evening Post*, June 5, 1948: 30–31.

46. M. A. Gold, "Causes of patients' delay in diseases of the breast," *Cancer*, 17 (1964): 564–577, 564, 576.

47. B. R. Shore, "The education of the public," 57.

48. However, in what seemed to be an acknowledgment that the ACS was losing its war to change physician attitudes, this same study noted that physicians were responsible for only 17 percent of patient delays in the 1923–1938 period but 27.8 percent of the delays in the 1946–1947 period. G. F. Robbins and J. F. Leach, 1947. "Surveys show cancer patients tend to avoid delays." *American Cancer Society News Service*, 3 (1947): 1.

49. J. B. Deaver, "Carcinoma of the breast" (speech read before Ohio County Medical Society, Wheeling, West Virginia, May 27, 1927), 4–5, Folder 127, Box 4, Series I, John B. Deaver Collection, College of Physicians of Philadelphia.

50. J. C. Bloodgood, "Benign lesions of female breast for which operation is not indicated."

51. J. C. Bloodgood, "The diagnosis of early breast tumors, based on the clinical history and pathology at the exploratory incision," *Journal of the American Medical Association*, 81 (1923): 875–882. As noted in Chapter 4, however, preoperative biopsies were rare events at Johns Hopkins during most of this period.

52. R. B. Greenough, "Early diagnosis of cancer of the breast," *Annals of Surgery*, 102 (1935): 233–238, 234.

53. J. C. Bloodgood, "The diagnosis of early breast tumors, based on the clinical history and pathology at the exploratory incision."

54. F. W. Foote, Jr., and F. W. Stewart, "Lobular carcinoma in situ: A rare form of mammary cancer."

55. J. C. Bloodgood, "Biopsy in breast lesions in relation to diagnosis, treatment and prognosis," *Annals of Surgery*, 102 (1935): 239–249.

56. N.J. Kilbourne, "If you have a lump in your breast," *Hygeia*, 13 (1935): 213.

57. Much of this material in this chapter previously appeared in my "Do not delay: Breast cancer and Time, 1900–1970." Milbank Quarterly, 79 (2001), 355–386. Reproduced with permission of Blackwell publishing.

7. "PROPHETS OF DOOM": SKEPTICS OF THE CANCER ESTABLISHMENT AT MID-CENTURY

1. Made for the American Cancer Society by the International Film Foundation, directed by Francis Thompson.

2. Made by the U.S. Public Health Service and the Department of Agriculture in cooperation with the American Association for the Control of Cancer, directed by W. Allen Luey.

3. See also another contemporary film in which "not delaying" resulted in a negative cancer diagnosis, the animated *Man Alive* (United Productions of America; American Cancer Society, 1952), which was nominated for an Oscar in the best short documentary category.

4. For a lively and exhaustive account of the rise and fall of the radical mastectomy, see B. Lerner, *Breast Cancer Wars* (Oxford and New York: Oxford University Press, 2001).

5. I. G. Tedesche, "Figures count," *Hygeia*, 26 (1948): 796–797, 796.

6. While many observers argued, as had been done since the early nineteenth century, that the increased crude cancer mortality was an artifact of longer lives brought about by other health improvements, virtually no one believed that cancer mortality was dropping. See N. L. Petrakis, "Historic milestones in cancer epidemiology," *Seminars in Oncology*, 6 (1979): 433–444, for a discussion of late-nineteenth-century and early-twentieth-century efforts to discern secular trends in cancer mortality. For example, Petrakis recounted efforts to adjust different age distributions so that different populations could be compared and early attempts in the United States to systematically sample deaths from cancer.

7. N. E. McKinnon, "Limitations in diagnosis and treatment of breast and other cancers: A review," *Canadian Medical Association Journal*, 73 (1955): 614–625, 616.

8. R. M. Janes, "A breast clinic," *Postgraduate Medicine*, 13 (1953): 513–518, 514.

9. In retrospect, skepticism about cancer statistics may have caused some unfortunate collateral damage, such as contributing to the belated consensus that lung cancer rates were rising and were due to smoking. N. L. Petrakis, "Historic milestones in cancer epidemiology."

10. W. F. Willcox, "On the alleged increase of cancer," *Publications of the American Statistical Association*, 15 (1917): 701–782, 757, 759.

11. W. M. Strong, "Is cancer mortality increasing?" *Journal of Cancer Research*, 6 (1921): 251–256, 256.

12. Lester Breslow, principal investigator, *A History of Cancer Control in the United States, 1946–1971*, prepared by the History of Cancer Control Project, UCLA School of Public Health, under contract to the National Cancer Institute (hereafter *A History of Cancer Control in the United States*), 500.

13. L. I. Dublin, E. W. Kopf, et al., *Cancer Mortality Among Insured Wage Earners and Their Families: The Experience of the Metropolitan Life Insurance Company Industrial Department 1911 to 1922* (New York: Metropolitan Life Insurance Company, 1925).

14. F. L. Hoffman, *San Francisco Cancer Survey Seventh Preliminary Report (Seventeenth, Eighteenth, Nineteenth and Twentieth Quarterly Reports)* (Newark: The Prudential Press, 1931), 170.

15. *A History of Cancer Control in the United States*, 10 (introduction).

16. L. I. Dublin, E. W. Kopf, et al., *Cancer Mortality Among Insured Wage Earners and Their Families,"* 16.

17. C. D. Haagensen, and A. P. Stout, "Carcinoma of the breast: I – Results of treatment," *Annals of Surgery*, 116 (1942): 801–815.

18. S. P. Reimann and F. H. Safford, "Statistical study of the influence of the educational campaign on the interval between discovery and consultation in mammary carcinoma, in *Report of the International Conference on Cancer, London –July17–20, 1928*, held under the auspices of the British Empire Cancer Campaign (London: John Wright & Sons, 1928), 562–569.

19. O. Marshino, "Breast cancer," *Hygeia*, 23 (1945): 176–201, 201.

20. G. C. Crile, Jr., *Cancer and Common Sense*, 8. One of Crile's many readers added to Crile's criticisms of cancer detection, that "like you, I am not impressed by the importance of the Cancer Detection Clinic as a means for early cancer although they certainly do pick up some. But the side product – finding hypertension and many other things about which we can do something is valuable. The medical profession has never been able to sell the idea of periodic health examinations. It is a rather dull business and has no glamor, but it has become more popular now that the bands are playing and the flags are flying." Frederick A. Coller to Crile, November 22, 1955, Box 13, *Cancer and Common Sense* scrapbook, Crile Papers, Cleveland Clinic archives.

21. First quote p. 60, second p. 84 in *A History of Cancer Control in the United States*. In Kaiser's own case, his expectations for cancer detection were high because his own thyroid cancer was picked up a young resident in a screening examination. In this same history, Kaiser concluded more generally that (p. 52) "I don't think that clinicians ever really felt that this cancer business … was really a function of the public health agencies." See Chapter 9 for more detail.

22. Joseph Bloodgood, in response to James Ewing, "The prevention of cancer," in *Cancer Control: Report of an International Symposium*, held under the auspices of the American Society for the Control of Cancer, Lake Mohonk, New York, September 20–24, 1926 (Chicago: The Surgical Publishing Company of Chicago, 1927), 165–184, quote is from p. 179.

23. Robert Thorpe to ACS, June 21, 1948, Box 94, Folder ACS 1948. Mary Lasker Papers, Columbia University.

24. D. Lewis and W. F. Reinhoff, Jr., "A study of the results of operations for the cure of cancer of the breast performed at the Johns Hopkins Hospital from 1889 to 1931," *Annals of Surgery*, 95 (1932): 336–400, 349, quoted in N. E. McKinnon, "Breast cancer mortality, Ontario, 1909–1947 : The lack of any decline and its significance," *Canadian Journal of Public Health*, 40 (1949): 257–269, 269.

25. J. Ewing, "The causal and formal genesis of cancer," *Report of the International Conference on Cancer, London – July 17–20, 1928*, 1–13.

26. H. S. N. Greene, "Identification of malignant tissues," *Journal of the American Medical Association*, 137 (1948): 1364–1366.

27. J. B. Deaver, Folder 177, Address – "Cancer control" [n.d.], Historical Collections, College of Physicians of Philadelphia.

28. I. MacDonald, "The individual basis of biologic variability in cancer," *Surgery, Gynecology, and Obstetrics*, 106 (1958): 227–229, 229.

29. I. MacDonald, "Biological predeterminism in human cancer," *Surgery, Gynecology, and Obstetrics*, 92 (1951): 443–452.

30. M. M. Black and F. D. Speer, "Biologic variability of breast carcinoma in relation to diagnosis and therapy," *New York State Journal of Medicine*, 53 (1953): 1560–1563, 1561.

31. E. J. Grace, "Simple mastectomy in cancer of breast," *American Journal of Surgery*, 35 (1937): 512–514.

32. I. MacDonald, "Biological predeterminism in human cancer," 444.

33. I. MacDonald, "Endocrine ablative procedures in disseminated mammary carcinoma," in *Proceedings of the Fourth National Cancer Conference, Minneapolis, Minnesota, September 13, 14, and 15, 1960*, 273–279, 285 (discussion).

34. I. MacDonald, "Biological predeterminism in human cancer," 448.

35. W. W. Park and J. C. Lees, "The absolute curability of cancer of the breast," *Surgery, Gynecology, and Obstetrics*, 93 (1951): 129–152. They cite Davis on p. 137.

36. Ibid., 133.

37. I. G. Williams, R. S. Murley, et al., "Carcinoma of the female breast: conservative and radical surgery," *British Medical Journal*, ii (1953): 787–796, 788.

38. R. G. Small and A. M. Dutton, "Survival of patients with carcinoma of the breast," *Journal of the American Medical Association*, 157 (1955): 216–219, 216.

39. I. MacDonald, "Biological predeterminism in human cancer."

40. W. W. Park and J. C. Lees, "The absolute curability of cancer of the breast," 136. Their bold reassertion was widely discussed and quoted. Ten years after this publication, a new generation of skeptics would cite this challenge and argue it remained undiminished: "I think the breast is a perfect example where almost all of out treatment is based on faith. I do not think there is even an answer to the questions posed by Park and Lees well over a decade ago. It is even very hard to demonstrate the effect of any therapy in breast cancer." A. M. Popma, "Cancer of the breast," in *Proceedings of the Fourth National Cancer Conference, Minneapolis, Minnesota, September 13, 14, and 15, 1960* (Philadelphia and Montreal: J. B. Lippincott, 1961), 737–739. (Quote is from Michael Shimkin on p. 739.)

41. I. MacDonald, "Endocrine ablative procedures in disseminated mammary carcinoma," in *Proceedings of the Fourth National Cancer Conference, Minneapolis, Minnesota, September 13, 14, and 15, 1960*, 273–279, 274.

42. N. E. McKinnon, "Breast cancer mortality, Ontario, 1909–1947," 262.

43. W. W. Park and J. C. Lees, "The absolute curability of cancer of the breast," 134.

44. L. J. Notkin, "The theory of biologic predeterminism: Its questionable usefulness and validity as a medical tool," *Canadian Medical Association Journal*, 81 (1959): 190–191.

45. D. P. Boyd, "Biological predeterminism [Editorial]," *Lahey Clinic Foundation Bulletin*, 18 (1969): 135–136, 136.

46. I. MacDonald, "The individual basis of biologic variability in cancer," 229.

47. Ibid., 228.

48. J. Foote, W. Frank and F. W. Stewart, "Lobular carcinoma in situ: A rare form of mammary cancer [Classics in Oncology]," *CA: A Cancer Journal for Clinicians*, 32 (1982 [orig. publ. 1941]): 234–237.

49. For a period after 1950 the norm for treating LCIS was "some form of mastectomy." R. V. P. Hutter, J. Foote, W. Frank, et al., "In situ lobular carcinoma of the female breast, 1939–1968," in *Breast Cancer: Early and Late: A Collection of Papers Presented at the Thirteenth Annual Clinical Conference on Cancer, 1968, at the University of Texas M. D. Anderson Hospital and Tumor Institute at Houston, Houston, Texas* (Chicago: Year Book Medical Publishers, 1970), 202.

50. Attributed to Stewart in E. F. Lewison, "Lobular carcinoma *in situ* of the breast: the feminine mystique," *Military Medicine*, 129 (1964): 115–123, 120.

51. J. B. Deaver, Addresses and Writings, 1904–1932, Historical Collection, College of Physicians of Philadelphia.

52. See Interview with Leopold Koss, *A History of Cancer Control in the United States* (p. 9), for all these details.

53. W. Ross, *Crusade: The Official History of the American Cancer Society* (New York, Arbor House, 1987), 86.

54. From John Dunn interview, *A History of Cancer Control in the United States*, 29.

55. N. E. McKinnon, "Limitations in diagnosis and treatment of breast and other cancers," 617, 620.

56. M. M. Black, T. H. C. Barclay, et al., "Association of atypical characteristics of benign breast lesions with subsequent risk of breast cancer," *Cancer*, 29 (1972): 338–343, 342.

57. C. D. Haagensen, C. Bodian, D. E. Haagensen, Jr., eds., *Breast Carcinoma: Risk and Detection* (Philadelphia: WB Saunders, 1981), 239.

58. Comment by Dr. Lees. "Significance of statistical analysis of end results in the treatment of breast cancer [round table discussion]," in *Proceedings of the Second National Cancer Conference*, Vol. I (New York: American Cancer Society, 1952), 107–145, 140–141.

59. Ibid.

60. N. E. McKinnon, "Breast cancer mortality, Ontario, 1909–1947, 259."

61. W. Kaempffert, "Does cancer run in families?" *Saturday Evening Post*, 217 (1945): 17.

8. BALANCING HOPE, TRUST, AND TRUTH: RACHEL CARSON

1. Nelle Nugent to Crile, April 10, 1987, Box 46, George Crile, Jr., Papers, Cleveland Clinic Foundation Archives, Cleveland, Ohio (hereafter, Crile Papers).

2. Crile to Nelle Nugent, April 30, 1987, Box 46, Crile Papers.

3. Portions of untitled screenplay, with Crile–Nugent correspondence, Box 46, Crile Papers.

4. Crile to Nelle Nugent, April 20, 1987, Box 46, Crile Papers.

5. L. Lear, *Rachel Carson: Witness for Nature* (New York: Henry Holt and Company, 1997), 184–185.

6. Freeman to Carson, January 9, 1960, Martha Freeman, ed., *Always, Rachel: The Letters of Rachel Carson and Dorothy Freeman, 1952–1964* (Boston: Beacon Press, 1994), hereafter *Letters*, 295.

7. Freeman also speculated about the role of stress, especially that of writing what would become *Silent Spring*, as a cause of Carson's duodenal ulcer. Their later correspondence about Carson's cancer would not contain any such speculation. Such psychosomatic reasoning was not a prominent part of the cultural construction of breast cancer during this era. Freeman to Carson, January 9, 1960, *Letters*, 296.

8. L. Lear, *Rachel Carson: Witness for Nature*, 367.

9. Carson to Crile, December 7, 1960, Box 46, Crile Papers. She wrote to friends Marjorie Spock and Polly Richards on April 12, 1960 that one of the two tumors was "suspicious enough to require a radical mastectomy." Box 16, The Lear/Carson collection, Charles E. Shain Library, Connecticut College, New London, CT.

10. Michael Healy to Crile, December 13, 1960, Box 46, Crile Papers.

11. L. Lear, *Rachel Carson: Witness for Nature*, 367. Lear cites the letter from Carson to Marjorie Spock and Polly Richards on April 12, 1960.

12. Carson to Crile, December 7, 1960, Box 46, Crile Papers.

13. See Carson to Paul Brooks, December 27, 1960, Box 16, The Lear/Carson collection, Charles E. Shain Library, Connecticut College, New London, CT. Also cited in L. Lear, *Rachel Carson: Witness for Nature*, 368.

14. G. Crile, Jr., *The Way It Was. Sex, Surgery, Treasure, and Travel, 1907–1987* (Kent, OH: Kent State University Press, 1992), 293.

15. George Crile, Jr., "The evolution of the treatment of breast cancer," 1, Box 4, Crile Papers.

16. Details in G. Crile, Jr., *The Way It Was*, 205–206.

17. From B. Crile, "Barney Crile oral history," *National Library of Medicine, History of Medicine Division* (1999), 25. Crile also argued that surgeons were reluctant to deviate from standard practice because of peer censure and threats of legal liability. George Crile, Jr., "The treatment of cancer. A dissenting view," Box 2, Crile Papers.

18. G. Crile, Jr., "A plea against blind fear of cancer," *Life*, October 31 (1955): 128–132. This article contained testaments by prominent surgeons supporting Crile's message.

19. G. Crile, Jr., *Cancer and Common Sense* (New York: Viking Press, 1955), 7.

20. Ibid., 45.
21. Ibid., 14.
22. Crile to Charles C. Lund, October 17, 1955, Box 28, Crile Papers.
23. G. Crile, Jr., *Cancer and Common Sense*, 52–53.
24. Crile to Charles C. Lund, October 17, 1955, Box 28, Crile Papers.
25. In 1991, for example, Crile wrote prominent clinical epidemiologist David Eddy, who was the son of one of Crile's Cleveland Clinic colleagues, "what is the meaning of 'sensitivity' and 'specificity'? I have seen these terms used but never understood them. Maybe there are more clinicians as dumb as I am." Crile to Eddy, January 8, 1991, Box 3, Folder "David Eddy," Crile Papers. These terms had become the standard quantitative measures for evaluating a diagnostic test. Crile was nevertheless able to observe insights earlier than others would make by statistical inference. For example, Crile observed that the perceived "increasing survival of treated cases" depended on "what is called cancer, Curing cancers that would not have been fatal if untreated does not alter the death rate from cancer in the population at large." Crile to Charles C. Lund, October 17, 1955, Box 28, Crile Papers.
26. G. Crile, Jr., *Cancer and Common Sense*, 73.
27. Ibid., 101.
28. Ibid., 105.
29. Ibid., 104.
30. Carson to Crile, December 7, 1960, Box 46, Crile Papers.
31. Carson to Crile, December 17, 1960, Box 46, Crile Papers.
32. Crile to Carson, December 22, 1960, Box 46, Crile Papers.
33. Crile to Michael Healy, December 16, 1960, Box 46, Crile Papers.
34. G. Crile, Jr., *The Way It Was*, 293.
35. Freeman to Carson, December 31, 1960, *Letters*, 325.
36. Carson to Freeman, January 17, 1961, *Letters*, 332.
37. Her rheumatologist, Dr. Crain, and other treating physicians, initially attributed her joint pain and large effusions to infection (she had a prior staphylococcus urine infection) and later as "settling in" to rheumatoid arthritis. L. Lear, *Rachel Carson: Witness for Nature*, 384 and Carson to Freeman, March 17, 1961, *Letters*, 361.
38. Carson initially wrote "for a day or two I felt the treatment was doing no good and would do none (and of course I know better now – the change is definite)." Carson to Freeman, March 4, 1961, *Letters*, 356. Carson later noted "definite shrinking." Carson to Crile, March 18, 1961, Box 102, folder 38, Rachel Carson Papers, Yale Collection of American Literature, Beinecke Rare Book and Manuscript Library, Yale University, New Haven, Connecticut (hereafter Rachel Carson Papers).
39. Details of Carson's medical experiences with arthritis were revealingly collected and summarized by Carson in a succinct summary she attached to a letter to Crile (Carson to Crile, March 23, 1960 – really 1961, Box 46, Crile Papers).
40. Carson to Freeman, February 15, 1961, *Letters*, 346.
41. "I am also feeling somewhat upset about this proposed treatment [gold]. Of course, I've already had a taste of having to submit to something I knew was dangerous and in theory undesirable [radiation] but there the alternative left no choice. Here

I feel I'd rather endure some arthritis and gamble with the bone marrow." Carson to Freeman, March 17, 1961, *Letters*, 362.

42. Carson to Crile, March 18, 1961, Rachel Carson Papers.

43. Carson to Crile, March 23, 1961, Box 46, Crile Papers. To Dorothy, Carson wrote that her friend at NIH had read her from the standard pharmacology text "an urgent statement that gold should not be administered to any person who has recently undergone a course of radiation! So there I had the answer to my own hunch. Yet this man, knowing perfectly well I'd just had radiation, was quite ready to give it to me. What this does to my already great cynicism about doctors you can perhaps imagine." Carson to Freeman, March 25, 1961, *Letters*, 365–366. The pharmacology text was L. S. Goodman, and A. Gilman, eds., *The Pharmacological Basis of Therapeutics*, 2nd edition (New York: Macmillan, 1955). Carson could not know that the authors of this often iconoclastic text were skeptical about the efficacy and the putative biological rationale of a good number of contemporary drugs.

44. Crile to Carson, March 24, 1961, Rachel Carson Papers.

45. In keeping with her more activist role in disease, she wrote Dorothy that she was going to the library to read about iritis. "That would at least give me an idea of whether there are other approaches than the one used by Dr. Wilber." Carson to Freeman, January 7, 1962, *Letters*, 393.

46. Carson to Freeman, January 6, 1962, *Letters*, 390.

47. Crile to Ralph Caulk, March 9, 1962, Box 46, Crile Papers.

48. Carson to Freeman, March 26, 1962, *Letters*, 399. Details on Biskind are from L. Lear, *Rachel Carson: Witness for Nature*, 320.

49. Carson to Freeman, March 28, 1962, *Letters*, 399.

50. Carson to Freeman, April 1, 1962, *Letters*, 401.

51. Carson to Freeman, April 10, 1962, *Letters*, 404.

52. Carson to Freeman, May 20, 1962, *Letters*, 405.

53. Carson to Freeman, October 23, 1962, *Letters*, 414.

54. Carson to Freeman, January 1, 1963, *Letters*, 425.

55. Carson to Crile, February 17, 1963, Rachel Carson Papers.

56. Carson to Freeman, January 1, 1963, *Letters*, 426.

57. Carson to Crile, February 17, 1963, Rachel Carson Papers.

58. Carson to Freeman, February 14, 1963, *Letters*, 435. Carson wrote Crile after Jane's death about how Jane had "been a tower of strength in my medical problems" and compared Jane's role to the way Carson and her mother had once followed a car ahead of them through 50 miles of unfamiliar North Carolina woods. "Jane was that kind of reassuring light to me. Now, without that light to follow, I admit my courage is somewhat shaken." Carson to Crile, February 17, 1963, Rachel Carson Papers.

59. Carson to Freeman, February 18, 1963, *Letters*, 436–437.

60. The discussion is related in a letter from Ralph Caulk to Crile, March 6, 1963, Box 46, Crile Papers.

61. Carson to Crile, February 17, 1963, Rachel Carson Papers.

62. Carson to Freeman, March 2, 1963, *Letters*, 439.

63. Carson to Crile, April 3, 1963, Box 46, Crile Papers. Dr. Ivy was a chief promoter of Krebiozen and scientific consultant to the Krebiozen Research Foundation (see below for more information).

64. Carson to Freeman, March 19, 1963, *Letters*, 442–443.

65. Carson to Freeman, April 1, 1963, *Letters*, 451.

66. In Europe and Canada, the sedative thalidomide caused thousands of children in the late 1950s and early 1960s to be born with birth defects, mostly deformed limbs. In the United States, thalidomide was never approved by the FDA. However, in the early 1960s thalidomide samples were distributed to numerous clinical "investigators," a common practice for a drug awaiting FDA approval. Moreover, the almost nonexisting record keeping for these investigator uses, also in line with the then common practice, rendered recalling thalidomide almost impossible when its devastating effects became clear. In the wake of this disastrous situation, Congress passed the Kefauver–Harris amendments in October 1962. The new legislation mandated FDA certification for all drugs undergoing clinical testing before market approval. It required filing plans for clinical testing with information about the nature of the drug and its method of manufacture, conducting toxicity studies and animal tests prior to clinical tests, and demonstrating the scientific qualifications of physicians who served as clinical investigators. It also required informed consent by patients participating in these clinical trials. Following the Kefauver–Harris legislation, interstate shipment of all experimental drugs that were not certified by the FDA – among them Krebiozen – was supposed to become illegal by June 7, 1963. When the FDA consequently started investigating Krebiozen in March 1963, patients who took Krebiozen and their families feared it would become unavailable. They started a public campaign that culminated in thousands picketing in a "Death Watch" in front of the White House in early June. P. S. Ward, "'Who will bell the cat?' Andrew C. Ivy and Krebiozen," *Bulletin of the History of Medicine*, 58 (1984): 42–44. Drawing attention to their situation, these activists created significant publicity for Krebiozen at a time when Carson was desperate for alternative treatment options.

67. Carson to Freeman, March 19, 1963, *Letters*, 442.

68. L. Lear, *Rachel Carson: Witness for Nature*, 426.

69. Crile to Carson, April 5, 1963, Box 46, Crile Papers.

70. The terms "remission" and "complete remission" have often served a parallel role to Halsted's sometimes evasive promise that surgery would prevent local recurrences. Both sets of formulations have a limited liability in their medical use but patients often read into them a hope for cure.

71. Crile to Carson, April 5, 1963, Box 46, Crile Papers.

72. Carson was greatly relieved by Crile's attitude toward Krebiozen. "I was afraid he'd be upset about the Krebiozen," she wrote Freeman. "He isn't at all, though, he isn't convinced it is the ultimate answer. But he is quite willing to have me try it now. This relieved my mind greatly." Carson to Freeman, April 7, 1963, *Letters*, 452.

73. Ralph Caulk to Crile, April 11, 1963, Box 46, Crile Papers.

74. Carson to Freeman, March 26, 1963, *Letters*, 445.

75. Carson to Freeman, May 2, 1963, *Letters*, 457.

76. The AMA has had a long campaign against medical "quackery" in cancer and other diseases since the nineteenth century. In the early twentieth century, the AMA established a "Propaganda Department" against quackery and health fraud. The newly established ASCC joined in an increasingly activist campaign against cancer quackery (Chapter 6). At mid-century the FDA added its regulatory power to the campaign. For a general history, see J. H. Young, *American Health Quackery* (Princeton: Princeton University Press, 1992).

77. Quote from Rachel Carson, "Undersea," *Atlantic Monthly* (September 1937). Carson noted that this was "purely a biologist's philosophy" that was "not wholly satisfying." Carson to Freeman, March 27, 1963, *Letters*, 446.

78. Carson to Freeman, March 27, 1963, *Letters*, 446–447.

79. Carson to Freeman, March 27, 1963, *Letters*, 447.

80. Carson to Freeman, September 10, 1963, *Letters*, 468.

81. Carson to Freeman, October 3, 1963, *Letters*, 475.

82. Carson to Freeman, October 31, 1963, *Letters*, 486.

83. Carson to Freeman, November 17, 1963, *Letters*, 495.

84. Carson to Freeman, November 27, 1963, *Letters*, 498.

85. Carson to Freeman, January 4, 1964, *Letters*, 511.

86. Carson to Freeman, January 9, 1964, *Letters*, 515.

87. Details from L. Lear, *Rachel Carson: Witness for Nature*, 478–480.

88. While definitely in the minority, physicians such as Thomas Gisborne, Worthington Hooker, and later Richard C. Cabot advocated that doctors be truthful even to terminally ill patients. See T. L. Beauchamp and R. R. Faden, "History of Informed Consent," in S. G. Post, ed., *Encyclopedia of Bioethics*, Vol. 3 (New York: The Free Press, 2004), 1272, and J. C. Jackson, *Truth, Trust and Medicine* (London and New York: Routledge, 2001), 17–20.

89. A search of *New York Times* articles from 1940 to 1965 with the full-text search engine Proquest Historical Newspapers for the keywords *truth, cancer, diagnosis,* and *patient* revealed mixed public attitudes about disclosing terminal diseases to patients. In 1942, Dr. Ralph Loyd spoke at the graduation ceremony of the New York Medical College and reminded the young doctors not to disclose the "awful truth" to patients in order not to "drive them into the hands of crooks and charlatans." "Medical college gives 81 degrees," *New York Times*, June 6, 1942, 16. Similarly, Dr. Leo Bartemeier in his address to the American Academy of General Practice in 1955 urged physicians not to disclose the truth about cancer to patients in order not to "distress them unduly." G. Hill, "Evasion of truth by doctor upheld," *New York Times*, March 29, 1955, 24. In contrast, in 1951 the *New York Times* reported about the practice in New York Cancer Detection Clinics to tell patients their diagnosis and prognosis. Patients felt relieved after their appointment, either knowing they didn't have cancer or having "the peace that comes from knowing something for a certainty and in knowing that something could and would be done about it and at once." "Topics of the Times," *New York Times*, April 3, 1951, 26. The *New York Times* also published a brief notice about an article in *The Heart and*

Chest Bulletin in which orthopedic surgeon Dr. M. C. Wilkinson and the Catholic priest Rev. Alphonsus Donnar urged doctors to disclose cancer diagnoses to their patients in order to give them a chance to prepare for death. "Writers urge truth for cancer victims," *New York Times*, August 26, 1959, 31. Finally, the *New York Times* reported about the mixed opinions among physicians about disclosure of cancer diagnoses a the annual meeting of the American Cancer Society in 1961. Walter Sullivan, "Specialists tell of cancer policy," *New York Times*, October 24, 1961, 25.

90. Five studies in the United States found that between 80 and 89 percent of cancer patients wanted to know the truth about their diagnoses. In comparison, a survey in Britain came up with more divided results, with 40 percent of patients saying doctors should tell a patient about his/her cancer, and 34 percent saying doctors should not. In contrast, two studies found that 69 percent and 88 percent of physicians respectively never or usually didn't tell their cancer patients about their diagnoses. A study of nurses in this period suggested that they were more comfortable with truth telling in terminal diagnosis than physicians. R. M. Veatch, "Truth-telling," in W. T. Reich, ed., *Encyclopedia of Bioethics*, Vol. 4 (New York: The Free Press, 1978), 1677–1682.

91. S. Standard, "Truth, an instrument in therapy," in S. Standard and H. Nathan, eds., *Should the Patient Know the Truth? A Response of Physicians, Nurses, Clergymen, and Lawyers* (New York: Springer, 1955), 24–25.

92. Barney Glaser and Anselm Strauss conducted extensive ethnographic research on dying in American hospitals in the early-to mid-1960s. They reported on the results of their 6-year NIH-funded study in their book *Awareness of Dying* in 1966. They distinguished four types of awareness of dying: closed awareness, suspected awareness, mutual pretense awareness, and open awareness. In closed awareness, the patient did not recognize his or her impending death even though everyone around him or her does; in suspected awareness, the patients suspected he might be dying and that others know about his diagnosis, and sought to validate his suspicion; in mutual pretense awareness, all sides knew about the terminal disease but pretended all others did not; and in open awareness, all sides knew and acted relatively openly about the terminal disease. In some sense, Carson appeared to have haltingly evolved through these last three stages in her years as cancer patient. B. G. Glaser and A. L. Strauss, *Awareness of Dying* (Chicago: Aldine, 1966), 6–7.

93. More recent surveys have revealed a dramatic shift in physicians' attitudes toward truth telling in the 1970s. The replication of an earlier study from the 1960s actually found a complete reversal of results for the 1970s: while in the 1961 sample only 10 percent physicians reported that they generally told their patients fatal diagnoses truthfully, in 1979 an almost unbelievable 97 percent physicians reported they told the truth about diagnoses. K. H. Brown, "Attitudes towards truth-telling," in W. T. Reich, ed., *Encyclopedia of Bioethics*, Vol. 3 (New York: The Free Press, 1995), 1221–1225.

94. For more details, see K. H. Brown, "Attitudes towards truth-telling."

95. According to L. Lear, *Rachel Carson: Witness for Nature* (p. 454, note 81), Carson explicitly presented pesticides in her June 1963 senate testimony as a "new kind of fallout" because of its wide (and harmful) dispersal from its point of application.

96. To underscore the different world of environmental activism in Carson's day, Lear notes that the first major purchase Carson made with the proceeds from *Silent Spring* was a mink coat. L. Lear, *Rachel Carson: Witness for Nature*, 469.

97. Crile to J. F. Raycroft, December 21, 1955, Box 46, Crile Papers.

98. SUPPORT investigators, "Controlled trial to improve care for seriously ill hospitalized patients," *Journal of the American Medical Association*, 274 (1995): 1591–1598. In this very large clinical trial of an intensive intervention to improve pain control and decision making at the end of life, family members in both the study and control group had significant and roughly equal amounts of regret about the way their relatives had been treated.

99. A very different analysis of historical change in truth telling is in E. Leopold, *A Darker Ribbon. Breast Cancer, Women, and Their Doctors in the Twentieth Century* (Boston: Beacon Press, 1999). Leopold explicitly contrasted the Crile–Carson doctor–patient relationship with Halsted's relationship with a breast cancer patient 40 years earlier. Leopold emphasized that although Carson's treatment options had (depressingly) changed little from the time of Halsted, her autonomy, decision-making, and relationship with Crile were far different than the experience of Halsted's patients. Leopold depicted Carson as ahead of her own time in the way she took ownership of her disease. Leopold also contrasted Sanderson's and others' dishonesty with the straightforward way Crile answered Carson's questions and was honest about the cancer diagnosis. As suggested earlier, however, the contrast between Crile and Carson's other doctors as well as Halsted may be overly stark, as Crile was less than explicit in discussions about prognosis.

100. Carson to Freeman, May 20, 1962, *Letters*, 405. See also B. Ehrenreich, "Welcome to Cancerland: A mammogram leads to a cult of pink kitsch," *Harpers Magazine*, November, 2001, 43–53.

9. THE RISE OF SURVEILLANCE

1. In conventional medical usage, a symptom is a subjective patient perception and a sign is an objective finding observed by a doctor. The distinction is often blurred in practice as well as being historically contingent. See my "When do symptoms become a disease?" *Annals of Internal Medicine*, 134 (2001): 803–808.

2. C. Howard, "A state cancer clinic could save your life," *Woman's Home Companion*, June (1950): 73–74.

3. See Louis I. Dublin's remarks at December 1, 1949 meeting of ACS Board of Directors in "ACS 1949 – Research Committee" Folder, Box 95, Mary Lasker Papers, Butler Library, Columbia University (hereafter Lasker Papers).

4. See D. D. Bromley, "What do you do about cancer?" *Woman's Home Companion*, 75 (1948): 4–8.

5. M. Mara, "Women's Field Army credited with fighting great fear of cancer." *Brooklyn Eagle*, March 30, 1945. Found in Box 93, Folder called "Cancer – ACS 1945 Campaign Publicity," Lasker Papers.

6. Albert S. Morrow, M.D. "Report on cancer detection clinics." Box 93, Folder "ACS-NYC 1946," Lasker Papers.

7. C. C. Little, "Education," in *Cancer: A Study for Laymen, Prepared for the Women's Field Army of the American Society for the Control of Cancer, Inc.* (New York and Toronto: Farrar and Rinehart, 1944), 109.

8. E. L'Esperance, "Cancer prevention clinics," *Quarterly Review*, 9 (1944): 5.

9. C. C. Little to T. Parran, October 4, 1936, Box 8, Folder 70. Thomas Parran Papers, University of Pittsburgh Archives.

10. Albert S. Morrow, M. D. "Report on cancer detection clinics." Box 93, Folder "ACS-NYC 1946," Lasker Papers.

11. "What do the American people know about cancer?" Box 93, Folder "ACS 1947 Campaign," Lasker Papers. It is unclear how many subjects were in this sample of a cross section of America.

12. J. Patterson, *The Dread Disease* (Cambridge: Harvard University Press, 1987).

13. Louis Dublin, "Address to the ACS board of directors." December 1, 1949. Box 95, Folder called "ACS 1949-research committee," Lasker Papers.

14. John Kilpatrick to James S. Adams, December 19, 1949. Box 95, Folder called "ACS 1949-research committee," Lasker Papers.

15. For example, Memorial Hospital's cancer detection clinic reported cancer detection rates of only 1–1.5 percent. A similar Philadelphia clinic reported only a 0.5 percent detection rate. Albert S. Morrow, M. D. "Report on cancer detection clinics." Box 93, Folder "ACS-NYC 1946," Lasker Papers.

16. MacFarlane blamed the failure of this early effort at cervical cancer screening ultimately on the male dominance in the medical profession. "By and large the male physician is interested in the big, the new, the spectacular," she noted. "He does not care too much about the medicine of the future which will emphasize prevention more than cure." MacFarlane believed that women physicians were better able to see further ahead. "By and large they are more patient, more painstaking and more aware that, in the last analysis, the prevention of disease is more important than cure." "The inside history of the periodic pelvic examination research (typed ms)." Box 2, Folder 23, Catherine MacFarlane Papers, Medical College of Pennsylvania archives (hereafter MacFarlane Papers).

17. B. Bailey, "An ounce of prevention: Today's cure for cancer," *Reader's Digest*, 45 (1944): 102–105.

18. These concerns were aired publically and privately among cancer activists and elite academic physicians. Maurice Winternitz, prominent pathologist and controversial dean of the Yale Medical School between 1920 and 1935, wrote an essay ("Statement regarding research in neoplastic diseases," found in Box 95, Folder "ACS 1949, January–April," Lasker Papers) in which he blamed the failure of cancer detection clinics on too much patient demand and doctors' poor diagnostic skills, laissez faire attitudes toward cancer, and greater interest in infectious disease.

19. Interview with John Dunn, April 1, 1976; in L. Breslow, *A History of Cancer Control in the United States, 1946–1971*, prepared by the History of Cancer Control Project for the National Cancer Institute, 18.

20. See Cancer Control Letter, U.S. Department of Health, Education, and Welfare, Public Health Service, National Cancer Institute, June 1, 1953. Box 119, Folder NCI, Lasker Papers.

21. American Cancer Society, *Cancer: The Problem of Early Diagnosis, For Professional Audiences* (New York: American Cancer Society, 1949), 8 (pamphlet prepared to accompany 1949 film of the same name), found in "Publicity" folder, Box 95, Lasker Papers.

22. Interview with Charles Cameron, *A History of Cancer Control in the United States*, 12.

23. After describing the development of different blood tests for cancer, one author wrote, "All these various serum reactions are attempting to do for the diagnosis of cancer what the Wasserman reaction is doing for the diagnosis of syphilis." E. Podolsky, *The War on Cancer* (New York: Reinhold Publishing, 1943), 39.

24. L. Fleck, *Genesis and Development of a Scientific Fact*, T. J. Trenn and R. K. Merton, eds., translated by F. Bradley and T. J. Trenn (Chicago: University of Chicago Press, 1979).

25. L. S. Goodman, M. M. Wintrobe, W. Dameshek, M. J. Goodman, A. Gilman and M. T. McLennan, "Nitrogen mustard therapy. Use of methyl-bis (beta-chloroethyl) amine hydrochloride and tris (beta-chloroethyl) amine hydrochloride for Hodgkin's disease, lymphosarcoma, leukemia and certain allied and miscellaneous disorders," *Journal of the American Medical Association*, 251 (1984): 2255–2261 (originally published in 1946). As a medical student at Yale in 1982, I listened to Gilman's first hand account, which stressed the group's initial hubris that they had found the "magic bullet" for cancer after a patient's complete remission, only to watch the disease reappear a short time later. This cycle has unfortunately repeated itself many times in the history of cancer chemotherapy.

26. A. Freund and G. Kaminer, "Zur Diagnose des Karzinoms," *Wiener klinische Wochenschrift*, 24 (1759–1764): 1911. Cited by D. De Moulin, *A Short History of Breast Cancer* (Boston: Martinus Nijhoff, 1983), 93.

27. NCI memo, "Cancer Diagnostic Tests," by Raymond F. Kaiser, June 16, 1955. Box 119, Folder "National Cancer Institute," Lasker Papers. Kaiser explained that the program would evaluate the many claims made about cancer blood tests using explicit criteria for efficacy. A workable cancer diagnostic test would produce positive results in 90 percent of true cases and less than 5 percent in noncancerous individuals. In addition the tests had to be simple and inexpensive.

28. "Screening program set up for cancer-finding tests," *Science News Letter*, September 25 (1948): 207.

29. "Early cancer diagnosis with electrical test 85% accurate," *Science News Letter*, May 2 (1942): 277. This test for stomach cancer measured electrical potential differences across the stomach membrane.

30. "Test blood for cancer," *Science News Letter*, January 1 (1949): 3. Article cites research using ant-trypsin antibodies, a clotting factor, to detect cancer.

31. "Atomic diagnosis of breast cancer is hope," *Science News Letter*, November 2 (1946): 281. This is a popular report based on an article in *Science* in which radioactive phosphorous was injected into the body and a Geiger counter was placed on breast. This test was not promoted as much as for early detection as for distinguishing preoperatively malignant from benign processes.

32. "Blood tests for cancer," *Science News Letter*, September 13 (1947): 163, and "Dye glows under rays to detect cancer tissue," *Science News Letter*, August 16 (1947): 101.

33. "Electrical cancer test," *Newsweek*, 19 (1942): 63.

34. W. L. Laurence, "New test for early cancer," *Reader's Digest*, 51 (1947): 41–42. Investigators were examing whether injections of blood from cancer patients into rats caused splenomegaly.

35. Memorandum (American Cancer Society, October 1954, Box 119, NCI 1954 folder, Lasker Papers) described "supervoltage x-ray for cancer diagnosis," which were to be used to diagnose lung cancer.

36. Sir Reginald Murley, "Earliest detection and management of cancer, Royal Society of Medicine," ms dated October 11, 1989, in Box 4, Folder "History of cancer breast, Crile and Murley," Crile Papers, Cleveland Clinic archives.

37. W. L. Laurence, "New test for early cancer," 42.

38. NCI memo, "Cancer Diagnostic Tests," by Raymond F. Kaiser, June 16, 1955. Box 119, Folder "National Cancer Institute," Lasker Papers.

39. *A History of Cancer Control in the United States*, 746.

40. Interview with Leopold Koss, *A History of Cancer Control in the United States*, 8. Koss related how the ACS was a society without a cause – unlike March of Dimes and the development of polio vaccines – and seized on the vaginal smear.

41. As with MacFarlane, there were many concerted efforts to aggressively diagnose or push screening for cervical cancer without the Pap technology. In Nazi Germany, for example, German activists promoted frequent pelvic examinations and colposcopy (a technique invented by Germans) as screening modalities for uterine and cervical cancer screening. R. N. Proctor, *The Nazi War on Cancer* (Princeton, Princeton University Press, 1999), 27, 32, 43. See also MacFarlane's January 30, 1946 speech to the Wayne County Medical Society, (Box 2, unlabeled binder, MacFarlane Papers), in which she stressed earlier German efforts, especially the work of East Prussian physician George Winter. MacFarlane noted, "Just before world war II, this campaign culminated in the passage of a law making it compulsory for every women in East Prussia to have a pelvic examination once a year."

42. M. J. Casper, and A. E. Clarke, "Making the Pap smear into the 'right tool' for the job: Cervical cancer screening in the USA, circa 1940–1995," *Social Studies of Science*, 28 (1998): 255–290.

43. W. Ross, *Crusade: The Official History of the American Cancer Society* (New York: Arbor House, 1987), 87. Ross is quoting the Holleb's recollections in an interview on September 13, 1984.

44. *A History of Cancer Control in the United States*, 601.

45. W. Ross, *Crusade: The Official History of the American Cancer Society*, 86. Ross is quoting the Holleb's recollections in a September 13, 1984 interview.

46. Interview with Charles Cameron, *A History of Cancer Control in the United States*, 5. Cameron recalled that Papanicolaou was trying in "his later years at Cornell," to get cytological material from the breast, "because after all our results were not very good even with radical treatments."

47. An analogous screening campaign in breast cancer would inherit the Pap smears problems as well. Early on, cancer officials observed that the introduction of the Pap smear had led to overdiagnosis of cervical cancer. In 1955, NCI official Ray Kaiser reported on the NCI funded field demonstration of Pap smears in Memphis, Tennessee, and noted that the rates of diagnosis of in situ cervical cancer were forty times higher than those found in morbidity studies of clinically diagnosed cervical cancer. Minutes of the National Advisory Cancer Committee, February 14–16, 1955, Box 119, Folder entitled "NCI," Lasker Papers.

48. The decline in cervical mortality in the United States started at least by the 1950s, before the mass uptake of PAP smears in the 1960s. See http://www.cdc.gov/mmwr/preview/mmwrhtml/rr4902a4.htm, accessed May 2006. For ethical and practical reasons, there has not been a clinical experiment studying the effect of the Pap versus no screening on cervical cancer mortality. To be sure, current expert opinion such as the U.S. Preventive Task force gives Pap screening its "A" (highest) level recommendation based largely on historical trends. See http://www.ncbi.nlm.nih.gov/books/bv.fcgi?rid-hstat3.section.4193, accessed on May 10, 2006.

49. Brief citations in M. J. Casper, and A. E. Clarke, "Making the Pap smear into the 'right tool' for the job" and W. Ross, *Crusade: The Official History of the American Cancer Society*, 90.

50. Ibid., 96. Ross claimed that three million women between 1947 and 1953 saw a movie about self-breast examination. 647 prints of the film were sold.

51. For example, Theodoric's *Cyrugia* (surgical treatise from 1267) reportedly includes an illustration of a women being taught to examine her breasts for an abscess. M. Yalom, *A History of the Breast* (New York, Ballantine Books, 1997), 211. Original citation is A. S. Lyons and R. J. Petrucelli, *Medicine: An Illustrated History* (New York: Harry N. Abrams, 1997), figures 490 and 498, 326–327.

52. "Progress in cancer control (typed ms)" Harrisburg, April 15, 1955. Box 2, binder labeled medical papers, MacFarlane Papers. MacFarlane produced breast self-examination leaflets with sensual illustrations and photos. The apparent message was that examining your breast was not dirty. Box 5, Folder 52, MacFarlane Papers.

53. SBE also responded to longstanding ideas about female modesty, including that breast examinations were women's business. This was also reflected in long held assumptions that female doctors should bear the responsibility for screening women for cancers. In one 1928 article, the male author speculates that a town of 100,000 inhabitants needs one "full time medical woman" to carry out breast examinations. A. Cooke, "Remarks on breast cancer," in *Report of the International Conference on*

Cancer, London, July 17–20, 1928, held under the auspices of the British Empire Cancer Campaign (London: John Wright & Sons, 1928), 572.

54. Interview with John Dunn, *A History of Cancer Control in the United States*, 19.

55. P. Strax, "Screening for breast cancer, *Clinical Obstetrics and Gynecology*, 20 (1977): 781–801, 797.

56. C. D. Haagensen, C. Bodian, and D. E. Haagensen, Jr., *Breast Carcinoma: Risk and Detection* (Philadelphia: Saunders, 1981), 386.

57. For a standard version of the history of mammography, see R. Egan, "Mammography and breast diseases," in L. Robbins, ed., *Golden's Diagnostic Roentgenology* (Baltimore: Williams and Wilkins, 1972), 19.1–19.9. Egan wrote that x-rays of the breast were "not a new procedure; some 75 articles on the subject had appeared in the literature, and the authors of the articles indicated varying degrees of accuracy with the procedure but usually stated doubt as to its value. Personal communication with a number of these earlier workers indicated that technical difficulties in obtaining satisfactory roentgenograms led to its abandonment in most instances."

58. Feig has a poorly reproduced image that purports to be the first radiograph of a breast, done on a surgical specimen by Dr. Albert Salomon in 1910 (p. 194, reference 9). S. A. Feig, "Mammographic screening: An historical perspective," *Seminars in Roentgenology*, 28 (1993): 193–203.

59. See, for example, R. B. Greenough, "Early diagnosis of cancer of the breast," *Annals of Surgery*, 102 (1935): 233–238.

60. W. Fray and S. L. Warren, "Stereoscopic roentgenography of the breasts: An aid in establishing the diagnosis of mastitis and carcinoma," *Annals of Surgery*, 95 (1932): 425–432. See also S. L. Warren, "A roentgenologic study of the breast," *American Journal of Roentgenology and Radium Therapy*, 24 (1930): 113–124.

61. W. R. Hendee, "History and status of x-ray mammography," *Health Physics*, 69 (1995): 636–648. The author offered (p. 636) the standard explanation for why Warren's 1930 report of success with diagnostic breast x-rays did not lead to changing practice: "After trying mammography with a few patients, most physicians became discouraged because the images were poor in quality and varied widely for reasons that were only partially understood."

62. R. Egan, "Mammography and breast diseases," 19.6.

63. W. Ross, *Crusade: The Official History of the American Cancer Society*, 98. See also "The role of mammography in the detection of breast cancer," *A History of Cancer Control in the United States*, 273–318. Warren was interviewed for this chapter and reported that his peers reacted with skepticism and apathy to his initial mammography reports. Warren called radiologic practice a "lonely business." NCI official Michael Shimkin, in this same chapter, stressed the status of surgeons and surgery, pointing out that palpation was a *surgical* technique and was therefore favored over something done by radiologists in a dark room.

64. Observation made in H. Ingleby and J. Gershon-Cohen *Comparative Anatomy, Pathology and Roentgenology of the Breast* (Philadelphia, University of Pennsylvania Press, 1960). According to the authors, Ries in 1931 showed it was unsafe to inject breast ducts. The authors also reported that injecting air into breast ducts

did not work and using contrast material appeared to raise the risk of tumors (see p. xv).

65. R. Leborgne, "Intraductal biopsy of certain pathologic processes of the breast," *Surgery*, 19 (1945): 47–54, 53.

66. One obituary (M. B. Hermel, "In memoriam: Jacob Gershon-Cohen, M. D., D. Sc. (Med.), 1899–1971," *American Journal of Roentgenology*, 112 (1971): 455.) noted the following as research areas for Gershon-Cohen: video diagnosis, the effect of tea on tooth cavities, the etiology of Cooley's anemia, and the viral etiology of cancer.

67. J. Gershon-Cohen, "Detection of unsuspected breast cancer by mammography," *Surgery Gynecology and Obstetrics*, 121 (1965): 97–101.

68. Note from Gershon-Cohen to Isador Ravdin (written on ibid.,), November 10, 1961. Box 16, ff 28, I. S. Ravdin Papers, University of Pennsylvania archives.

69. See J. Gershon-Cohen, "Imperative changes in detection methods for breast cancer," *Southern Medical Journal*, 64 (1971): 387–391.

70. See J. Gershon-Cohen, "Detection of unsuspected breast cancer by mammography," 97–101 ("brief respite" quote on p. 98) and H. Ingleby and J. Gershon-Cohen, *Comparative Anatomy, Pathology and Roentgenology of the Breast*.

71. "If a universal cancer test were to be announced tomorrow, the necessity of finding the lesion would only aggravate the present problem of early cancer detection (p. 478)." J. Gershon-Cohen, H. Ingleby, et al., "Analysis of 2,514 examinations during early phases of an x-ray survey of breast," *Surgery, Gynecology, Obstetrics*, 106 (1958): 478–480. This is a report of a screening study of over 2,000 women funded by NIH.

72. Ibid., 479. In this same report, Gershon-Cohen et al. showed deference to family physicians who referred patients to the study and reassured them that participation would not result in losing clinical control of their patients.

73. J. Gershon-Cohen, M. B. Hermel, et al., "Detection of breast cancer by periodic x-ray examinations: A five-year survey," *Journal of the American Medical Association*, 176 (1961): 1114–1116.

74. J. Gershon-Cohen, H. Ingleby, et al., "Analysis of 2,514 examinations during early phases of an x-ray survey of breast," 479.

75. Ibid.

76. Detecting precancers by x-ray was generally greeted with skepticism, although with technological changes and the diffusion of screening mammography x-rays would eventually lead to an exponential rise in in-situ diagnoses (see Chapter 11). "There are some enthusiastic radiologists who claim that carcinoma in situ can be recognized by mammography," one radiologist noted in 1964. "In my opinion this is the 'triumph of hope over experience' and I have not found x-ray examination of the breast especially rewarding in the diagnosis of this particular disease." E. F. Lewison, "Lobular carcinoma *in situ* of the breast: the feminine mystique," *Military Medicine*, 129 (1964): 115–123, 118.

77. Interview with Lewis Robbins, *A History of Cancer Control in the United States*, 15.

78. P. Strax, ed., *Control of Breast Cancer Through Mass Screening* (Littleton, MA: PSG Publishing, 1979), 170.

79. I. S. Ravdin to Gershon-Cohen, November 22, 1957, Box 16, ff 28, University of Pennsylvania archives, I. S. Ravdin Papers. Highlighting Gershon-Cohen's marginality and idiosyncratic situation, 65 percent of his subjects were Jewish. J. Gershon-Cohen, H. Ingleby, et al., "Mammographic screening for breast cancer: Results of a ten-year survey," *Radiology*, 88 (1967): 663–667.

80. I. S. Ravdin to Gershon-Cohen, October 19, 1955. Box 16, ff 28, I. S. Ravdin Papers, University of Pennsylvania archives.

81. Interview with Lewis Robbins, *A History of Cancer Control in the United States*, 15.

82. Gershon-Cohen reportedly started experimenting with thermography as "soon as infrared-sensing devices were declassified by the military." He was the first president of national thermography society. M. B. Hermel, "In memoriam: Jacob Gershon-Cohen, M. D."

83. J. Gershon-Cohen, "Imperative changes in detection methods for breast cancer," figure 4. Technological innovation in breast imaging took off in the 1960s and has continued since, although the mammogram has yet to be dislodged in clinical practice. ACS activist W. L. Ross predicted in 1968 that on the horizon for breast cancer screening were liquid crystals painted on breasts to detect heat from cancers, ultrasound, and the laser beam. W. L. Ross, "A look into the past and into the future in cancer of the breast," *Cancer*, 23 (1969): 762–766.

84. R. Egan, "Mammography and breast diseases." Egan's technological innovations also increased the radiation exposure to the breast. This was noted at the time but did not attract much attention because it was not yet generally appreciated that perfectly normal women undergoing screening were being exposed (and thus there was an argument for a much lower threshold of acceptable risk) and the thrust of technological innovation at the time was on increasing the sensitivity of the test, not reducing risk. Another problem with Egan's innovations was that women's breasts needed to be compressed. In W. R. Hendee, "History and status of x-ray mammography."

85. Interview with Lewis Robbins, *A History of Cancer Control in the United States*, 17.

86. W. L. Ross, "A look into the past and into the future in cancer of the breast." Ross recalled (p. 764) that "from 1961 to the present a total of 1,200 radiologists and 700 x-ray technologists have been trained in mammography. During 1967 alone, 250 radiologists and 160 technicians were trained in 9 centers supported by the Cancer Control Program at a cost of over $600,000."

87. R. Egan, "Experience with mammography in a tumor institution. Evaluation of 1,000 studies," *Radiology*, 75 (1960): 894–900. Details on the reception of mammography in R. Egan, "History of Mammography," in *Mammography and Breast Diseases* (Baltimore: Williams & Wilkins, 1970), 1936–1939.

88. Egan wrote that he changed the name from *roentgenography of the breast* to *mammography* "with full knowledge that the latter was a misnomer, but this allowed some degree of disassociation with the former term." R. Egan, "Mammography and breast diseases," in L. Robbins, ed., *Golden's Diagnostic Roentgenology*, 190–199, 196.

89. L. W. Bassett and R. H. Gold, "The evolution of mammography [Progress in Radiology]," *American Journal of Radiology*, 150 (1988): 493–498.

90. R. L. Egan, "Mammography, an aid to diagnosis of breast carcinoma," *Journal of the American Medical Association*, 182 (1962): 101–105.

91. R. L. Clark, and L. C. Robbins, "Editorial: Mammography (Egan) in cancer of the breast," *American Journal of Surgery*, 109 (1965): 125–126. "Most radiologists familiar with the use of mammography in apparently well women see no opportunity to use this procedure as it stands today for the routine screening of the general population (p. 126)."

92. R. L. Clark, M. M. Copeland, et al., "Reproducibility of the technique of mammography (Egan) for cancer of the breast," *American Journal of Surgery*, 109 (1965): 127–133, 132–133.

93. R. Egan, "Mammography and breast diseases," 197.

94. Minutes of a breast cancer conference in 1961 (A. M. Popma, "Cancer of the breast," in *Proceedings of the Fourth National Cancer Conference, Minneapolis, Minnesota, September 13, 14, and 15, 1960* (Philadelphia and Montreal: J. B. Lippincott, 1961), 737–739, 739.

95. G. M. Stevens, and J. F. Weigen "Mammography survey for breast cancer detection: A 2-year study of 1,223 clinically negative asymptomatic women over 40," *Cancer*, 19 (1966): 51–59, 51.

96. H. Marks, *The Progress of Experiment: Science and Therapeutic Reform in the United States, 1900–1990* (Cambridge: Cambridge University Press, 1997). The attention to clinical trials was itself preceded by institutional innovations in regulating research and marketing.

97. S. Shapiro, P. Strax, et al., "Periodic breast cancer screening," in *Presymptomatic Detection and Early Diagnosis*, C. L. E. H. Sharp and H. Keen, eds. (London: Pitman Medical Publishing, 1968), 203–236.

98. L. E. Weeks, ed., *Sam Shapiro in First Person : An Oral History* (Ann Arbor: American Hospital Association, 1988), 42.

99. S. Shapiro, P. Strax, et al., "Periodic breast cancer screening," 203–236.

100. S. Shapiro, P. Strax, and L. Venet, "Periodic breast cancer screening in reducing mortality from breast cancer," *Journal of the American Medical Association*, 215 (1971): 1777–1785.

101. According to some estimates, Shapiro and colleagues ended up so excluding about 853 women in the study group and 336 from the control group. See http://www.bringoutyourbest.com/index.cfm?fuseaction-new.view&id-263, accessed in November, 2005 and G. Kolata and M. Moss, "X ray vision in hindsight," *New York Times*, February 11, 2002, A18.

102. S. Shapiro, P. Strax, and L. Venet, "Periodic breast cancer screening in reducing mortality from breast cancer."

103. A review panel analyzing results in 1977 estimated that mammography made an independent contribution to one third of the morality benefit. L. Breslow, L. B. Thomas, et al., "Final reports of National Cancer Institute ad hoc working groups on mammography screening for breast cancer and a summary report of their joint

findings and recommendations," *Journal of the National Cancer Institute*, 59 (1977): 467–537.

104. P. Strax, ed., *Control of Breast Cancer Through Mass Screening* (Littleton, MA: PSG Publishing, 1979), 200.

10. CRISIS IN PREVENTION

1. (1): "The mammography muddle [Editorial]," *New York Times*, May 12, 1977; (2): P. Strax, ed., *Control of Breast Cancer Through Mass Screening* (Littleton, MA: PSG Publishing, 1979), 207; (3) Morton Goodman, p. 161, (4) Rose Kushner, p. 183, and (5) Sam Thier, p. 278, *Consensus Development Meeting on Breast Cancer Screening, September 14–16, 1977*, U.S. Department of Health, Education, and Welfare, 1977 (hereafter, *Consensus Development Meeting on Breast Cancer Screening*).

2. W. Ross, *Crusade: The Official History of the American Cancer Society* (New York: Arbor House, 1987), 99.

3. R.A. Rettig, *Cancer Crusade: The Story of the National Cancer Act of 1971* (Princeton: Princeton University Press, 1977). Section 409 of the act established a cancer control program under the NCI with a separate appropriation. See also Institute of Medicine background paper, M. McGeary "The National Cancer Program: Enduring Issues." http://www.iom.edu/?id-13984, accessed on May 15, 2006.

4. S. Shapiro, P. Strax, and L. Venet, "Periodic breast cancer screening in reducing mortality from breast cancer," *Journal of the American Medical Association*, 215 (1971): 1777–1785.

5. From Minutes of BCDDP Special Meeting for Discussion of Project Protocol, January 9, 1974. Given to John C. Bailar III in response Freedom of Information Act search request (hereafter Bailar files).

6. "Report of the Working Group to Review the National Cancer Institute-American Cancer Society Breast Cancer Detection Demonstration Projects," *Journal of the National Cancer Institute*, 62 (1979): 639–709. (Hereafter, "Report of Working Group to Review BCDDP.")

7. D. Armstrong, "The medical aspects of the Framingham Community Health and Tuberculosis Demonstration," *International Journal of Epidemiology*, 34 (2005): 1183–1187 (reprint of 1917 report).

8. For a critical analysis of such assumptions, see R. A. Aronowitz, "Situating health risks," in R. Stevens, C. Rosenberg, and L. R. Burns, eds., *History and Health Policy in the United States: Putting the Past Back In* (New Brunswick, NJ: Rutgers University Press, 2006), 153–175.

9. The 29 centers were at 27 locations as 2 locations sponsored 2 separate mammography programs. It took one and half years to award all the contracts. "Report of Working Group to Review BCDDP."

10. Minutes of the meeting of the BCDDP's Protocol Committee, University of Oklahoma Medical School, November 14, 1974, Bailar files.

11. J. A. H. Lee to Bailar, June 30, 1973, Bailar files.

12. Sidney Cutler to Nathaniel Berlin, August 7, 1973, Bailar files.

13. From "Comments on the National Breast Cancer Demonstration project" made after three site visits to possible participating institutes by Marvin Zelen, March 1973, Bailar files.

14. Malcolm C. Pike to William Pomerance, December 16, 1974, Bailar files.

15. J. C. Bailar, "Mammographic screening: A reappraisal of benefits and risks," *Clinical Obstetrics and Gynecology*, 21 (1978): 1–14.

16. Arthur Holleb to Nathaniel Berlin, October 3, 1973, Bailar files. For his part, Holleb was apparently ignorant of the basic methodological and interpretive issues raised by a screening trial. According to the minutes of one of the early discussions of the progress of BCDDP, "Dr. Holleb asked about definition of 'prolonged survival,' 'postponement of death,' 'preclinical duration of disease,' 'slow growing and fast growing disease,' etc. He indicated that he did not understand the meaning of these terms." From Minutes of BCDDP Special Meeting for Discussion of Project Protocol, January 9, 1974. Bailar files.

17. Arthur Holleb to Nathaniel Berlin, October 3, 1973, Bailar files.

18. L. H. Baker, "Breast cancer detection demonstration project: Five-year summary report," *CA: A Cancer Journal for Clinicians*, 32 (1982): 194–225.

19. The case detection rate was very high on initial examination in BCDDP, reported as 5.54 cases per 1,000 women screened. The HIP rate was only 2.73/1000. "Report of Working Group to Review BCDDP."

20. Meeting agenda, BCDDP meeting of Project Directors, January 8, 1974. Bailar files.

21. John Bailar to Kenneth Olson, March 21, 1973. From Attachment titled "Questions for study: Breast cancer detection demonstration units." Bailar files.

22. BEIR Committee (The Advisory Committee on the Biological Effects of Ionizing Radiation). BEIR-I: *The Effects on Populations of Exposure to Low Levels of Ionizing Radiation*, Division of Medical Sciences, the National Academy of Sciences, National Research Council, Washington, DC, 1972. Extrapolating from the Japanese tragedy was difficult, however, because the baseline rate of breast cancer was much lower in Japan than in the United States.

23. See, for example, B. J. Ostrum, W. Becker, et al., "Low-dose mammography," *Radiology*, 109 (1973): 323–326. The politics of the fear of medical x-rays has a long and sometimes ironic history. For example, German socialist physicians in the 1930s caricatured Nazi fears of health damage from medical x-rays as "racial scaremongering." R. N. Proctor, *The Nazi War on Cancer* (Princeton: Princeton University Press, 1999), 87.

24. L. Breslow, L. B. Thomas, et al., "Final reports of National Cancer Institute ad hoc working groups on mammography screening for breast cancer and a summary report of their joint findings and recommendations," *Journal of the National Cancer Institute*, 59 (1977): 467–537.

25. BCDDP radiologists were able to reduce average radiation exposure from mammography from 3.1R surface rads to 1.2R by the third year of the project. "Report of Working Group to Review BCDDP."

26. Interview with John Bailar, April 19, 1999.

27. J. C. Bailar, "Mammography: A contrary view," *Annals of Internal Medicine*, 84 (1976): 77–84.

28. A. Geffen, "Risks versus benefits of mammography," in L. Venet, ed., *Breast Cancer: A Practical Guide to Diagnosis and Treatment* (New York and London: SP Medical and Scientific Books), 33–42.

29. S. A. Feig, "Hypothetical breast cancer risk from mammography," *Recent Results in Cancer Research*, 90 (1984): 1–10, 8.

30. P. Strax, ed., *Control of Breast Cancer Through Mass Screening*, 226.

31. Breslow, L. B. Thomas, and A. C. Upton, "Final reports of National Cancer Institute ad hoc working groups on mammography." See also [Proposed] Benefits and Risk Statement Consent Form (n.d.), found in Bailar files. Patients were informed of the potential radiation risk and were told that physicians believed that the benefits outweigh the risk. But no attempt was made to give patients any estimate of benefit and risk, so it was not clear how such statements helped patients make their own informed decision about mammography.

32. A. I. Holleb, "Restoring confidence in mammography [Editorial]," *CA: A Cancer Journal for Clinicians*, 26 (1976): 376–378.

33. J. C. Bailar, *Consensus Development Meeting on Breast Cancer Screening*, 49.

34. ACS, "Mammography 1982: A statement of the American Cancer Society," *CA: A Cancer Journal for Clinicians*, 32 (1982): 226–231, 227.

35. J. C. Bailar, "Mammographic screening: A reappraisal of benefits and risks," 5.

36. Ibid., 13.

37. "Report of Working Group to Review BCDDP."

38. Donald Friedrickson. *Consensus Development Meeting on Breast Cancer Screening*, vi.

39. Sidney Wolfe. *Consensus Development Meeting on Breast Cancer Screening*, 188.

40. *Consensus Development Meeting on Breast Cancer Screening*, 232–233. Bross argued that there had been a cover-up about the radiation risks posed by mammography.

41. Phillip Strax. *Consensus Development Meeting on Breast Cancer Screening*, 226.

42. John Bailar. *Consensus Development Meeting on Breast Cancer Screening*, 51.

43. John Bailar. *Consensus Development Meeting on Breast Cancer Screening*, 146.

44. Brian MacMahon. *Consensus Development Meeting on Breast Cancer Screening*, 244.

45. Cochrane said of the need of additional RCTs of mammography: "Is it really ethical not to do these trials, when the results are so important to the future particularly of women?" *Consensus Development Meeting on Breast Cancer Screening*, 388.

46. John Bailar. *Consensus Development Meeting on Breast Cancer Screening*, 52.

47. Phillip Strax. *Consensus Development Meeting on Breast Cancer Screening*, 155.

48. Dr. C. Smart. *Consensus Development Meeting on Breast Cancer Screening*, 130–131.

49. Rose Kushner. *Consensus Development Meeting on Breast Cancer Screening*, 184.

50. John Bailar. *Consensus Development Meeting on Breast Cancer Screening*, 58.

51. D. S. Greenberg, "Perils in a cancer screening project," *Washington Post*, October 10, 1978.

52. A. I. Holleb, "Those '66' cases of 'misdiagnosed' breast cancer [Editorial]," *CA: A Cancer Journal for Clinicians*, 29 (1979): 63–64.

53. Dr. Milton Elkin argued, "I wouldn't call it a risk if you detect lesions early and somebody beyond that detection gums it up." To which Dr. Virgil Loeb retorted, "But you can't dismiss the implications – if we are going to agree that screening is important, we can't just stop with the screen. We have to be responsible for what occurs as a result of the screening." *Consensus Development Meeting on Breast Cancer Screening*, 288.

54. MacMahon agreed to sign onto the consensus about screening only if this phrase was added. *Consensus Development Meeting on Breast Cancer Screening*, 261.

55. James Deluca. *Consensus Development Meeting on Breast Cancer Screening*, 268.

56. Sam Thier. *Consensus Development Meeting on Breast Cancer Screening*, 259, 249, 278.

57. "Report of Working Group to Review BCDDP," 653.

58. Ibid., 648.

59. Ibid., 701, 704.

60. Robert Egan. *Consensus Development Meeting on Breast Cancer Screening*, 156.

61. Most recently and prominently, O. Olsen and P. Gotzsche, "Cochrane review on screening for breast cancer with mammography," *The Lancet*, 358 (2001): 1340–1342.

11. BREAST CANCER RISK: "WAITING FOR THE AXE TO FALL"

1. M. Hacker, "Journal Entries," in H. Raz, ed., *Living On the Margins* (New York: Persea Books, 1999), 235.

2. Attributed to Fran Visco, C. Read, *Preventing Breast Cancer – The Politics of an Epidemic* (London: Pandora, 1995), 21.

3. Breast Cancer Facts and Figures 2004, American Cancer Society. From http://www.cancer.org/downloads/STT/CAFF2003PWSecured.pdf, http://www.cancer.org/downloads/STT/CAFF_finalPWSecured.pdf, accessed in December 2005.

4. See Chapter 1, note 1.

5. E. Marshall, "Search for a killer: Focus shifts from fat to hormones," *Science*, 259 (1993): 618–621, 618. This "inexorable rise in risk" is frequently referred to as an "epidemic," despite its chronic and noninfectious nature. Some observers have questioned this usage on the grounds that the increased incidence is most likely an unfortunate and unintended consequence of women's improved social and health status, such as greater reproductive choice and better nutrition. See D. Plotkin, "Good news and bad news about breast cancer," *The Atlantic Monthly*, June (1996): 53–76.

6. L. A. G. Ries, M. P. Eisner, C. L. Kosary, B. F. Hankey, B. A. Miller, L. Clegg, A. Mariotto, E. J. Feuer, and B. K. Edwards, eds., *SEER Cancer Statistics Review, 1975–2002* (Bethesda, MD: National Cancer Institute), http://seer.cancer.gov/csr/1975_2002/, based on November 2004 SEER data submission, posted to the SEER web site 2005, Tables 1V-5 and 1V-6. SEER stands for the Surveillance, Epidemiology and End Results program of the NCI, which uses state-of-the-art sampling and survey methodology to arrive at their estimates of incidence and

mortality. SEER incidence statistics are necessarily best estimates of *diagnosed* cases, and as such reflect the normal patterns of detection and diagnosis in American communities.

7. For a cautious analysis of SEER and other data showing a probable causal association between increased screening and increased incidence of in situ and localized disease, see B. A. Miller, E. J. Feuer, et al., "The increasing incidence of breast cancer since 1982: Relevance of early detection," *Cancer Causes Control*, 2 (1991): 67–74.

8. For example, it is possible that the incidence of "destined to harm" cancer has been increasing so rapidly that it has "hid" the expected impact (decreased incidence) from treatment of noninvasive cancers. In order for this to have happened, the "natural" increase in invasive breast cancer (what would have been recorded if non-invasive cancers had not been diagnosed and treated, assuming for sake of simplicity, that each case of treated noninvasive cancer resulted in the prevention of one case of invasive cancer) would have had to be double the observed increase, i.e., there would have been a two-thirds rather than a one-third increase of invasive cancers between 1975 and 2002. One candidate among known risk factors to have driven such a large increase in incidence is the greater use of hormone replacement therapy during this period. While I do not want to reject this possibility out of hand and I could be proven wrong, I do not think there has been enough demographic and lifestyle change to cause such a massive increase in destined-to-harm disease.

9. S. Zackrisson, I. Andersson, L. Janzon, J. Manjer, and J. P. Garne, "Rate of overdiagnosis of breast cancer 15 years after end of Malmö mammographic screening trial: follow-up study," *British Medical Journal*, 332 (2006): 689–92.

10. 18 percent (Gilbert Welch) and 30 percent (Peter C. Gotzsche). See http://bmj.bmjjoburnals.com/cgi/eletters/bmj.38764.572569.7Cv1, accessed on April 5, 2006.

11. See G. Welch, *Should I Be Tested for Cancer?* (Berkeley: University of California Press, 2004), 87.

12. In my experience over the past 20 years, most clinicians have generally distinguished between LCIS and DCIS in this manner. However, there has also been disagreement, controversy, and difficult-to-interpret data. For recent data suggesting much less difference between LCIS and DCIS, see C. I. Li, K. E. Malone, B. S. Saltzman, and J. R. Daling, "Risk of invasive breast carcinoma among women diagnosed with ductal carcinoma in situ and lobular carcinoma in situ, 1988–2001," *Cancer*, 106 (2006): 2104–2112. In this analysis of SEER data, LCIS was associated with *higher* incidence of invasive cancer than DCIS, both in the same and opposite breast. As a result, the authors suggest that "LCIS may be a precursor rather than just an ambiguous risk factor for invasive breast cancer."

13. V. L. Ernster, J. Barclay, et al., "Incidence of and treatment for ductal carcinoma in situ of the breast," *Journal of the American Medical Association*, 275 (1996): 913–918.

14. O. Olsen and P. Gotzsche, "Cochrane review on screening for breast cancer with mammography," *The Lancet*, 358 (2001): 1340–1342.

15. See D. A. Berry, K. A. Cronin, S. K. Plevritis, D. G. Fryback, L. Clarke, M. Zelen, J. S. Mandelblatt, A. Y. Yakovlev, J. D. F. Habbema, and E. J. Feuer, "Effect of screening and adjuvant therapy on mortality from breast cancer," *New England Journal of Medicine*, 353 (2005): 1784–1792. It is important to keep in mind that these groups started with the assumption that clinical trials had shown mammography to be effective in reducing mortality from breast cancer – an assumption contested by observers, such as Olsen and Goetze above. Some news reports of this "thought experiment" touted it as additional proof of screening mammography's efficacy, a circular conclusion since this was one of the shared assumptions of the study.

16. R. A. Rettig, *Cancer Crusade: The Story of the National Cancer Act of 1971* (Princeton: Princeton University Press, 1977), 286.

17. I am skeptical that we will ever find an important local-environmental determinant of breast cancer that explains either the rising incidence (much of which may itself be due to increased diagnosis and lowered diagnostic thresholds) or geographic variation (which may be explained by the composition of the population more than the physical environment). One reason is that the incidence among males, who might be expected to have rising incidence rates of breast cancer if there were increased exposures to causal environmental toxins, has been stable. Some efforts to link the physical environment to breast cancer via synthetic estrogen exposure, however, are intriguing and plausible, but there has not yet been much convincing (to me) aggregate data to support the linkage. In terms of action, I am generally sympathetic with efforts to promote a burden of proof on those who introduce untested chemicals into the environment and share Richard Peto's view that "environmentalists with biased judgments and a quasi-religious certainty of right will fight more battles than any reasonable sceptic would do, and even if their victories confer 10 or 100 times less benefit on humanity than they imagine, they will in the long run probably do more good than harm – unless they materially reduce food production, distort research priorities, or direct attention." R. Peto, "Distorting the epidemiology of cancer: The need for a more balanced overview," *Nature*, 284 (1980): 297–300, 300.

18. G. Kolata, "L. I. cancer found to be explainable," *New York Times*, December 19, 1992, 29. For some residents and activists, the attribution of geographic clustering to the demographic characteristics of people who constitute a place is equivalent to blaming the already victimized. Cathy Read paraphrased some bitter Long Island activists' caricature of the CDC study's conclusion as, "they [Long Island women] were suffering breast cancer because they were rich and Jewish." C. Read, *Preventing Breast Cancer: The Politics of an Epidemic* (London: Pandora, 1995), 71.

19. J. Patterson, *The Dread Disease* (Cambridge, MA: Harvard University Press, 1987), 139. See also D. Cantor, "Cancer," in W. F. Bynum and R. Porter, eds., *Companion Encyclopedia of the History of Medicine*, Vol. 1 (London and New York: Routledge, 1993), 537–561.

20. A. M. Brandt, "Behavior, disease, and health in the twentieth-century United States: The moral valence of individual risk," in A. M. Brandt and P. Rozin, eds.,

Morality and Health: Interdisciplinary Perspectives (New York: Routledge, 1997), 53–77, 70.

21. "Some of the many views of mammography." *New York Times*, February 05, 2002, F3.

22. Mary Ann Napoli, quoted in G. Kolata, "Stand on mammograms greeted by outrage," *New York Times*, January 28, 1997, C1, C8.

23. L. Schwartz, S. Woloshin, F. J. Fowler, and H. G. Welch, "Enthusiasm for cancer screening in the United States," *Journal of the American Medical Association*, 291 (2004): 71–78.

24. B. Fisher, "The evolution of paradigms for the management of breast cancer: A personal perspective," *Cancer Research*, 52 (1992): 2371–2383.

25. Sixty percent of women from 1986 to 1993 were diagnosed with localized disease in the U.S. American Cancer Society, *Breast Cancer Facts and figures* (Atlanta: American Cancer Society, 1997), 14.

26. For an incisive critique, see B. Ehrenreich, "Welcome to cancerland: A mammogram leads to a cult of pink kitsch," *Harpers*, November (2001): 43–53. I have not told the important story of disease advocacy, in part because it largely occurred in the years after 1977, when my narrative of specific developments ends. See, for example, B. Lerner, "No shrinking violet: Rose Kushner and the rise of American breast cancer activism," *Western Journal of Medicine*, 174 (2001): 362–365, for a description of one of the earliest and most important patient advocates.

27. Attributed to Dawn Chastain, in a collection of writings about the breast cancer experience, in I. Yalof, ed., *Straight From the Heart: Letters of Hope and Inspiration From Survivors of Breast Cancer* (New York: Kensington, 1996), 12.

28. A. W. Jaffee, "The Good Mother" in H. Raz, ed., *Living on the Margins*, 50.

29. For a full analysis of the difference between individual and group decision-making in medicine, see D. A. Asch and J. C. Hershey, "Why some health policies don't make sense at the bedside," *Annals of Internal Medicine*, 122 (1995): 846–850.

30. The promotion of mass prevention has also shared a useful and purposeful ambiguity with Halsted's promotion of the complete operation and his uniform, disciplined approach to treatment. In both cases, there has been a willingness to accept limited endpoints in evaluating and communicating about efficacy (see Chapter 10 in which the number of detected cancers was construed a valid endpoint for BCDDP).

31. "Some of the many views on mammography," *New York Times*, February 5, 2002, F3.

32. See http://bcra.nci.nih.gov/brc/start.htm, accessed on October 20, 2005. The instructions are directed at health care professionals, but lay persons are not excluded.

33. W. C. Black, R. F. Nease, et al., "Perceptions of breast cancer risk and screening effectiveness in women younger than 50 years of age," *Journal of the National Cancer Institute*, 87 (1995): 720–731. Women in this study also understood, incorrectly, that breast cancer is nearly always rapidly fatal.

34. B. Fisher, "The evolution of paradigms for the management of breast cancer: A personal perspective," 2374.

35. Ibid., 2375.

36. Kushner's awareness of this ambiguity helped her make a decision not to receive chemotherapy, a decision also motivated by her belief that there were few data supporting its use in her case. At the time of her memoir, she had survived her disease and it seemed like a wise reading of the ambiguity. She later would die of metastatic disease. R. Kushner, "Is aggressive adjuvant chemotherapy the Halsted radical of the' 80s?" *CA: A Cancer Journal for Clinicians*, 34 (1984): 345–351.

37. This is a fast moving field. A 2002 consensus review, for example, concluded that the evidence for efficacy among high-risk women was "fair," the evidence for harm was "good," and that high-risk women should discuss the situation with their doctor since it was reasonable for some women to take medications. See U.S. Preventive Services Task Force, "Chemoprevention of breast cancer: recommendations and rationale," *Annals of Internal Medicine*, 137 (2002): 59–67. Curiously (and suggestive of the need for critical cultural *and* evidence-based review), the major negative trials of preventive use of antiestrogens were done in Europe.

38. Given Fisher's model above, many observers believe that "chemoprevention" is a misnomer; these drugs are treating *disease* that is clinically invisible with current technology.

39. While I stand by my assessment of current facts, viewed from my particular clinical and historical vantage point, it is entirely possible that I am committing a serious error of omission here. See my discussion of Gladwell in note 42, in which I describe how cultural arguments in the face of conflicting data misled some observers from what later appeared to be true.

40. R. A. Aronowitz, "Situating risk," in C. Rosenberg, R. Stevens, and R. Burns., eds., *American Health Care History and Policy* (New Brunswick, NJ: Rutgers University Press, 2006).

41. N. Krieger, I. Lowy, R. A. Aronowitz, et al., "Hormone replacement therapy, cancer, controversies, and women's health: Historical, epidemiological, biological, clinical, and advocacy perspectives," *Journal of Epidemiology and Community Health*, 59 (2005): 740–748.

42. It is curious, given the great magnitude of breast cancer fears, that reducing heart disease and osteoporosis risk trumped breast cancer risk for many policy makers and women during this period. A lot can be explained by claims – using the language of relative risk – of net quantitative benefit for HRT made on the basis of observational clinical trials. But to some extent the promotion of HRT also reflected a curious backlash against presumed exaggeration of breast cancer risk by zealous advocates. Malcolm Gladwell made this explicit in a *New Yorker* article in which he attacked the opposition to HRT use among breast cancer advocates. Gladwell attacked prominent breast cancer activist, surgeon, and popularizer Susan Love for overstating the risks (and understating the benefits) of HRT, especially for developing breast cancer. According to Gladwell, the risk of breast cancer from HRT was "probably not huge and is certainly nowhere close to canceling out the benefits of estrogen in fighting heart disease." Gladwell extended his attack to Love's skepticism "of modern medicine – of the idea that medical salvation can come in the

form of a pill." Love's false consciousness, unfortunately for Gladwell but thankfully for women who had turned to her popular book on sex hormones, turned out to be pretty much right on target. M. Gladwell, "The estrogen question," *The New Yorker*, June 9, 1997, 54–61.

43. In the entire HRT saga, the issue was the preventive use of these medications, not their use to treat menopausal symptoms.

44. J. E. Rossouw,, G. L. Anderson, et al., "Risks and benefits of estrogen plus progestin in healthy postmenopausal women: Principal results from the women's health initiative randomized controlled trial," *Journal of the American Medical Association*, 288 (2002): 321–333.

45. R. A. Aronowitz, "Situating health risks."

46. The seminal essay on the time and cultural boundedness of efficacy is: C. Rosenberg, "The therapeutic revolution: Medicine, meaning, and social change in nineteenth-century America," in *Explaining Epidemics and Other Studies in the History of Medicine* (Cambridge: Cambridge University Press, 1992), 9–31.

47. A. N. Papaioannou, *The Etiology of Human Breast Cancer: Endocrine, Genetic, Viral, Immunologic and Other Considerations* (New York: Springer, 1974), V.

48. W. S. Halsted, "The results of radical operations for the cure of carcinoma of the breast," *Annals of Surgery*, 46 (1907): 1–19, 15.

49. Patients frequently feel frustrated by the lack of a clear medical recommendation in some situations while embracing shared decision-making in others. One breast cancer patient wondered after her surgeon refused to make a clear recommendation about what to do, because, she imagines, he fears a lawsuit if things go badly, "why it is not considered malpractice for a doctor to refuse to share his wisdom." E. Greene, "Telling," in H. Raz, ed., *Living on the Margins*, 277.

Index

Made in the USA
Columbia, SC
27 August 2020